Samir A. Melki • Jason Brenner
Wassef Chanbour
Editors

Refractive Surgery Atlas

Surgical techniques and complications

Springer

Editors
Samir A. Melki
Massachusetts Eye and Ear
Harvard Medical School
Brookline, MA, USA

Jason Brenner
Boston Vision
Brookline, MA, USA

Wassef Chanbour
University of Minnesota
Minneapolis, MN, USA

ISBN 978-3-031-60660-1 ISBN 978-3-031-60661-8 (eBook)
https://doi.org/10.1007/978-3-031-60661-8

This Springer imprint is published by the registered company Springer Nature Switzerland AG
The registered company address is: Gewerbestrasse 11, 6330 Cham, Switzerland

To all my fellows who constantly inspire me through their boundless curiosity and thirst for knowledge.

—Samir A. Melki

To my teachers at Boston Vision. To my parents Ahmad and Sahar, whose love and guidance have shaped me into the person I am today. To my beloved wife Lulwa, whose unwavering support and encouragement have fueled my passion for writing. And to my precious daughter Yasma, who is the inspiration behind every word written in this book.

—Wassef Chanbour

To my wife Allison who helped put me through medical school, raise our children, and is the keystone to our family.

—Jason Brenner

Foreword

With gratitude and great admiration, I am honored to introduce the outstanding work of the *Refractive Surgery Atlas: Surgical Techniques and Complications* by Samir Melki, MD, PhD, Wassef Chanbour, MD, and Jason Brenner, MD. This comprehensive book is a testament to the remarkable progress achieved in refractive surgery, providing a guide to surgical techniques while addressing the complexities and challenges of managing potential complications.

Refractive surgery has undergone tremendous advancements, revolutionizing how we correct vision and liberating countless individuals from dependence on corrective lenses. The advent of laser vision correction has been remarkable, driven by the relentless pursuit of safety and efficiency. Moreover, refractive surgery is on the path to being considered a specialty of medicine with ophthalmology as a prerequisite, as defined by the World College of Refractive Surgery and Visual Sciences (www.wcrsvs.org).

Within these pages, esteemed experts in the field have meticulously documented and curated an extensive collection of surgical techniques, ensuring readers acquire the knowledge and skills required to navigate the intricate world of refractive surgery. This atlas is a comprehensive guide for experienced surgeons and aspiring ophthalmologists and provides valuable insights for researchers and scholars interested in this rapidly evolving field. One of the distinguishing features of this atlas is its unwavering focus on the understanding of complications. While refractive surgery offers immense benefits, it is not without risks. Recognizing this, the authors have dedicated significant attention to preventing and managing potential complications arising during or after surgical interventions. By shedding light on the nuances of difficulties, they empower practitioners to approach these challenges confidently, ensuring the highest level of patient care and safety.

I sincerely appreciate the authors and contributors who have dedicated their time, knowledge, and passion to creating this remarkable atlas. Their unwavering commitment to advancing the field of refractive surgery is evident in every chapter, making this volume an indispensable resource that will undoubtedly shape the future of ophthalmic surgery.

I am honored to contribute to this work by describing a case of iatrogenic ectasia after SMILE. This was the first (and still the only) case of ectasia that I generated after laser vision correction. Paradoxically, I dedicate my research to preventing such complex and unfortunate complications. Nevertheless, the lessons learned using the "black-box thinking" mindset have been fundamentally relevant for my evolution as a refractive surgeon-scientist. I recommend this work and invite you to the learning journey through the *Refractive Surgery Atlas: Surgical Techniques and Complications*. May this atlas inspire and empower you to provide the best possible care for your patients.

The Federal University of the State of Rio de Janeiro
International Society of Refractive Surgery (ISRS)
Refractive Surgery Alliance (RSA)
Rio de Janeiro, Brazil

Renato Ambrósio Jr

Preface

The *Refractive Surgery Atlas* starts with an introduction that provides an overview of the most commonly used refractive surgical techniques. The subsequent chapters delve into the intraoperative and postoperative complications that can arise from LASIK and PRK surgeries, combining detailed descriptions of potential complications with strategies for preventing and treating them.

In addition to LASIK and PRK, *Refractive Surgery Atlas* also covers other types of refractive surgeries, such as phakic intraocular lenses, SMILE, and incisional surgeries. Each surgery is discussed in detail, with explanations on their indications and their potential risks and benefits.

One of the unique features of this book is the case-based approach used to present normal and abnormal changes encountered during and following refractive surgeries.

Overall, *Refractive Surgery Atlas* is an essential resource for anyone interested in refractive surgery. Whether you're a surgeon, an optometrist, a medical student, or a resident, this book provides comprehensive information that will help you identify potential complications and make the right decisions to manage them.

Boston, MA, USA — Samir A. Melki
Boston, MA, USA — Jason Brenner
Minneapolis, MN, USA — Wassef Chanbour

Contents

Editors and Contributors

About the Editors

Samir A. Melki, MD, PhD is the founder and director of the Boston Vision and Boston Eye Group. He is also a clinical instructor at Harvard Medical School and assistant in ophthalmology at the Massachusetts Eye and Ear Infirmary. He was medical director for ophthalmology at the UK Specialist Hospitals. He completed his ophthalmology residency at Georgetown University Hospital, where he was elected as chief resident. This was followed by a fellowship in Corneal and Refractive Surgery at the Massachusetts Eye and Ear Infirmary, where he served as chief fellow. His areas of interest include refractive surgery, complex cataract surgery, and ocular surface reconstruction.

Jason Brenner, MD started his education at Lafayette College where he obtained a Bachelor of Science in biology with a minor in medical ethics. After his undergrad, he attended medical school at George Washington University School of Medicine in Washington, D.C. He then completed his residency training at Temple University Hospital in Philadelphia, where he was also chief resident.

He is a board-certified ophthalmologist, specializing in cornea, refractive, and anterior segment surgery. He did his fellowship under the supervision of Dr. Melki, at the Boston Eye Group and is currently one of the primary refractive surgeons at Boston Vision. He is also an associate staff at Beth Israel Deaconess Medical Center in Boston. As a cornea specialist, his primary interests are LASIK, Visian ICL surgery, femtosecond-assisted cataract surgery, sutured intraocular lenses, anterior segment reconstruction, and corneal transplants.

Wassef Chanbour, MD is an assistant professor at the University of Minnesota. After obtaining the medical degree from the Lebanese University in Beirut, he completed the ophthalmology residency at the Beirut Eye and ENT Specialist Hospital. He is specialized in cornea and refractive surgery, and his fellowship training was at Beth Israel Deaconess Medical Center and Boston Vision, under the guidance of Dr. Samir Melki. His practice includes all patients with different medical and surgical corneal and anterior segment diseases. He treats adults and children with the latest surgical techniques including endothelial keratoplasties in addition to the latest refractive procedures including LASIK, ICL, and femtosecond-assisted cataract surgery.

Contributors

Renato Ambrósio Jr Department of Ophthalmology, Federal University the State of Rio de Janeiro (UNIRIO), Rio de Janeiro, Brazil

Jad F. Assaf Faculty of Medicine, American University of Beirut Medical Center, Beirut, Lebanon

Shady T. Awwad Department of Ophthalmology, American University of Beirut Medical Center, Beirut, Lebanon

Jason Brenner Boston Vision, Department of Ophthalmology, Harvard Medical School, Boston, MA, USA

Yara Bteich Department of Ophthalmology, American University of Beirut Medical Center, Beirut, Lebanon

Wassef Chanbour Department of Ophthalmology and Visual Neurosciences, University of Minnesota, Minneapolis, MN, USA

Lulwa El Zein Department of Ophthalmology, Mayo Clinic, Rochester, MN, USA

Louise Pellegrino Gomes Esporcatte Department of Ophthalmology, Federal University of São Paulo, São Paulo, Brazil

Perla Ibrahim, MD Cornea and Refractive Surgery Fellow, Boston Vision and Beth Israel Deaconess Medical Center, Boston, MA, USA

Soosan Jacob Dr. Agarwal's Refractive and Cornea Foundation, Cataract and Glaucoma Services, Dr. Agarwal's Group of Eye Hospital and Eye Research Centre, Chennai, India

Francesca Kahale Mass Eye and Ear Infirmary, Boston, MA, USA

Guy M. Kezirian World College of Refractive Surgery and Visual Sciences, Scottsdale, AZ, USA

Aydano P. Machado Department of Ophthalmology, Federal University of São Paulo, São Paulo, Brazil

Kevin G. Makhoul KU Eye Center, University of Kansas Medical Center, Kansas City, KS, USA

Karen Matar Cole Eye Institute, Cleveland Clinic Foundation, Cleveland, OH, USA

Alexander Melki UCLA, Los Angeles, CA, USA

Samir A. Melki Boston Vision, Department of Ophthalmology, Harvard Medical School, Boston, MA, USA

Reeda Bou Said Department of Ophthalmology, Mayo Clinic, Rochester, MN, USA

Marcella Q. Salomão Department of Ophthalmology, Federal University of São Paulo, São Paulo, Brazil

Cases Contributors

Shady T. Awwad, MD Department of Ophthalmology, American University of Beirut Medical Center, Beirut, Lebanon

Mohammad Dastjerdi Rutgers New Jersey Medical School, Newark, NJ, USA

Juliana Freitas, MD Conselho Brasileiro de Oftalmologia, São Paulo, Brazil

Willem-Martin Gerber, MD Durbanville, Cape Town, South Africa

Arun Gulani, MD Gulani Vision Institute, Jacksonville, FL, USA

Joshua H. Hou, MD University of Minnesota, Minneapolis, MN, USA

Jimmy Hu, MD New York Eye and Ear Infirmary at Mt. Sinai, New York, NY, USA

Deborah S. Jacobs, MD Mass Eye and Ear, Boston, MA, USA

Soosan Jacob, MS, FRCS, DN Dr. Agarwal's Refractive and Cornea Foundation, Cataract and Glaucoma Services, Dr. Agarwal's Group of Eye Hospital and Eye Research Centre, Chennai, India

Roger Kardawi, MD Milford Franklin Eye Center, Franklin, MA, USA

Johnny Khoury, MD NVISION Eye Centers, Ontario, CA, USA

Catherine Liu, MD Brigham and Women's Hospital, Boston, MA, USA

Matthew McCauley, MD Berkeley Eye Center, Houston, TX, USA

Majid Moshirfar, MD Department of Ophthalmology and Visual Sciences, University of Utah School of Medicine, Moran Eye Center, Salt Lake City, UT, USA

Dan Ohman, MD Orebro University Hospital, Orebro, Sweden

Ravi Patel, MD Jacksonville, FL, USA

Roy Rubinfield Georgetown University, Washington, DC, USA

Brian Shafer, MD Chester County Eye Care, Perelman School of Medicine, University of Pennsylvania, Philadelphia, PA, USA

Bogdan Spiru, MD The Institute for Refractive and Ophthalmic Surgery (IROC), Zurich, Switzerland

Suphi Taneri, MD Augenzentrum am St. Franziskus Hospital Münster, Münster, Germany

Abbreviations

AC	Anterior chamber
AI	Artificial intelligence
AK	Arcuate keratotomy
ART-max	Ambrósio relational thickness-maximum
ASN	Acute stromal necrosis
AS-OCT	Anterior segment optical computed tomography
BCL	Bandage contact lens
BCVA	Best corrected visual acuity
BL	Bowman's layer
CAIRS	Corneal allogenic intrastromal ring segments
CBI	Corneal Biomechanical Index
CCT	Central corneal thickness
CXL	Collagen cross-linking
DALK	Deep anterior lamellar keratectomy
DLK	Diffuse lamellar keratitis
EBMD	Epithelial basement membrane dystrophy
Epi-ON CXL	Epithelium-ON collagen cross-linking
FS-ICRS	Femtosecond-assisted intracorneal ring segment implantation
ICL	Implantable collamer lens
ICRS	Intrastromal corneal ring segments
IOL	Intraocular lens
LALEX	Laser-assisted lenticular extraction with a small incision
LASIK	Laser-assisted in situ keratomileusis
LRI	Limbal relaxing incisions
LVC	Laser vision correction
OBL	Opaque bubble layer
OCT	Optical coherence tomography
OZ	Optical zone
PK	Penetrating keratoplasty
PRFI	Pentacam random forest index
PRK	Photorefractive keratectomy
PTA	Percent of tissue altered
PTK	Phototherapeutic keratectomy
RK	Refractive keratectomy
RSB	Residual stromal bed
SMILE	Small incision lenticule extraction
TBI	Tomography and biomechanical index
UCVA	Uncorrected visual acuity
VGB	Vertical gas breakthrough

Acknowledgements

We wish to thank the contributing authors of this book, whose hard work has resulted in a more up-to-date text. We are deeply grateful to the doctors who generously shared their expertise and clinical cases, making this book a rich resource for medical professionals and students alike. Your contribution to this book, through your photographs and compelling clinical cases, is invaluable and will undoubtedly make a difference in the lives of many patients. Thank you for being a vital part of this project.

This book was not funded by any external sources.

1 Introduction

Jason Brenner, Wassef Chanbour, and Samir A. Melki

Refractive surgery has undergone tremendous transformation in the last 20 years. While modern refractive surgical techniques have improved safety and reliability over prior generations, they still have their own variety of challenging intraoperative and postoperative complications.

"Refractive Surgery Atlas: Surgical Techniques and Complications" is a review guide to the latest surgical techniques and complications in refractive surgery. This book will function first as a step-by-step intraoperative description of the surgical procedures, second as a visual reference encompassing not only common but also rare complications that can arise intra-operatively and following surgery, and third, the book follows a case-based approach offering practical tips for preventing and managing these complications.

The book is written by leading experts in the field of refractive surgery and is aimed at residents and fellows in training, ophthalmologists, optometrists, and other medical professionals who are interested in expanding their knowledge and skills in this area. It is an invaluable tool for both experienced surgeons and those new to the field covering both common and uncommon complications that can be encountered following surgery.

Most of the presented data comes from real life cases that were managed at Boston Vision, one of the busiest refractive surgery practices in the New England area where more than 40,000 cases have been performed over the last 30 years primarily by author Dr. Samir Melki but also by Dr. Jason Brenner. In addition, many of the top US refractive specialists have contributed photographs and cases that they have encountered during their years of practice.

Each chapter will discuss a different pathologic entity, it will include a summary of the most recent updates (pathophysiology, presentations, risk factors, preventions, and management…) followed by example pictures showing these pathologies. Pictures will be combined into cases that will include patient history, clinical description of the pictures, management and learning points. The case studies provide real-world examples of how these complications are managed in the clinical setting. In the end of each chapter, we will include take home messages that summarizes the learning aspects of the aforementioned cases.

J. Brenner (✉) · S. A. Melki
Boston Vision, Department of Ophthalmology, Harvard Medical School, Boston, MA, USA
e-mail: brenner@bostonvision.com; melki@bostonvision.com

W. Chanbour
Department of Ophthalmology and Visual Neurosciences, University of Minnesota, Minneapolis, MN, USA
e-mail: chanb013@umn.edu

S. A. Melki et al. (eds.), *Refractive Surgery Atlas*, https://doi.org/10.1007/978-3-031-60661-8_1

Surgical Techniques

2

Wassef Chanbour, Samir A. Melki, and Jason Brenner

Surface Ablation Techniques

Photo Refractive Keratectomy (PRK)

Step 1: Epithelial ablation:, it can be performed with corneal brush, alcohol, blade, or trans epithelial ablation (Figs. 2.1 and 2.2).

Step 2: Laser stromal ablation (Fig. 2.3).

Step 3: Mitomycin application (Fig. 2.4).

Step 4: Bandage contact lens placement.

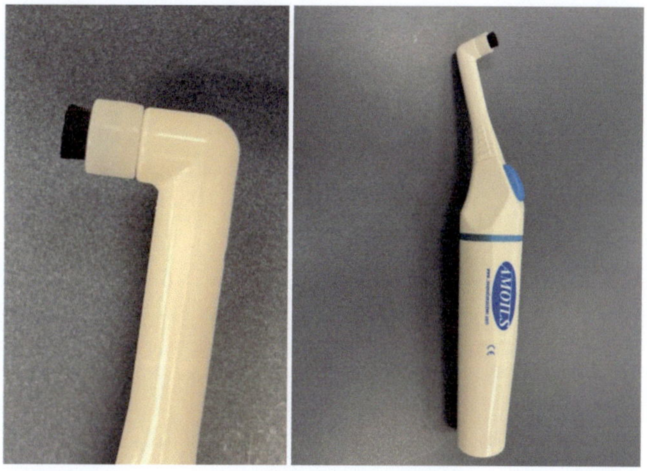

Fig. 2.1 Corneal brush used for epithelial ablation. Brush size: Myopic: 6.5 mm; Hyperopic: 9.0 mm; Hyperopic XL: 9.5 mm. (Innovative Excimer Solutions©, Inc. *Courtesy of Ravi Patel, MD*)

W. Chanbour (✉)
Department of Ophthalmology and Visual Neurosciences, University of Minnesota, Minneapolis, MN, USA
e-mail: chanb013@umn.edu

S. A. Melki · J. Brenner
Boston Vision, Department of Ophthalmology, Harvard Medical School, Boston, MA, USA
e-mail: melki@bostonvision.com; brenner@bostonvision.com

S. A. Melki et al. (eds.), *Refractive Surgery Atlas*, https://doi.org/10.1007/978-3-031-60661-8_2

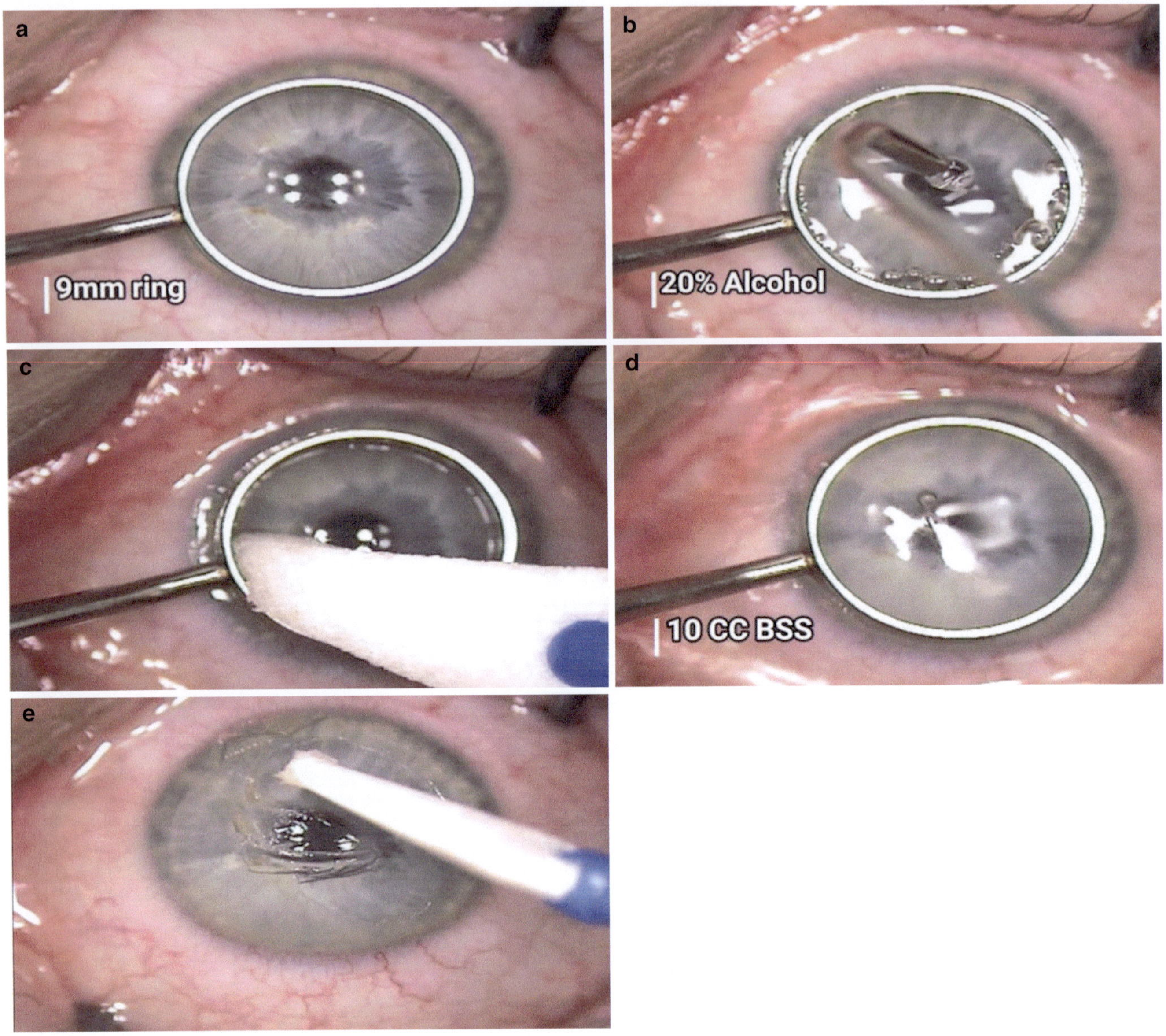

Fig. 2.2 Steps of epithelial ablation with alcohol. Cone (8.5–9.5 mm) applied to the cornea (**a**) . 20% alcohol added in the cone (**b**). Removal of Alcohol with weck-cel after 40 s (**c**). Irrigation of all the surface with BSS (**d**). Epithelial scraping with instrument or weck-cel (**e**)

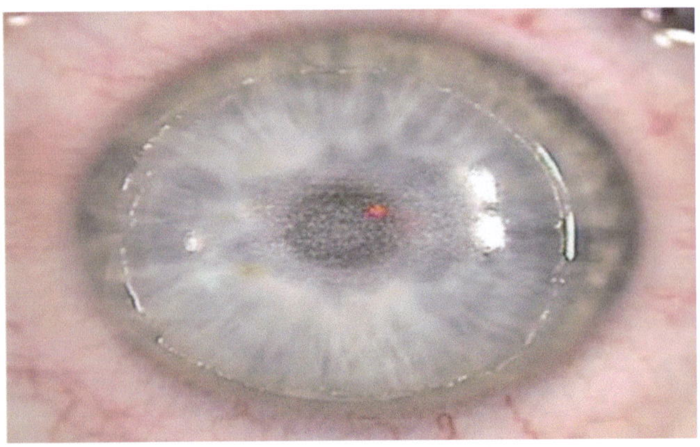

Fig. 2.3 Centered laser with activated stromal ablation

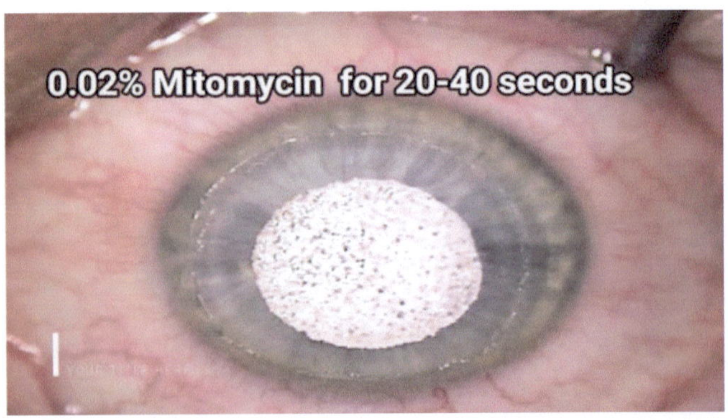

Fig. 2.4 Sponge soaked with 0.02% mitomycin placed over the ablation zone

Variants of PRK

Laser Subepithelial Keratomileusis LASEK

A spatula is used to separate a flap of full-thickness epithelium from the underlying Bowman's layer. The epithelium is delicately folded back leaving a small "hinge," which is usually located superiorly or temporally (Fig. 2.5).

Epi-LASIK

The microkeratome is modified with a dull blade and thin applanation plate to mechanically remove the epithelial flap without the use of alcohol.

Epi-LASEK

Epi-LASEK is similar to Epi-LASIK except that alcohol is added with the goal of facilitating creation of the epithelial flap.

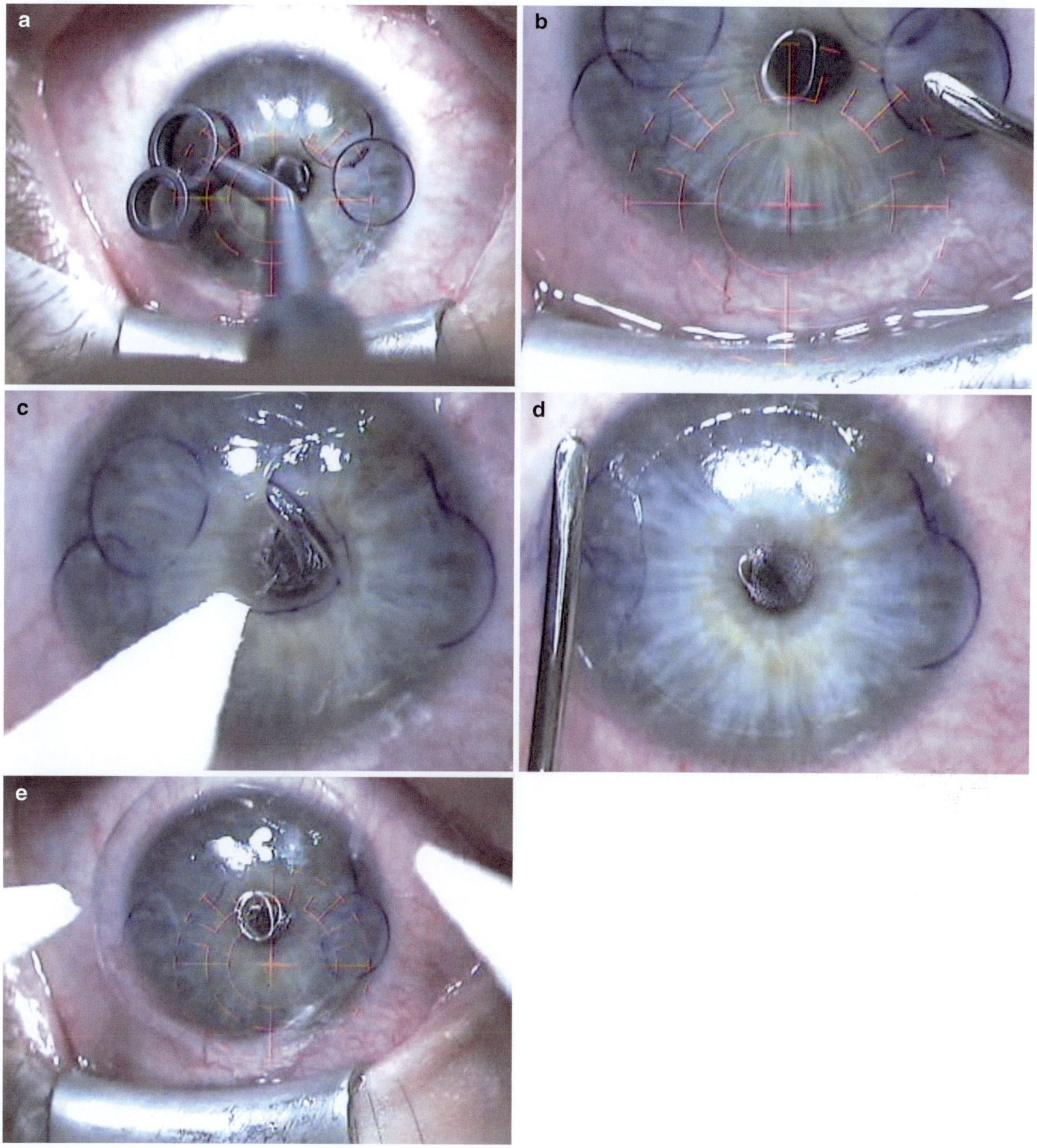

Fig. 2.5 Steps of LASEK surgery. Epithelial marking (**a**). Alcohol application (5 s) followed by dissection of an epithelial flap with a spatula (**b**). Weck-cel used to slide the epithelium out of the treatment zone (**c**). Epithelium folded temporally (**d**). Following the laser treatment, epithelium is repositioned back to original position and a BCL is placed on the cornea (**e**)

Femtosecond LASIK

See Figs. 2.6 and 2.7.

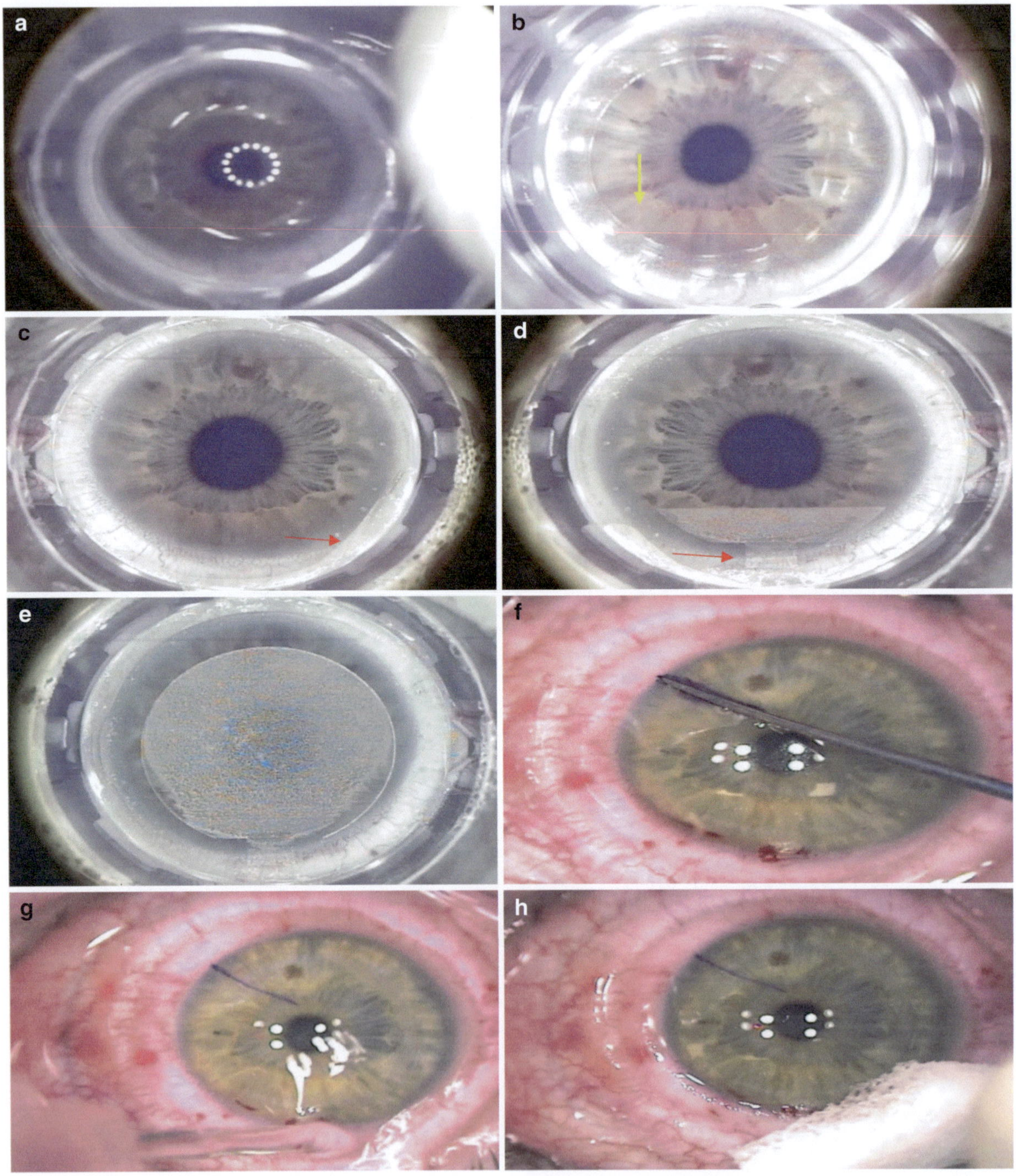

Fig. 2.6 Steps of femtosecond LASIK surgery. WaveLight® Alcon refractive suite was used for this case. Suction ring placed with the cornea centered (**a**). Applanation cone lowered with partial corneal applanation (*yellow arrow*) (**b**). Complete corneal applanation, soft docking is noted as peripheral air is present on top of the conjunctiva (*red arrow*) (**c**). Superior channel *(red arrow)* created with ongoing Femtosecond Flap cut (**d**). Compete Flap creation with ongoing side cut (**e**). Marking of the flap edge with a straight metal instrument (**f**). Surface irrigation with normal saline to remove debris (**g**). Drying the surface with weckcel (**h**). Flap lifter used to identify and engage the flap (**i**). Flap dissection until the superior hinge (**j**). Inferior partial flap dissection (Not to dissect beyond the edge) (**k**). Complete dissection of the remaining attached area followed by flap lift (**l**). Drying the stromal interface with a weckcel (**m**). Laser treatment (**n**). Hydrating the interface to facilitate flap reposition (**o**). Flap repositioning (**p**). Surface irrigation to remove debris (**q**). Irrigation under the flap to remove debris (**r**). Soothing the surface with the cannula to remove remaining interface fluid (**s**). Drying the flap edge to see a complete silver ring with equal gutter on both sides (**t**)

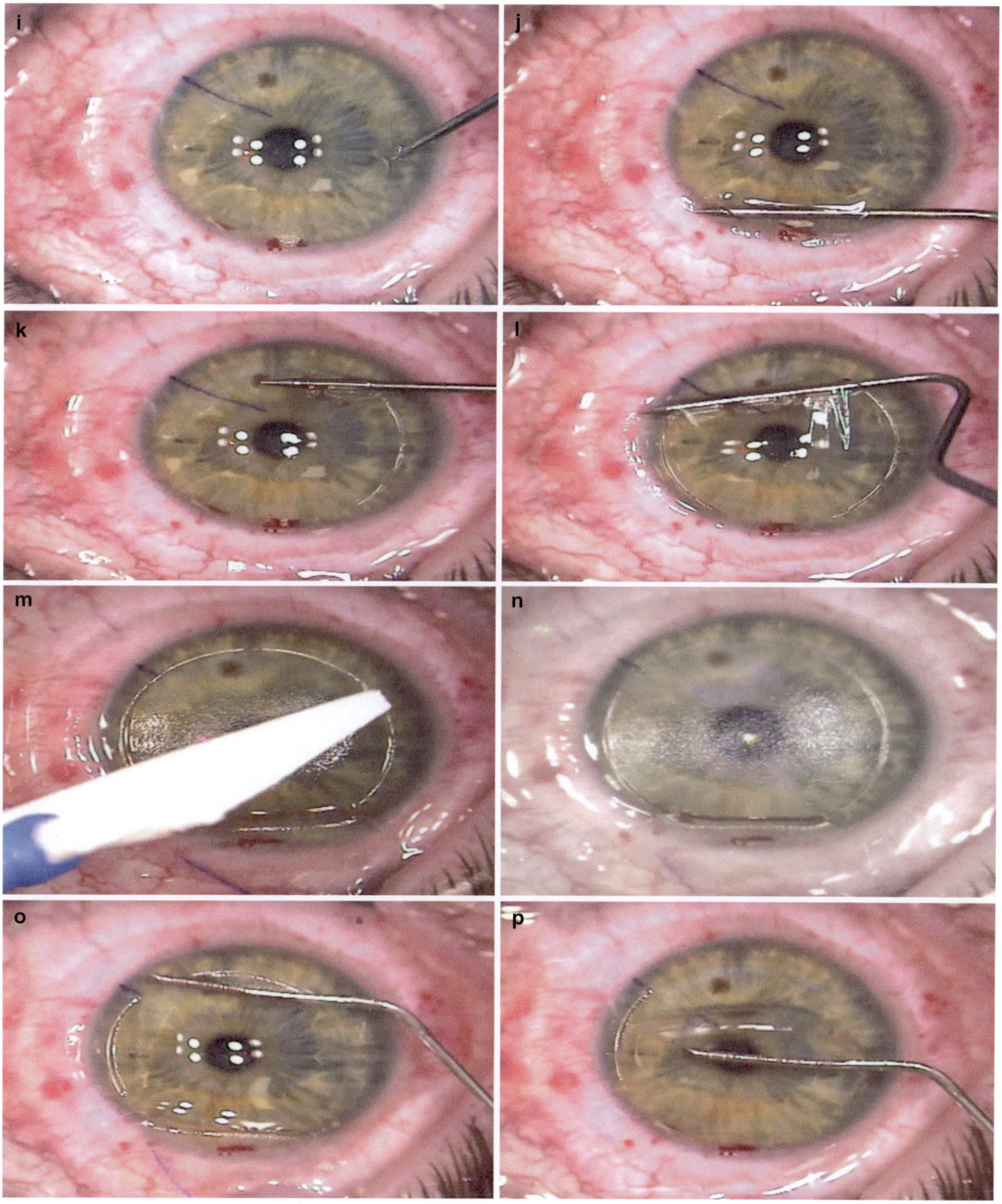

Fig. 2.6 (continued)

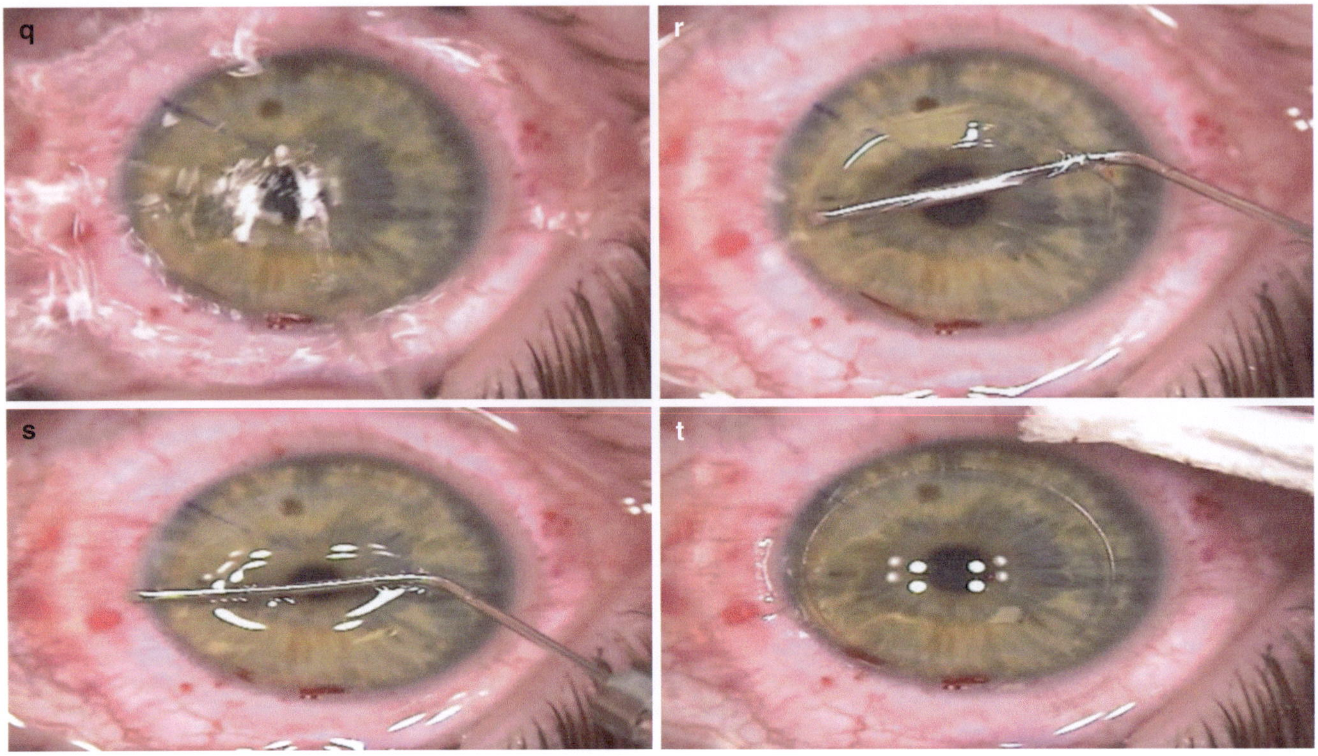

Fig. 2.6 (continued)

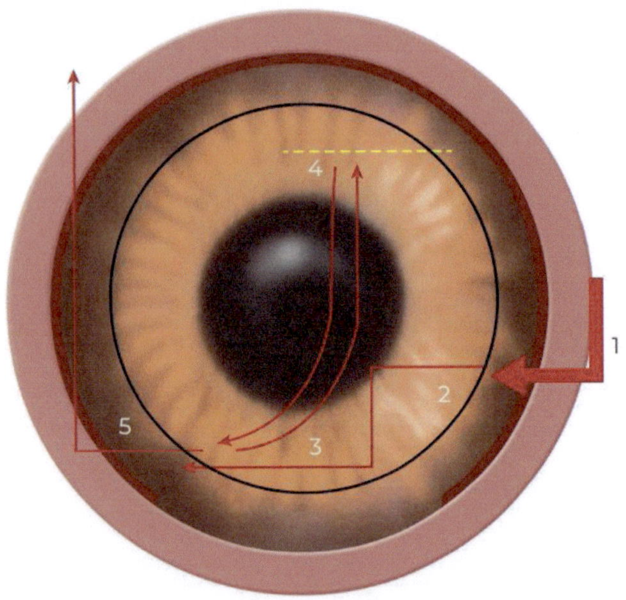

Fig. 2.7 Consecutives steps for flap dissection. Note that step 1 requires a downward movement to enter the gutter before proceeding into the horizontal movement to dissect the flap in step 2

Microkeratome LASIK

Suction ring is centered to the cornea and vacuum is activated followed by keratome insertion and activation to create a flap (Fig. 2.8). (The rest of the procedure is similar to Femtosecond LASIK).

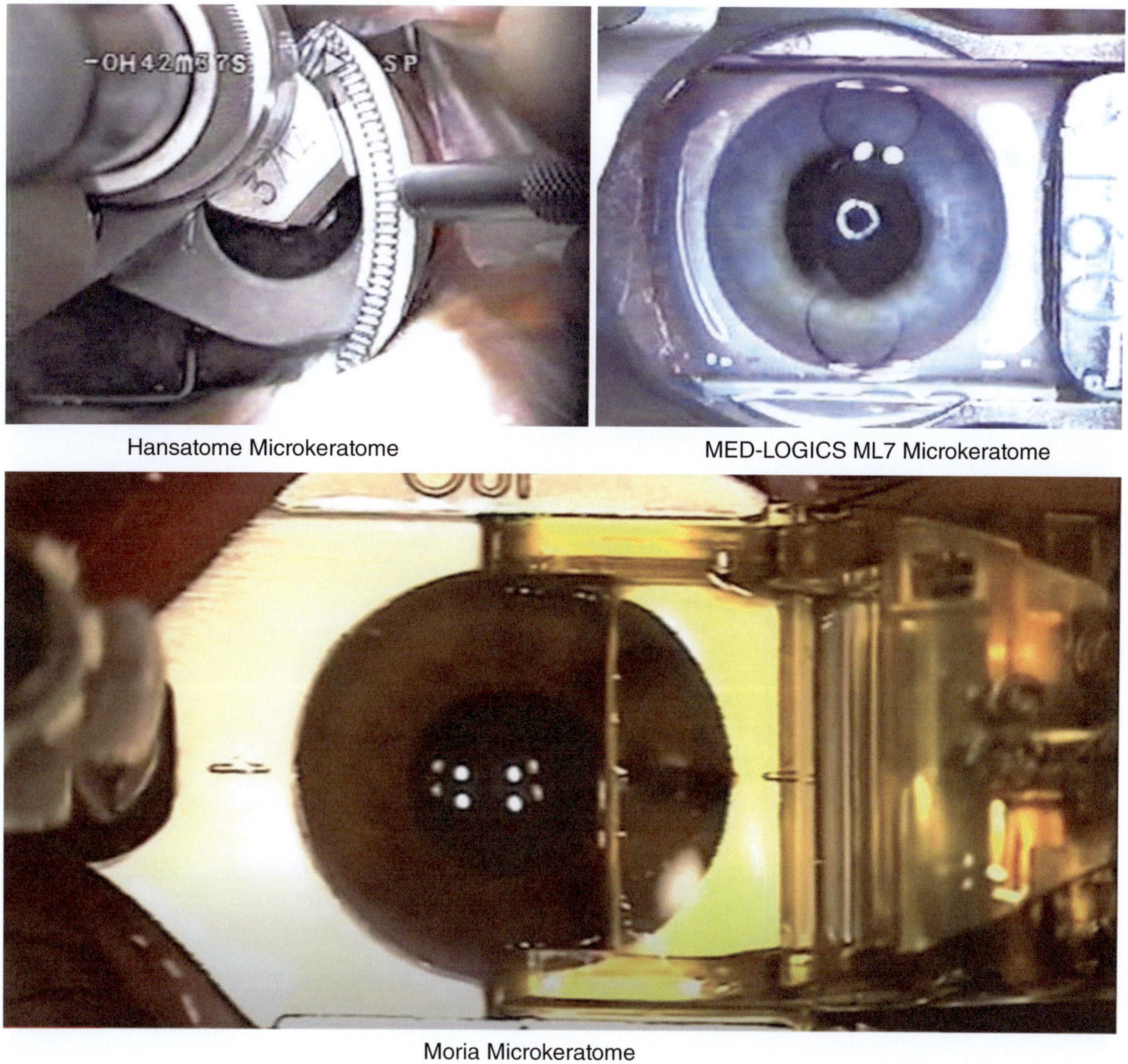

Fig. 2.8 Microkeratomes flap creation. (**a**) Hansatome microkeratome. (**b**) MED-LOGICS ML7 microkeratome. (**c**) Moria microkeratome

Small Incision Lenticule Extraction (SMILE)

See Fig. 2.9.

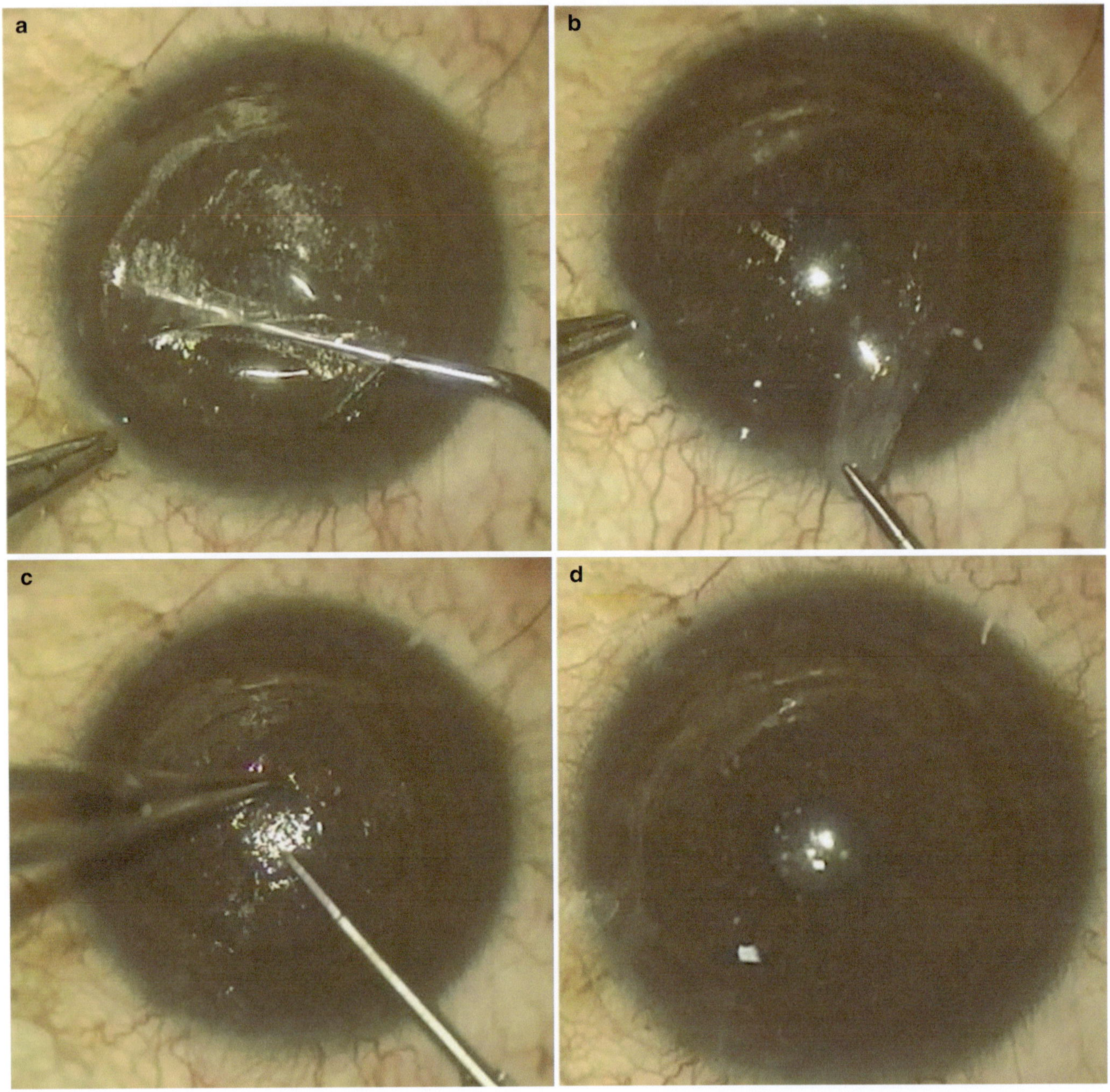

Fig. 2.9 Steps of SMILE surgery. Femto-second laser application creating lenticule cut (underside of the lenticule) lenticule side cut, cap cut and cap opening incision (**a**). Anterior lamellar plane (cap cut) is delineated through the incision using a dissector (**b**). Posterior lamellar plane (lenticule cut) is delineated using dissector (**c**). Anterior lamellar plane is dissected using spatula (**d**). Posterior lamellar plane is dissected using spatula (**e**). SMILE lenticule is extracted with micro forceps (**f**). Extracted lenticule is examined to verify complete lenticule (**g**). Cornea seen at end of surgery (**h**). (*Courtesy of Dr. Soosan Jacob, MS, FRCS, DN, Dr. Agarwal's Refractive and Cornea Foundation, Chennai, India*)

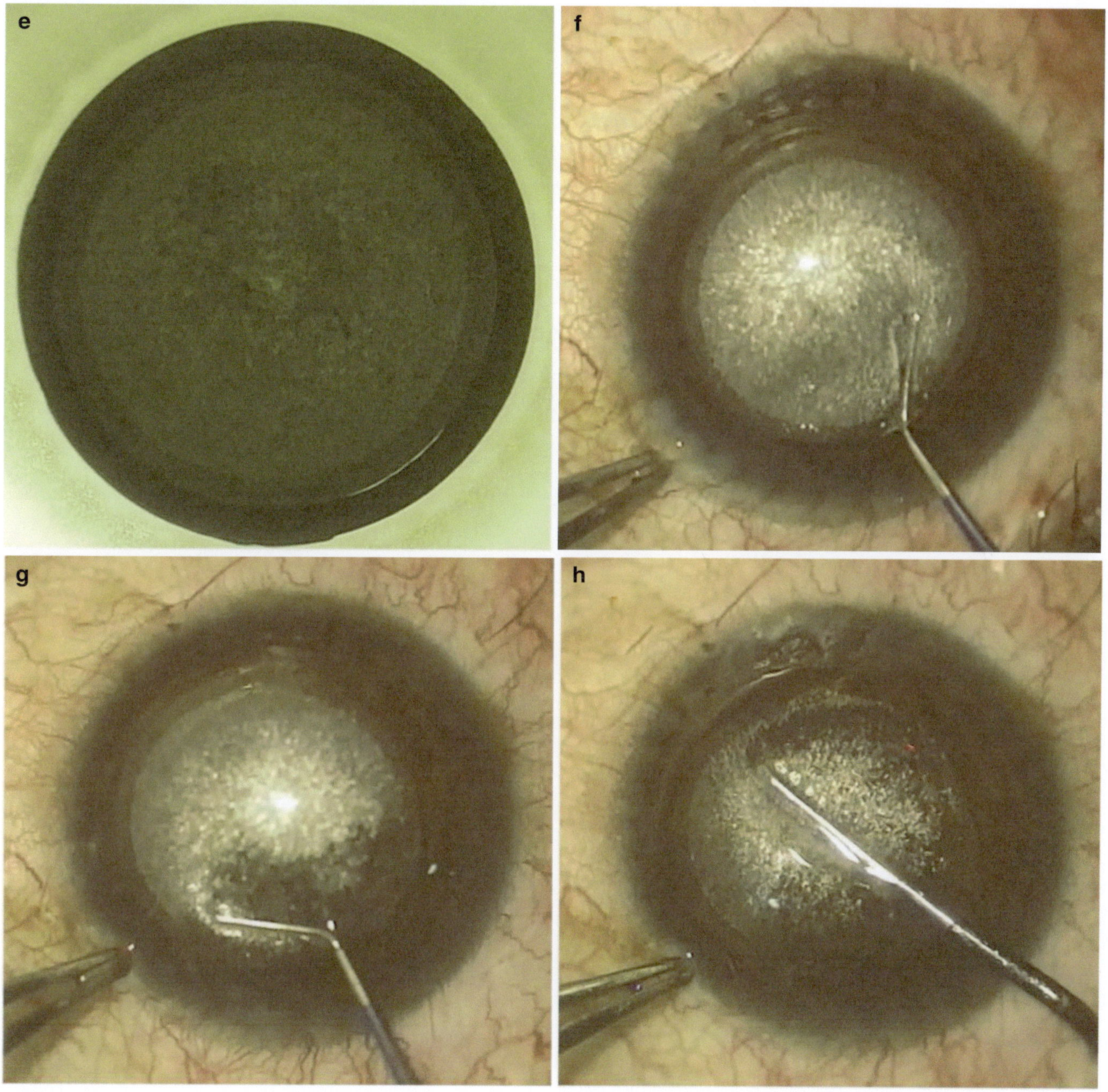

Fig. 2.9 (continued)

Femtosecond Limbal Relaxing Incisions (LRI)

CATALYS™ Precision Laser System is used for this case (Fig. 2.10).

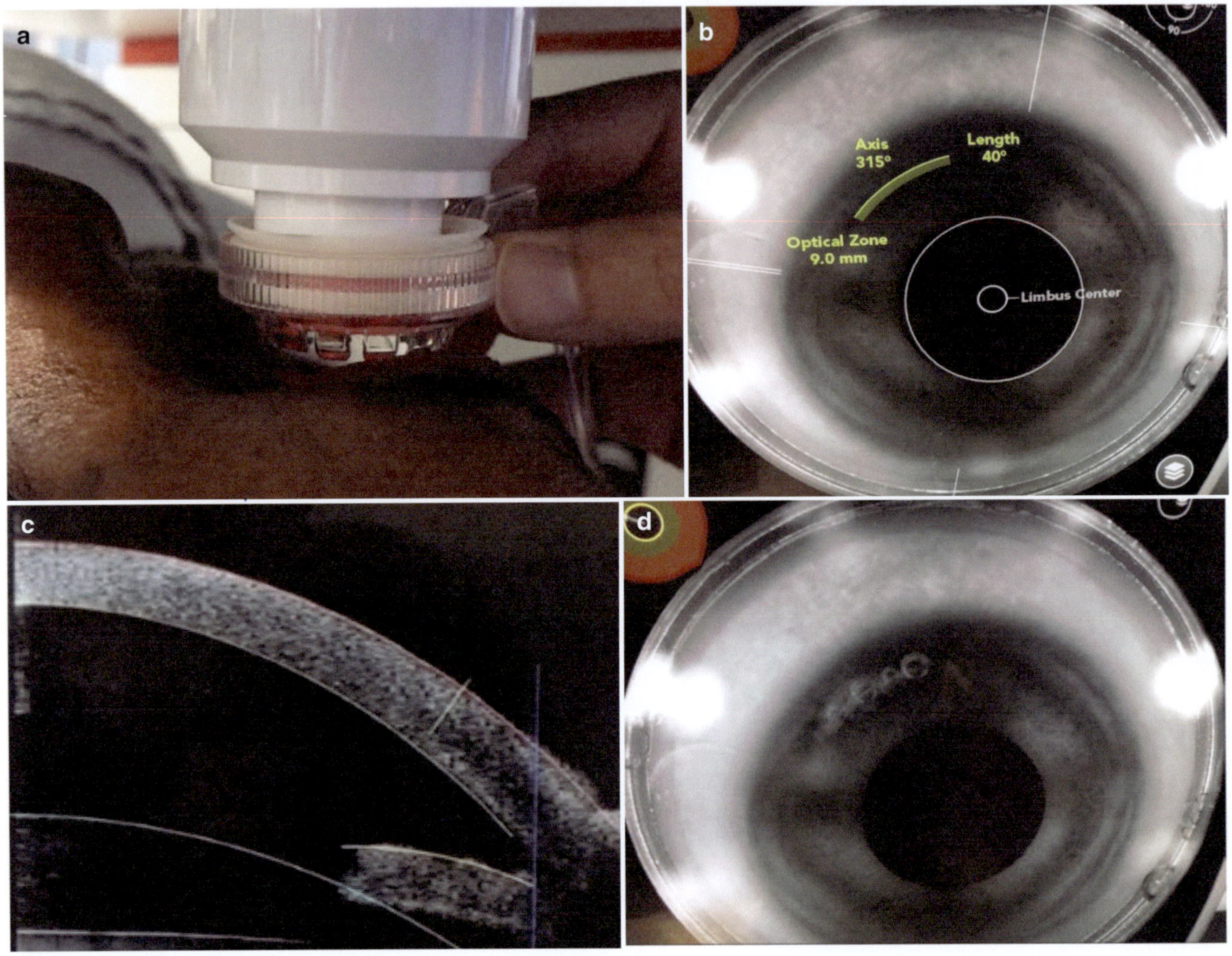

Fig. 2.10 Steps of femtosecond LRI surgery. Sucction device applied with liquid optics interface application (**a**). LRI position on the cornea (**b**). OCT cut of the cornea showing the depth of the planned LRI treatment (**c**). Whitening and bubbles formation at the area of the femtosecond cut (**d**)

Manual Arcuate Keratotomy

See Fig. 2.11.

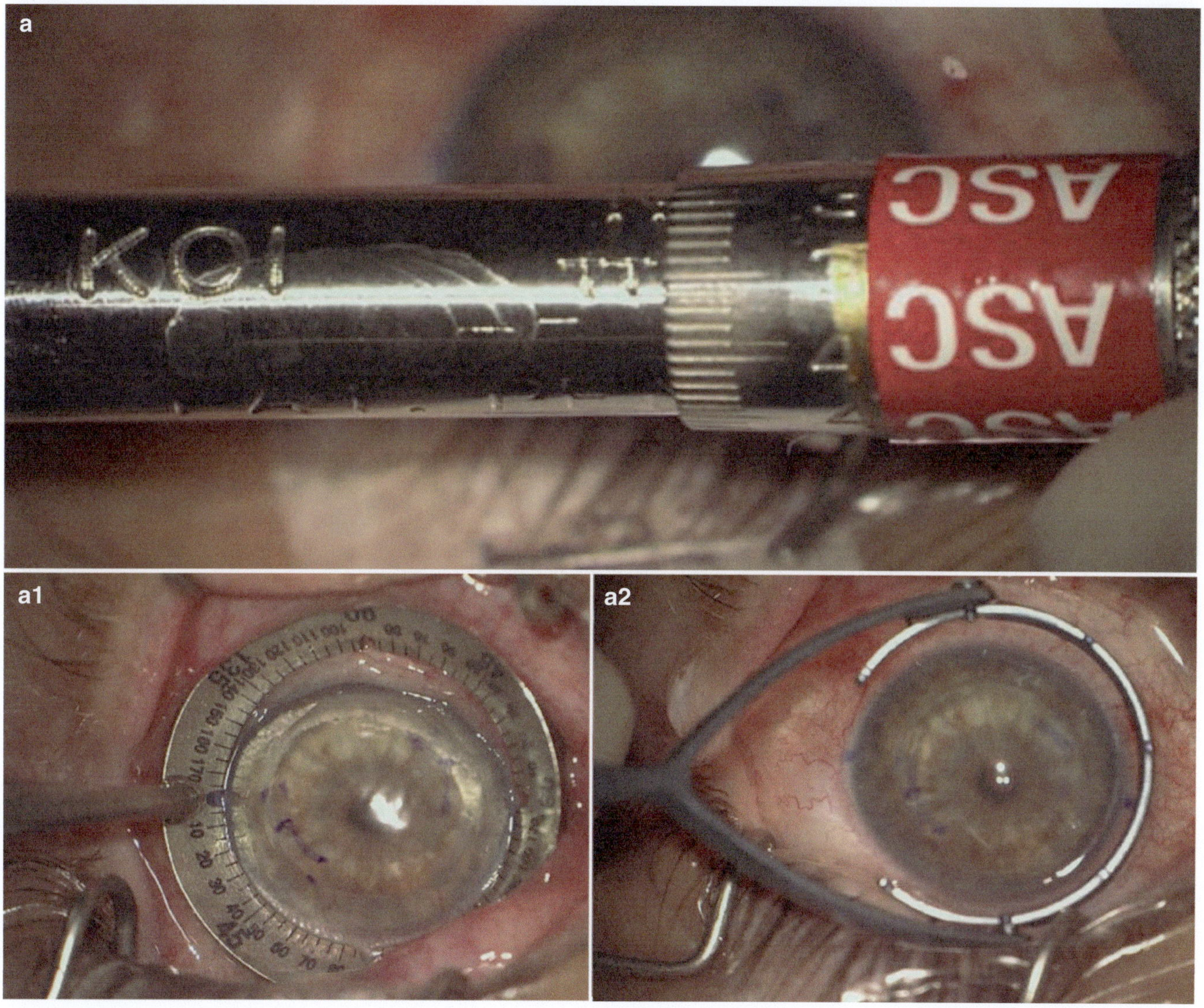

Fig. 2.11 Steps of manual arcuate keratotomy. Diamond blade used for mannual corneal dissection, setting the depth between 60 and 90% of the corneal pachymetry (**a**). Corneal markings of the arcs to be dissected (**a1**). Globe fixation ring used to prevent movements (**a2**). Diamond blade incisions (**a3**). Dissection of the incisions using Sinskey hook (**a4**). Keratoscopy prior to incisions showing oval ring indicating high astigmatism (**b**). Keratoscopy following incisions showing smaller degree of irregularity (**c**)

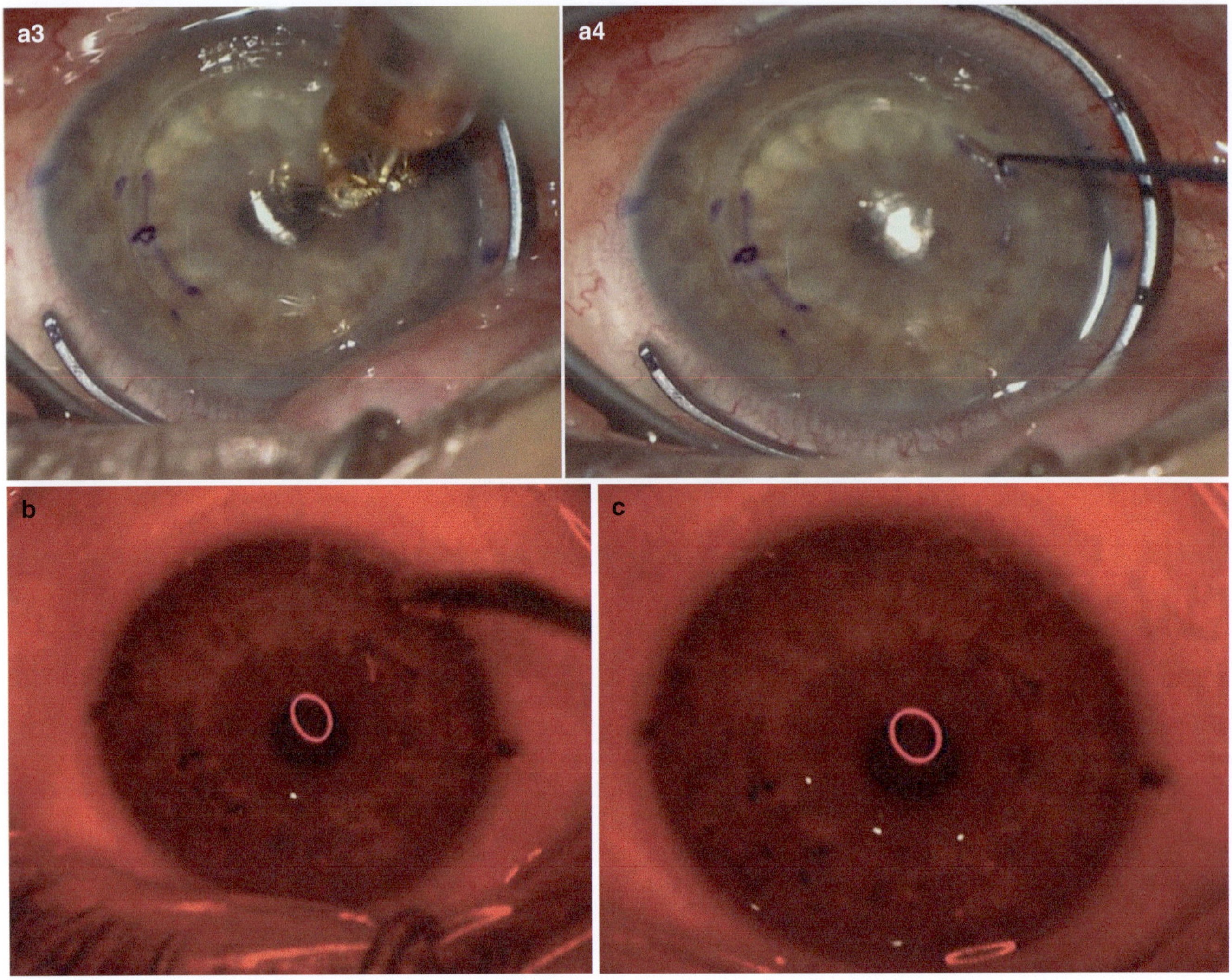

Fig. 2.11 (continued)

Intrastromal Corneal Ring Segments (ICRS)

iFS® (Intralase femtosecond) advanced femtosecond laser is used for this case (Fig. 2.12).

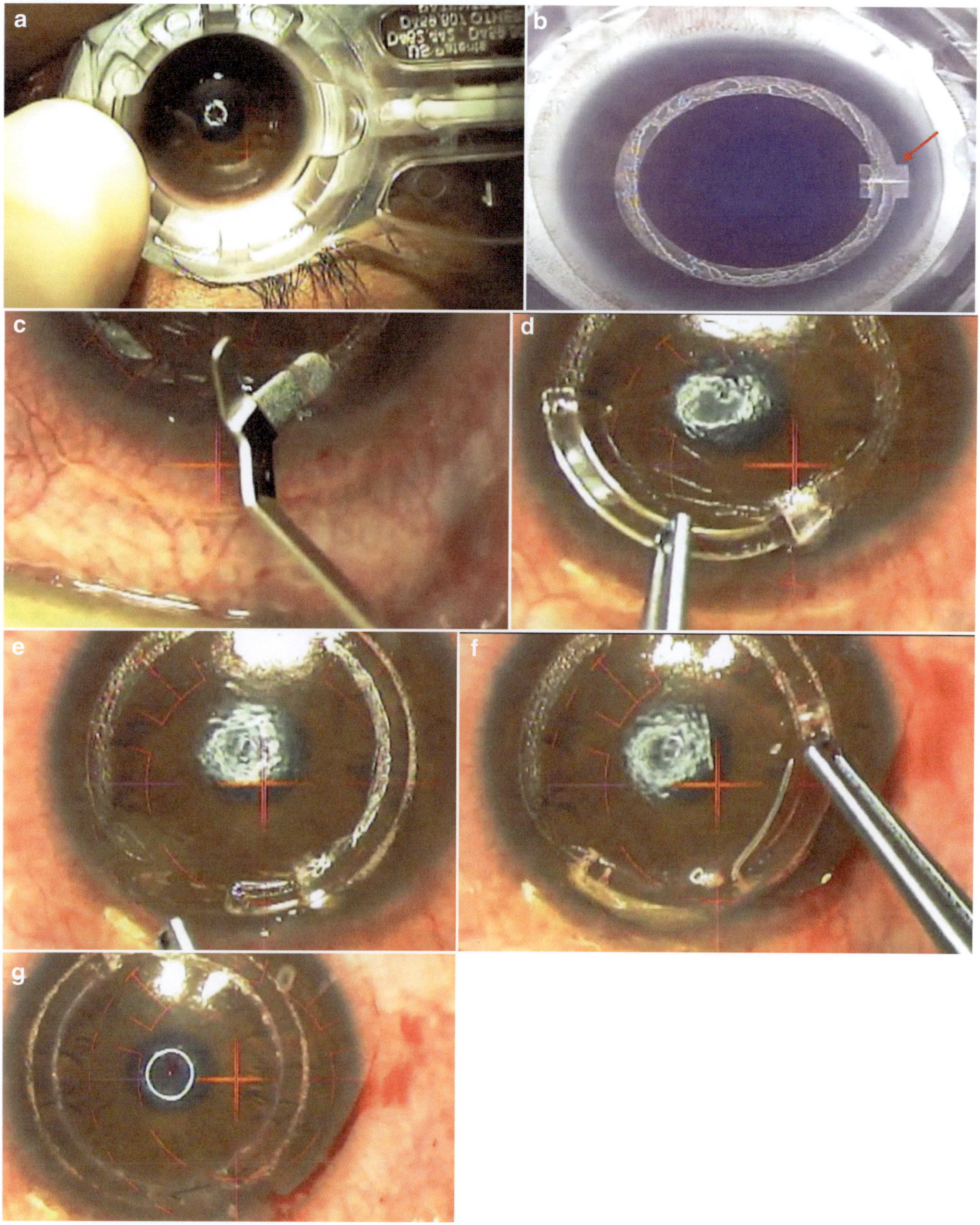

Fig. 2.12 Steps of ICRS implantation. Suction ring application (**a**). 360° Tunnel creation with femtosecond at preselected depth, radius and width. Incision can be noted with the (*red arrow*) (**b**). Dissector used to identify the tunnels through the incision (**c**). ICRS insertion into the tunnels created by femtosecond (**d**). ICRS can be seen inserted partially in the cornea (**e**). Insertion of the second segment on the opposite side (**f**). Both ICRS segments are inserted and a suture can be seen closing the incision to prevent migration of the segments (**g**)

Implantable Collamer Lens (ICL)

See Fig. 2.13.

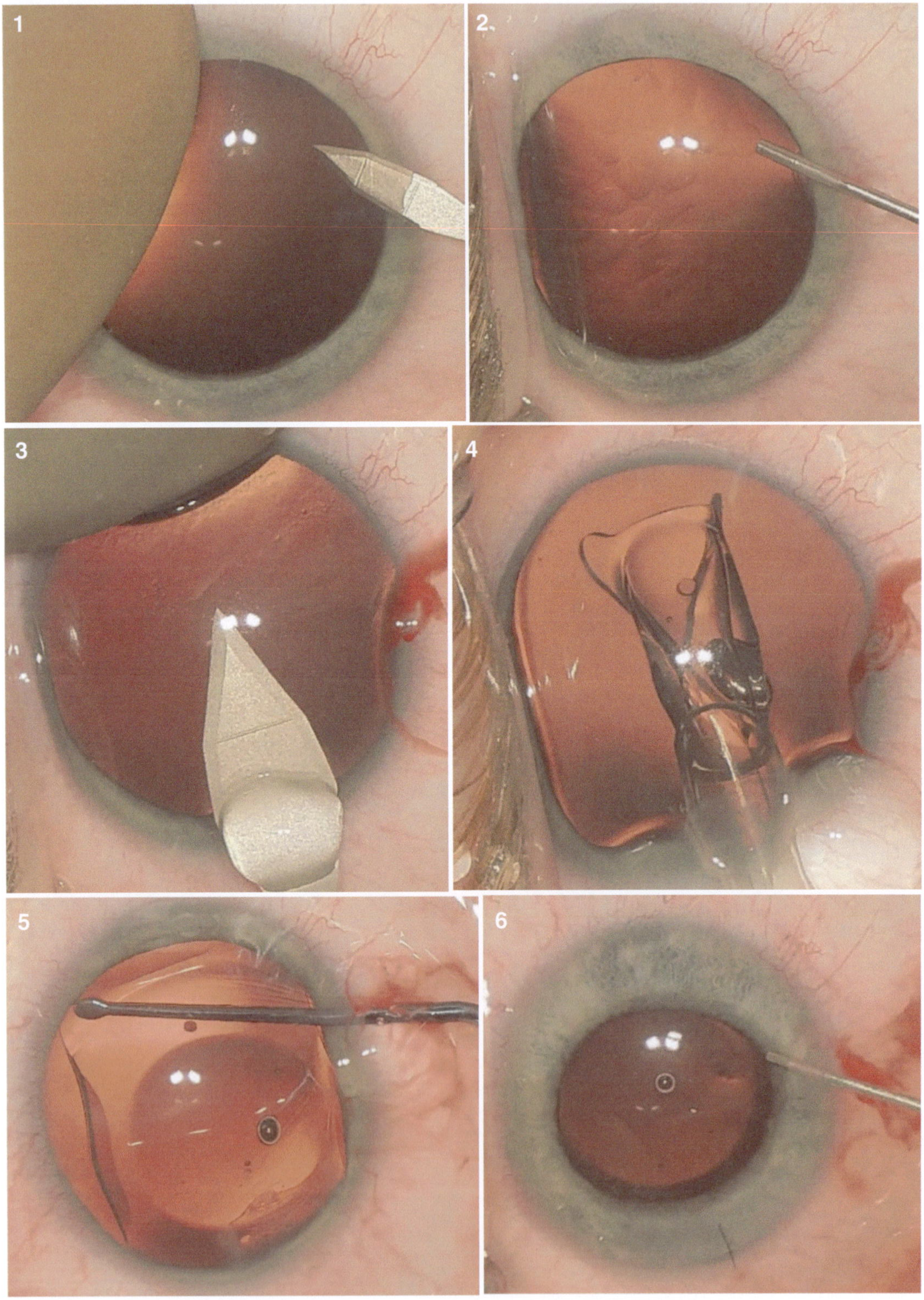

Fig. 2.13 Steps of ICL implantation. Side port incision (**a**). Dispersive viscoelastic injection in the anterior chamber (AC) methylcellulose 20 mg/mL (Ocucoat; Bausch & Lomb, Rochester, New York) is recommended by the ICL manufacturer (Staar Surgical Co, Monrovia, California, USA) (**b**). Clear temporal incision of 3.0 mm (**c**). ICL injection in the AC (**d**). Positioning the haptics behind the iris (**e**). Closure of the main wound with 10-0 nylon (optional) and irrigation of the viscoelastic with BSS (**f**)

Flap Related Complications

3

Karen Matar, Samir A. Melki, Jason Brenner, and Wassef Chanbour

See Table 3.1.

Case: During the LASIK side cut incisions, conjunctiva was noted to be extending into the incision area inferiorly (*red arrow*), the surgeon proceeded with the case without complications (Fig. 3.1).

Management: If the complication was noticed before creating the flap, the suction should be reapplied again.

Core message: The side cut incision may not be complete if the conjunctiva reached the treatment zone.

Case: Intraoperative pictures taken, showing femtosecond LASIK flap creation and the pupil is not well centered (Fig. 3.2a). The edge of the flap is seen close to the pupillary border (*red arrow*) (Fig. 3.2b).

Management: Pupil-centered laser ablation can result in unexpected visual outcomes if the flap edge bypasses the 6 mm optical zone treatment. In this case the procedure can be aborted and PRK may be performed later.

Core message: Misaligned suction ring can lead to a decentered flap. If possible, the treatment can be performed with a smaller optical zone or PRK may be done.

Case: During flap lift and dissection, the surgeon accidentally creates a linear tear in the flap (*arrowheads*) (Fig. 3.3).

Management: The laser treatment was performed, and the edges of the flap were reapproximated successfully. The patient final UCVA was 20/20.

Core message: If the tear occurred during the flap lift, the surgeon could elect to proceed with the surgery and put the flap back approximating the edges of the tear.

Case: During femtosecond LASIK surgery, a foreign body was noted at the interface (*red arrow*) (Fig. 3.4a), the flap lifting was not possible due to a central adhesion to the stromal bed (Fig. 3.4b).

Table 3.1 Recommended settings for flap creation

Flap settings	Measurement
Diameter	9–9.5 mm in hyperopic treatment
	8–9 mm in myopic treatment
Depth	100–130 μm
Hinge location	Superior (90°)
Hinge angle	40–50°
Hinge width	3.5–5 mm
Side cut angle	70–110°

Spot size, spot separation, and energy are better used according to manufacturer recommendations and adjusted as needed

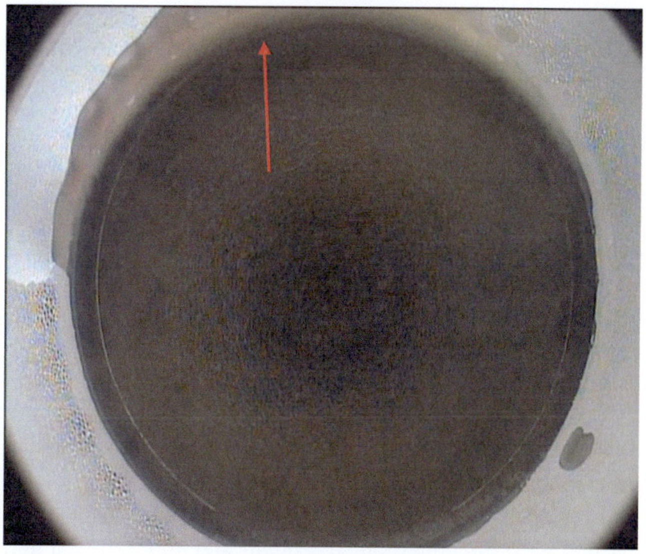

Fig. 3.1 Conjunctival suction. (*Courtesy of Suphi Taneri MD, Augenzentrum am St. Franziskus Hospital Münster, Münster, Germany*)

K. Matar
Cole Eye Institute, Cleveland Clinic Foundation, Cleveland, OH, USA

S. A. Melki (✉) · J. Brenner
Boston Vision, Department of Ophthalmology, Harvard Medical School, Boston, MA, USA
e-mail: melki@bostonvision.com; brenner@bostonvision.com

W. Chanbour
Department of Ophthalmology and Visual Neurosciences, University of Minnesota, Minneapolis, MN, USA
e-mail: chanb013@umn.edu

S. A. Melki et al. (eds.), *Refractive Surgery Atlas*, https://doi.org/10.1007/978-3-031-60661-8_3

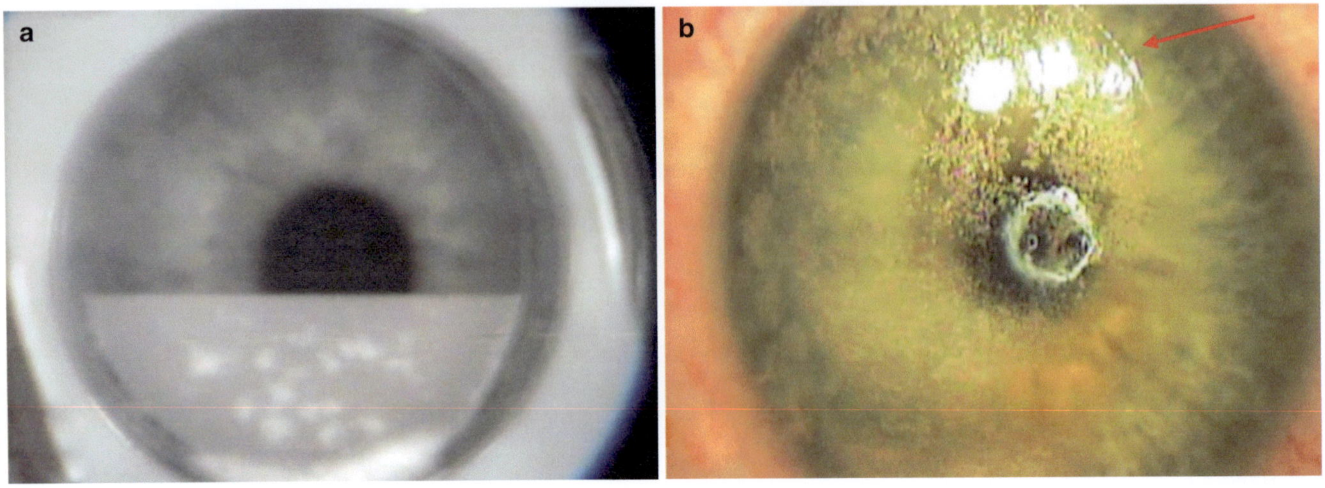

Fig. 3.2 Decentered flap

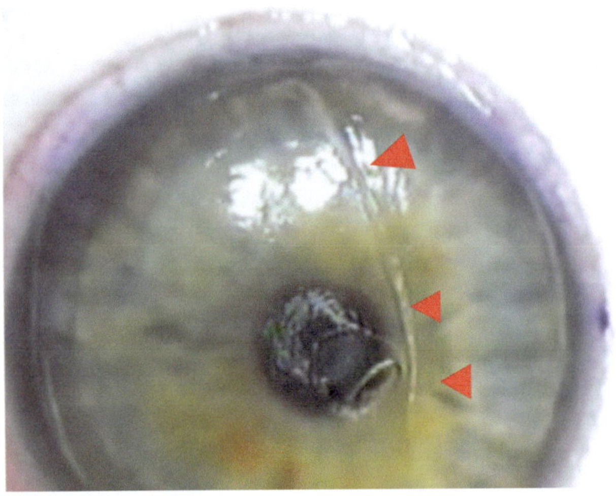

Fig. 3.3 Crescent flap

Management: Flap was repositioned, and the patient had a PRK at a later time.

Core message: Debris should always be removed from the interface before performing the femtosecond cut.

Case: During a slit-lamp exam 5 min following a non-complicated LASIK procedure, the flap was found to be completely dislocated (Fig. 3.5).

Management: Urgent flap repositioning under microscope.

Core message: Same day and day 1 slit lamp exam are necessary to detect and manage flap emergencies.

Case: During a femtosecond LASIK procedure, a free cap occurred (Fig. 3.6a). The completely dislodged flap can be seen marked with ink (Fig. 3.6b).

Management: Intact free flap can be placed on wet surgical pad with the epithelial side down and kept covered and moist. Once the laser ablation is performed, the flap was centered back in its original position (Fig. 3.6c), it was rotated to align the corneal marks (Fig. 3.6d) and allowed to air dry for >5 min. A contact lens should be placed in the end of the procedure. Alternatively, one or multiple 10–0 nylon sutures can be used to secure the flap in place in patients with high risk of dislocation. (Squinting, sensitive to pain or with history of rubbing their eyes.) (Fig. 3.6e).

Core message: Flap marking is a must before lifting any flap.

Case 1: Incomplete flap due to loss of suction with microkeratome LASIK. Flap lift was not possible due to proximity to the hinge (Fig. 3.7a).

Case 2: Following a femtosecond LASIK cut, the surgeon was not able to dissect the flap beyond this point (Fig. 3.7b).

Management:

Case 1: Manual dissection of the flap with a blade while trying to keep the same lamellar plane. Laser ablation was performed within the originally planned optical zone without complications (Fig. 3.7c).

Case 2: Flap was not lifted, and the procedure was aborted. Patient underwent surface refractive surgery a few weeks later (Fig. 3.7d).

Core message: Careful dissection of the flap with a blade can be performed when the area of flap-stroma attachment is small.

Case: Following a femtosecond cut, the surgeon was unable to dissect a wide area consisting of an incomplete side cut. The flap lifter could not get through the flap on the nasal side (Fig. 3.8a).

Management: A scissors was used to cut the flap edge (Fig. 3.8b). The procedure was then completed without complications (Fig. 3.8c).

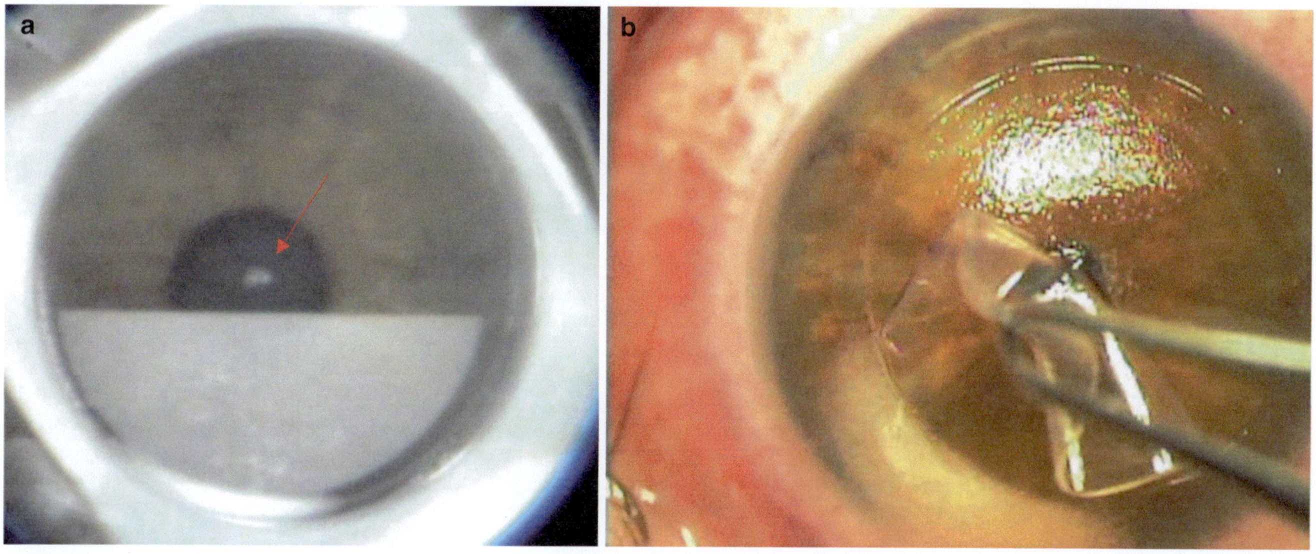

Fig. 3.4 Interface debris

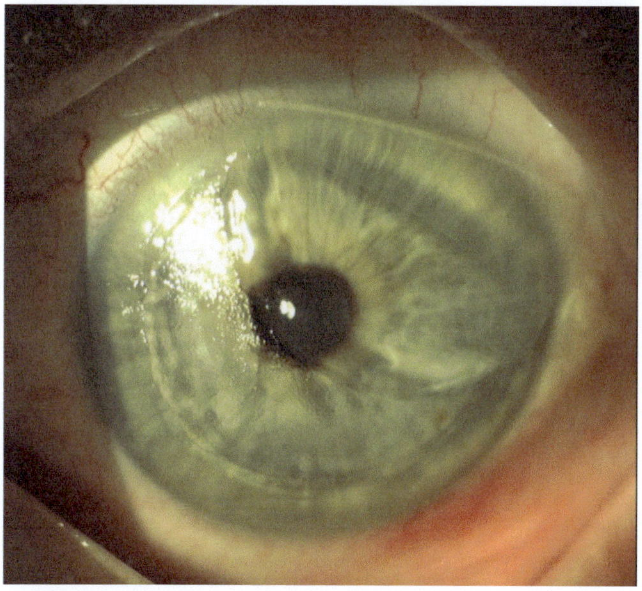

Fig. 3.5 Post-operative dislodged flap

Core message: Cutting the edge of the flap should be performed with one single large snip to avoid flap edge irregularities and epithelial ingrowth. This technique can be used when the incomplete area is extensive (about 45 degrees) and the ring forceps could induce a flap tear.

Case 1: Incomplete flap construction due to loss of suction mid-way across the planned cut (Fig. 3.9a).

Case 2: Loss of suction occurring at two-thirds the distance across the planned cut (Fig. 3.9b).

Management: Suction ring was reapplied and the second cut was created using the same cone at the same depth (Fig. 3.9c, d).

Core message: Same applanation cone should be used to create a flap when there is a loss of suction during LASIK.

Case: A very thin flap was lifted following a microkeratome cut (Fig. 3.10a).

Management: The laser ablation was performed, the flap was repositioned properly, and the contact lens was placed (Fig. 3.10b).

Core message: Thin flaps occur mostly with microkeratome and it is prone to causing folds, therefore a contact lens should be placed.

Case: During the microkeratome cut, the suction was lost but the treatment was completed. When the flap was lifted, a piece remained attached inferiorly to the stromal bed (*black arrow*) (Fig. 3.11a).

Management: No laser ablation as the edge was close to the visual axis. The flap was repositioned (Fig. 3.11b) and bandage contact lens was placed. PRK was performed later.

Case: Two patients were examined following a complicated microkeratome LASIK surgery (Fig. 3.12).

Exam: Central buttonholes can be seen on the first post operative day in patient 1 (Fig. 3.12a). Localized stromal inflammation is noted around the edge of the buttonhole in patient 2 (Fig. 3.12b).

Management: Epithelium healed during the first week leaving a grade 1 corneal scar at 2 months postop (Fig. 3.12c).

Case: During flap lift, the dissector created a hole close to the hinge and distant from the flap edge (*red arrow*)

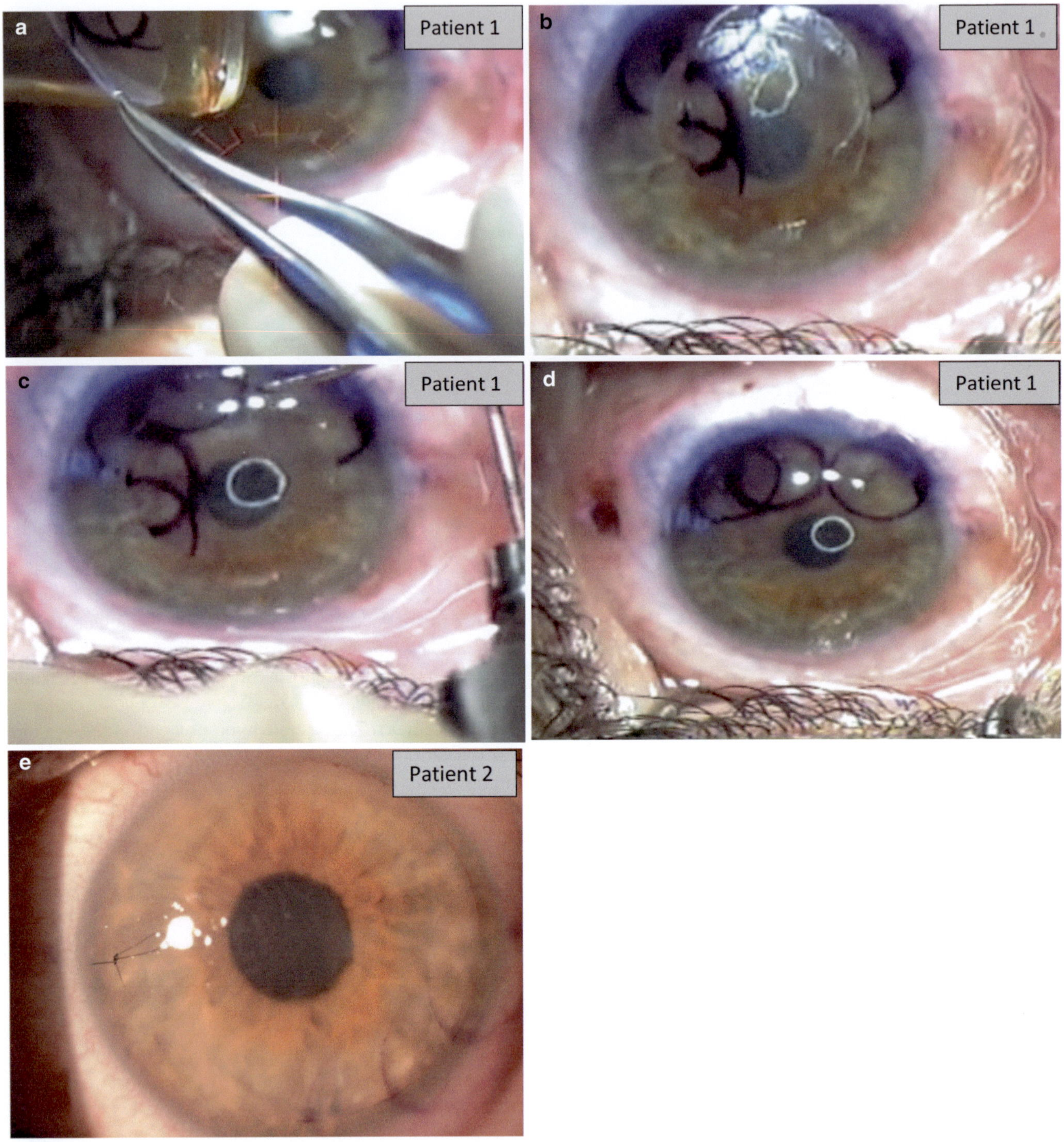

Fig. 3.6 Free cap

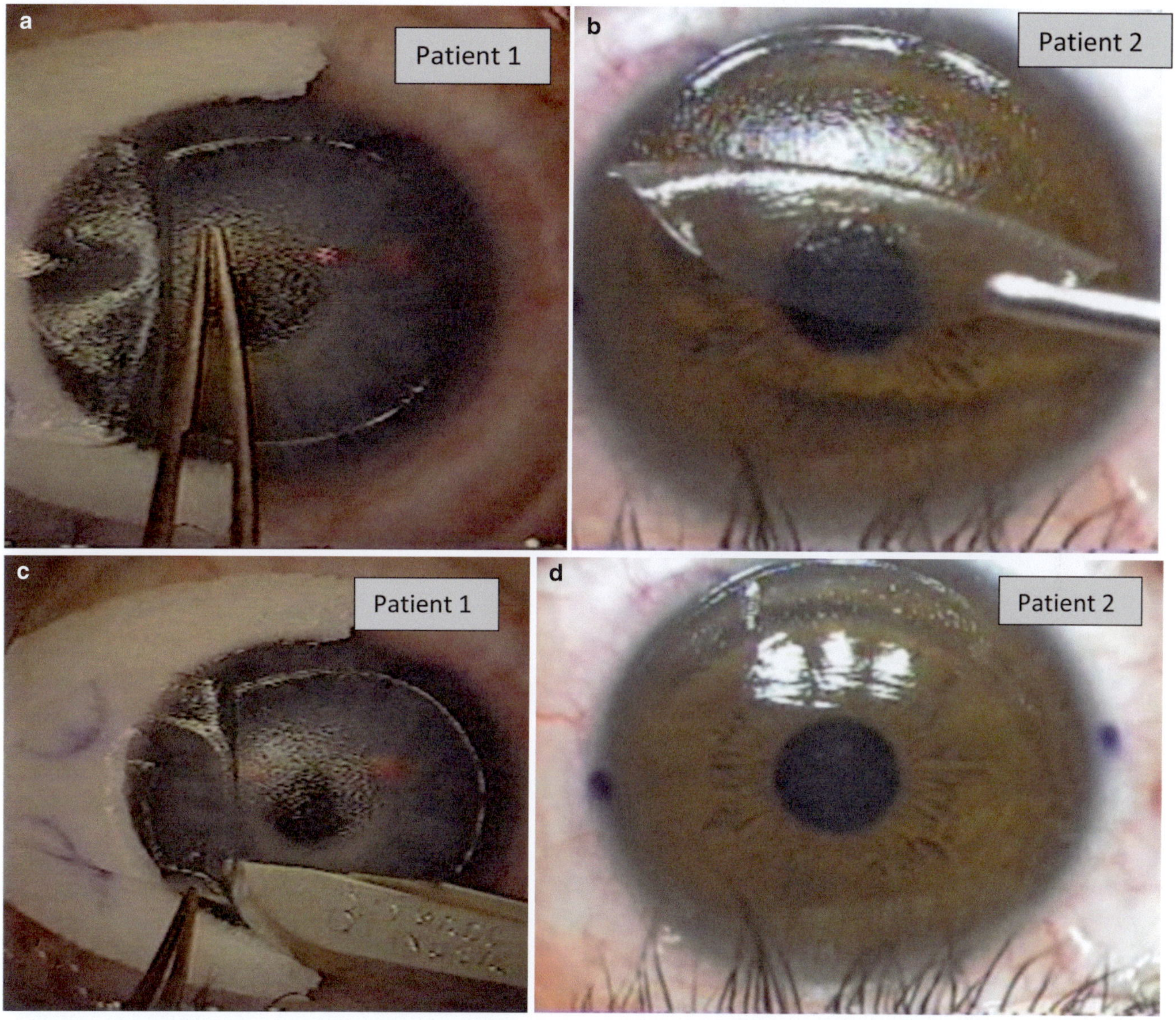

Fig. 3.7 Incomplete flap

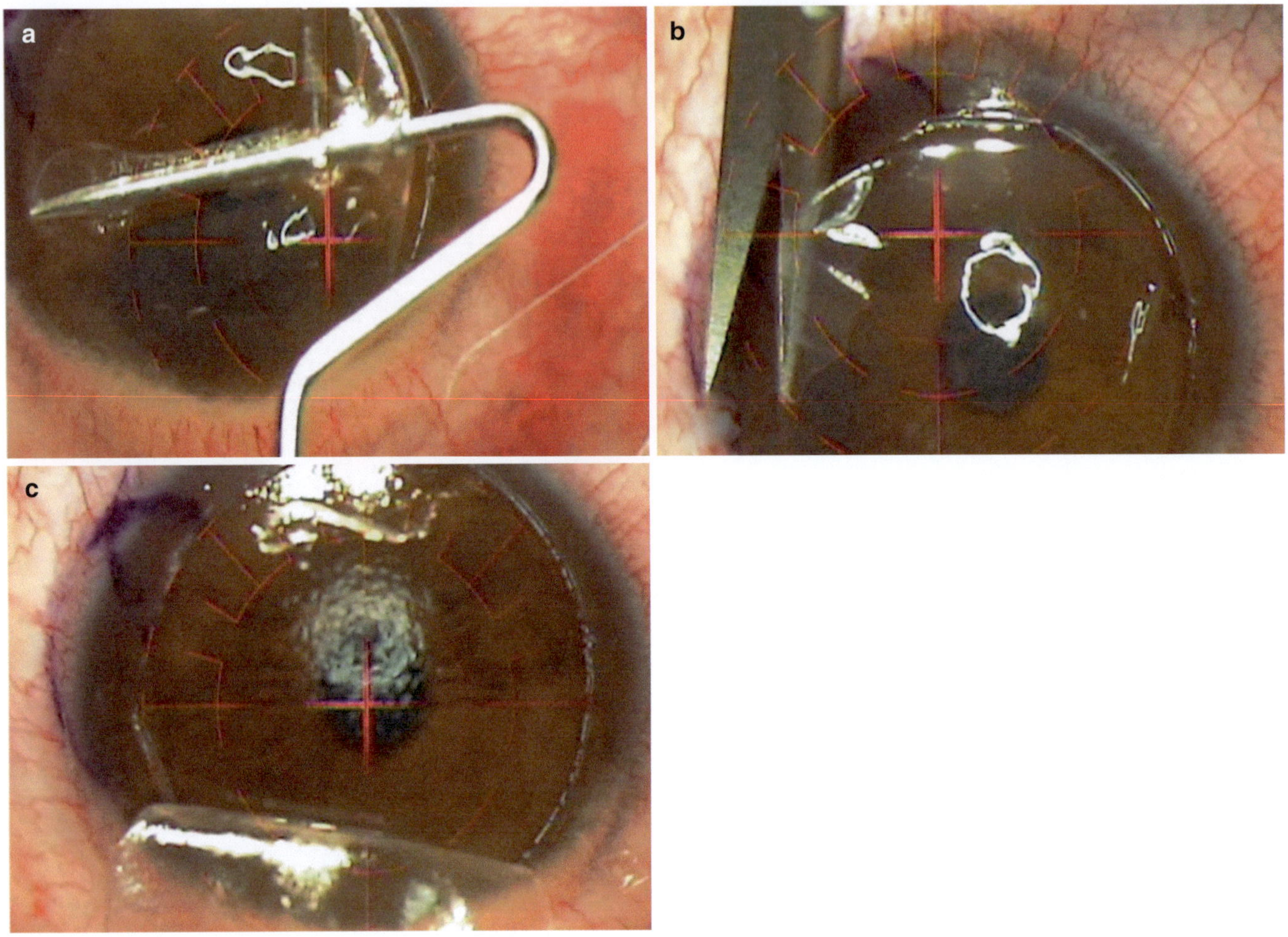

Fig. 3.8 Incomplete side cut

(Fig. 3.13a), while dissecting the flap tear extended paracentrally (*black arrow*) (Fig. 3.13b).

Management: The surgeon dissected the flap through the other side (Fig. 3.13c), the laser ablation was performed, and the flap was repositioned (Fig. 3.13d).

Core message: The flap edge should be reached by the dissector from one side of the hinge to the other side, the tip of the instrument should be always directed downwards to avoid creating holes in the flap.

Case: During flap dissection and lift, the surgeon was using excessive traction when dissecting the flap (Fig. 3.14a), the flap was torn, and an oblique line can be seen at the location of the tear (*red arrow*) (Fig. 3.14b).

Management: Flap dissection should be aborted. The flap was repositioned and a contact lens applied for protection.

Core message: When the flap is adherent to the stroma, gentle dissection in small increments with the tip of the dissector helps release the adhesions.

If the surgeon encounters an incomplete side cut with an area with minimal adhesions, a ring forceps can be used to dissect the area in a flap-rhexis fashion and complete the flap lift (Fig. 3.15).

Take-Home Message

- When the conjunctiva is folded into the applanation interface, the applanation should be reapplied again. In case of recurrence, stretching the conjunctiva may be performed by applying posterior pressure on the speculum.
- Surgeon should never dissect the flap forcefully.
- Debris should always be removed from the femtosecond applanation interface.
- Never attempt to release central flap-stromal adhesions.
- A blade can be used to dissect the flap-stromal interface in case of residual small tags.
- LASIK should be aborted if the flap is not lifted from the central 6 mm optical zone.
- Sutures and BCLs can be used if there is a free cap.
- Ring forceps, tying forceps, or scissors can be used to complete the flap if the side cut was incomplete.

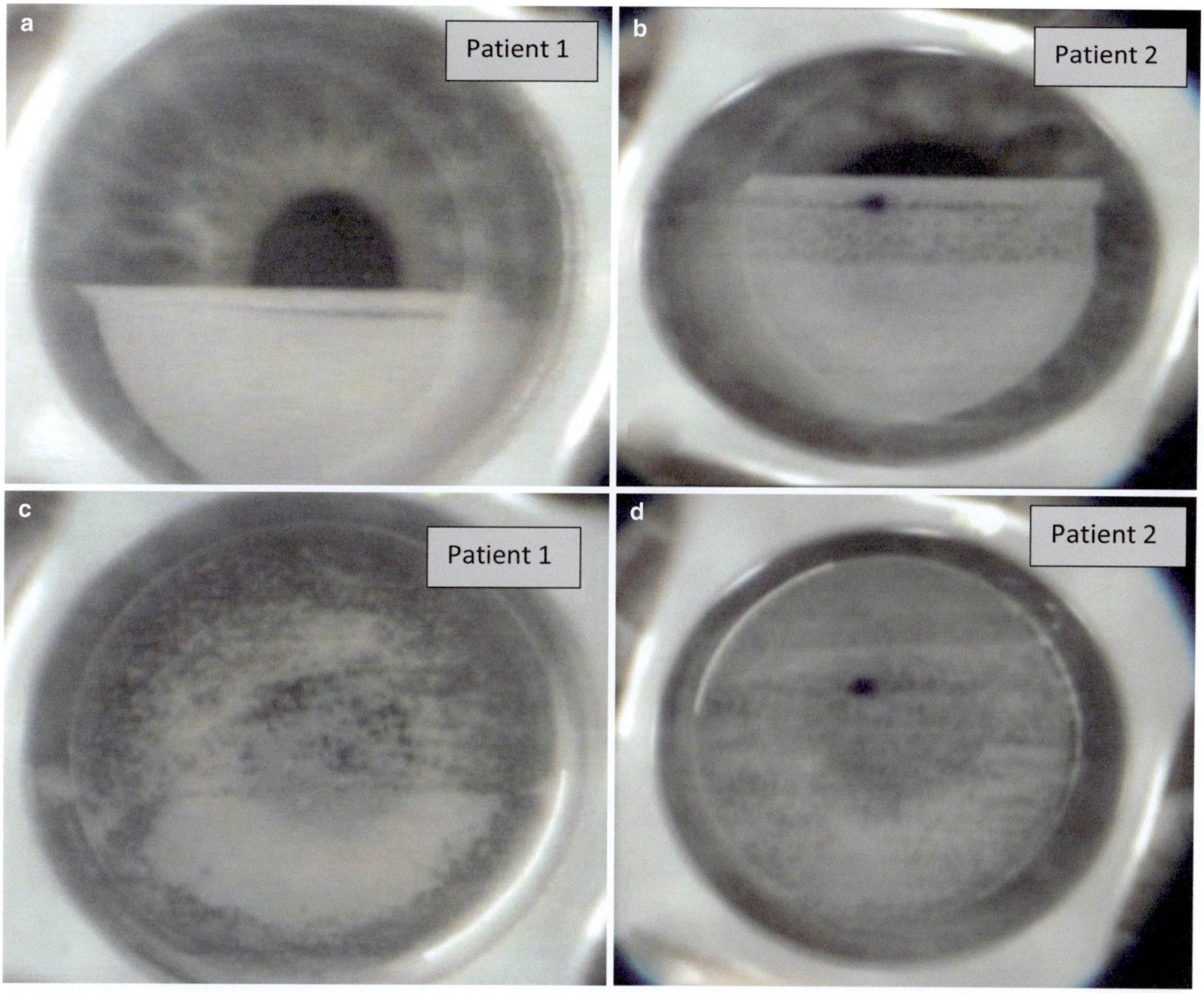

Fig. 3.9 Loss of suction

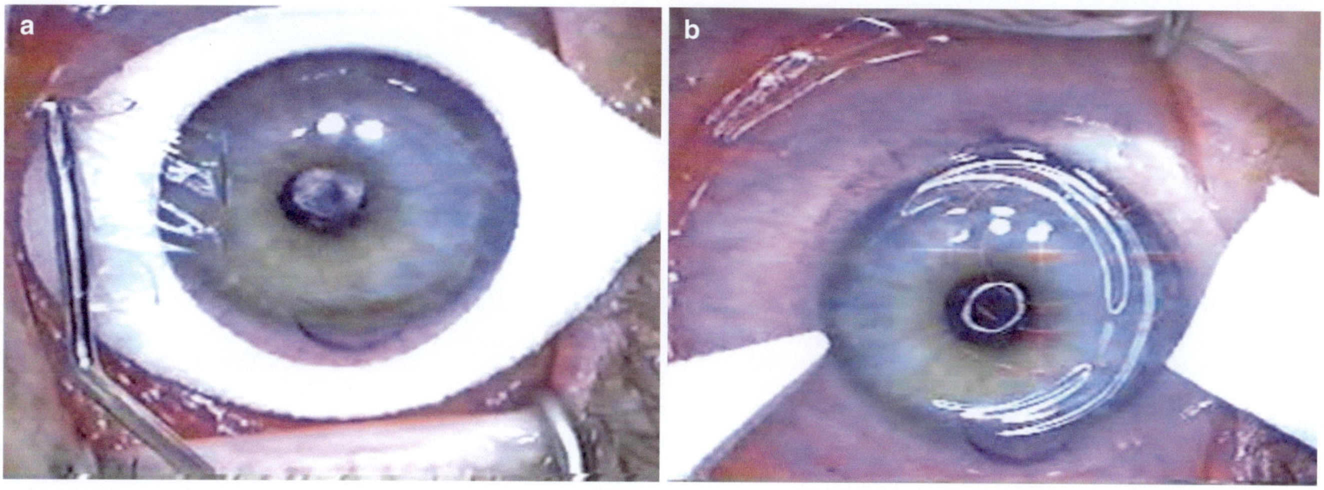

Fig. 3.10 Thin incomplete flap

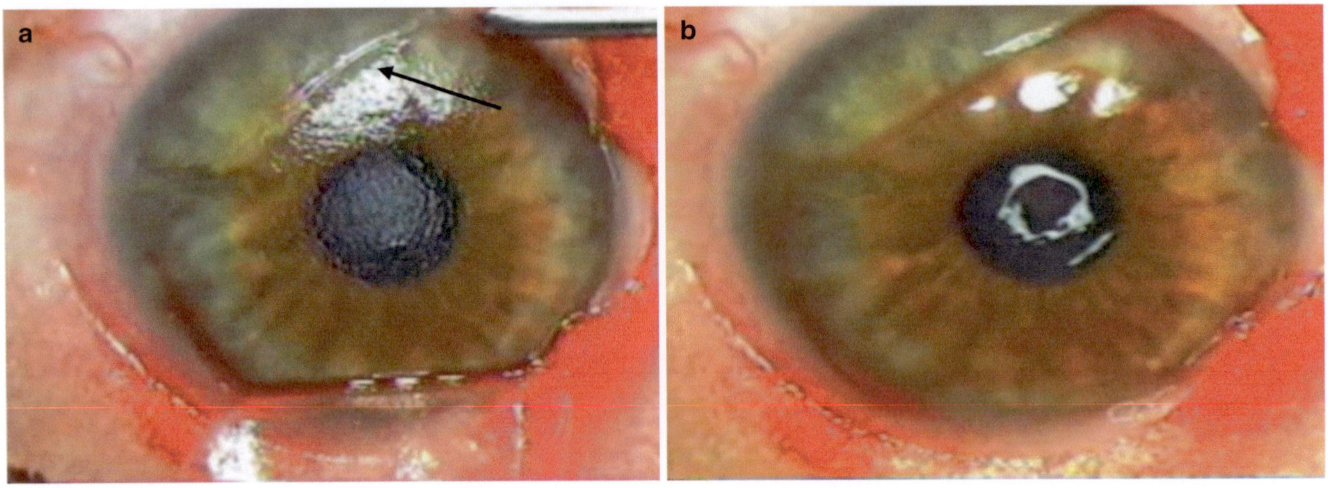

Fig. 3.11 Partial flap

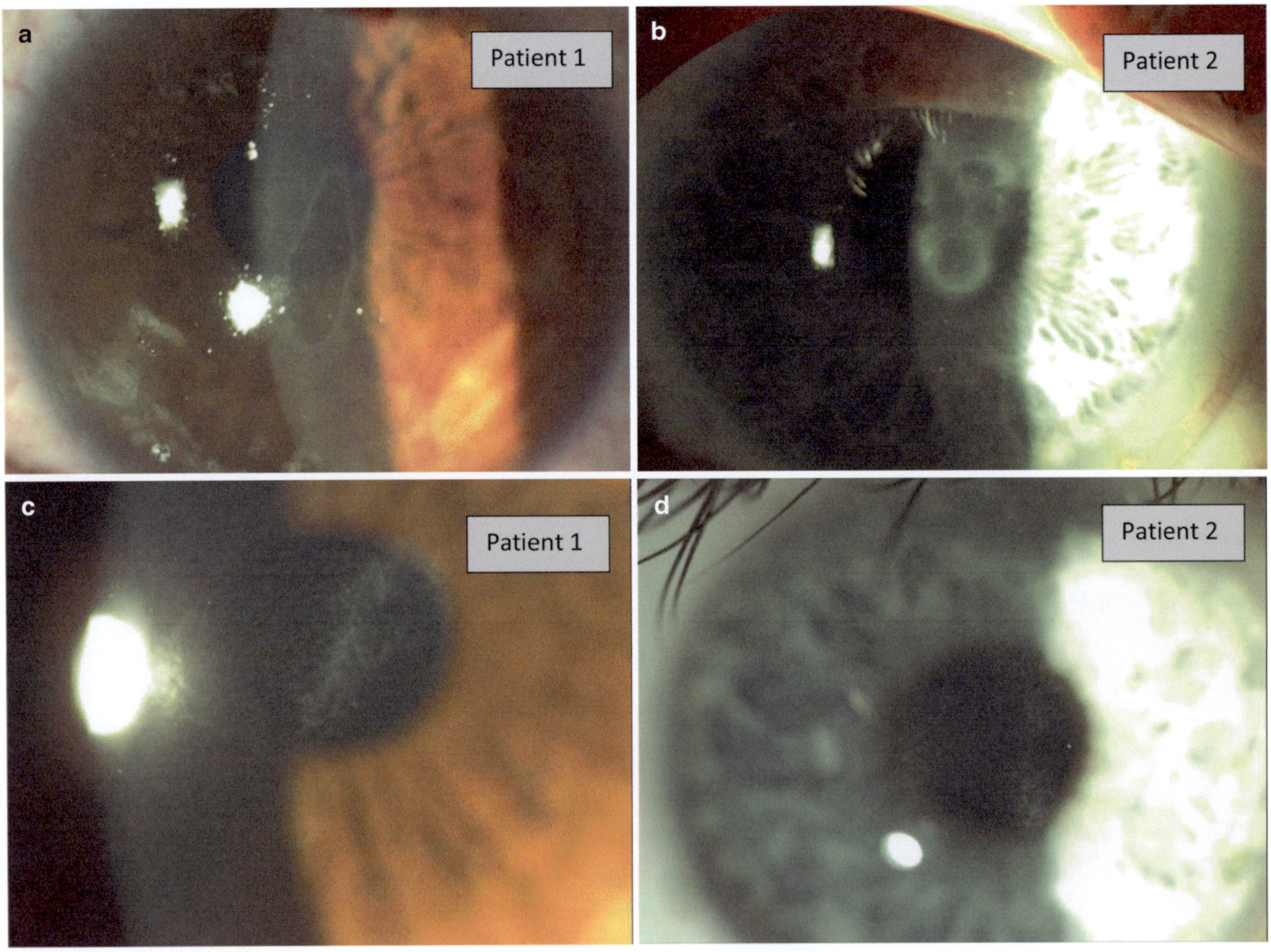

Fig. 3.12 Central buttonhole

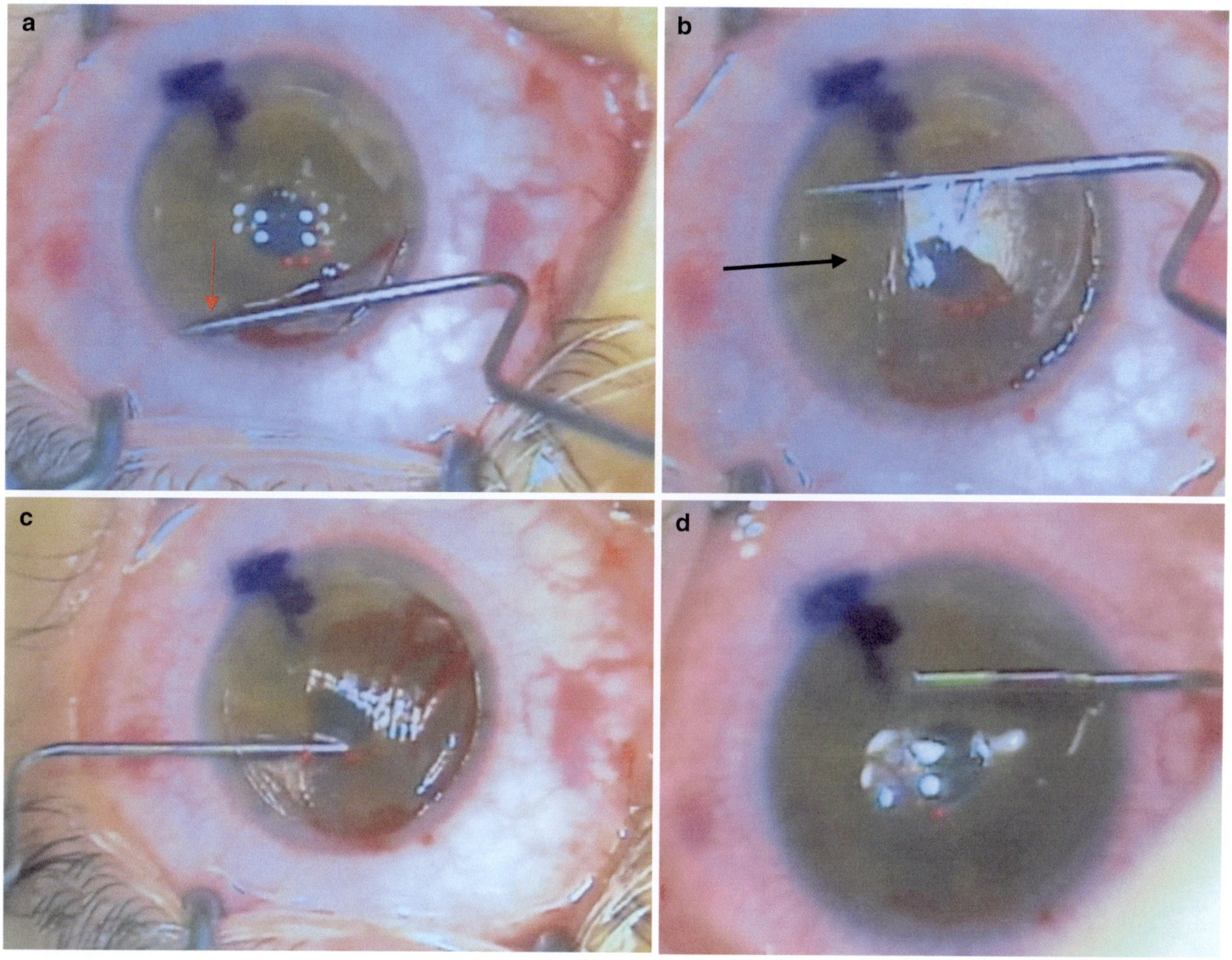

Fig. 3.13 Central flap laceration

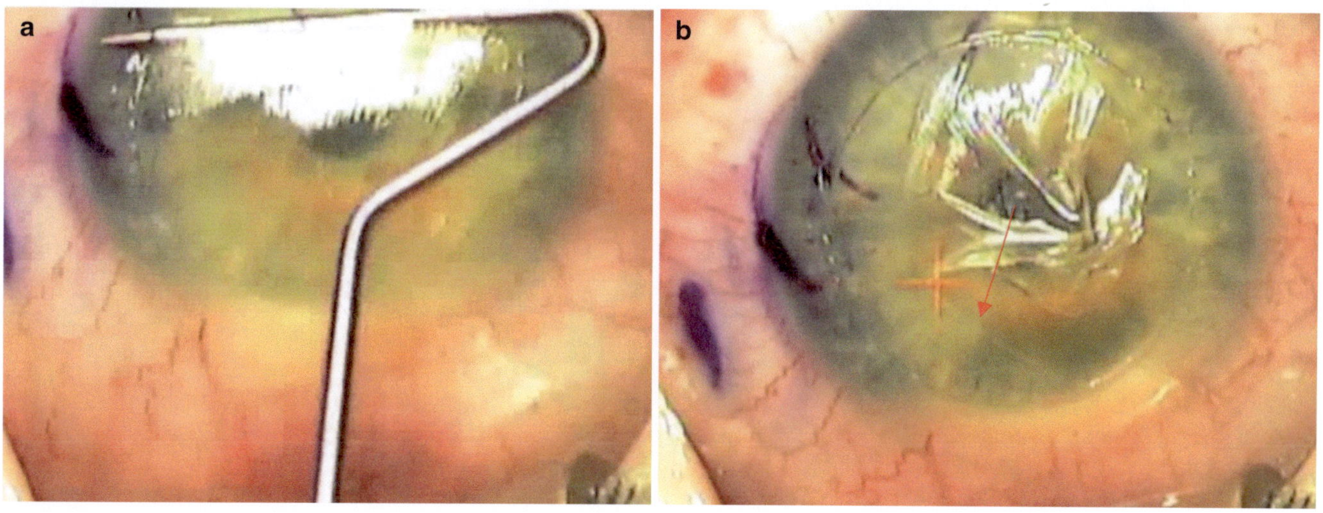

Fig. 3.14 Torn flap

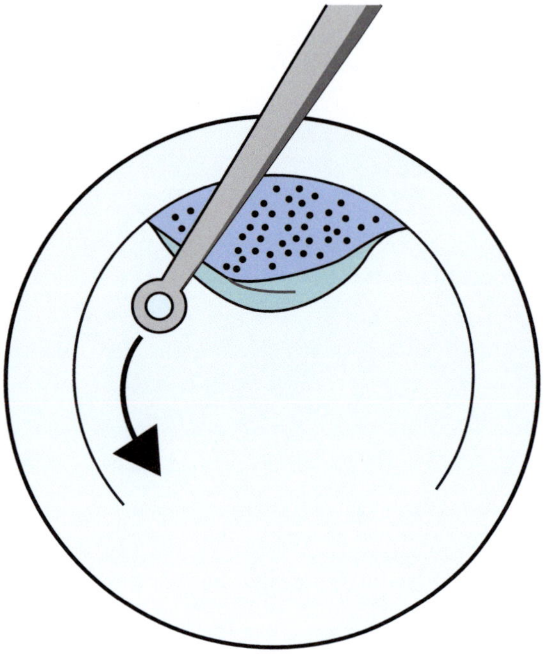

Fig. 3.15 Dissection technique for incomplete side cut

4 Gas Related Events in Lasik

Jason Brenner, Wassef Chanbour, and Samir A. Melki

See Table 4.1.

Cases:

(Fig. 4.1a): Small paracentral island of OBL.

(Fig. 4.1b): Large peripheral OBL.

(Fig. 4.1c, d): Diffuse OBL covering the visual axis of the same patient.

Management: When the OBL is large and covering the pupil, it may interfere with the pupil tracker. Rubbing the stoma with a sharp dissector is enough to remove the OBL (Fig. 4.1e).

Case: Slit lamp exam few minutes following a LASIK surgery. VGB can be noted superiorly with an air bubble located under the epithelium extending into the deep stroma. The patient has a history of cataract surgery with superior corneal incision (Fig. 4.2).

Core message: Corneal scars from previous incisions, trauma, or infection can induce VGB.

Case: Central VGB formed during femtosecond cut; it has a black appearance (Fig. 4.3a); the epithelial bullae can be seen at the location of the VGB (Fig. 4.3b).

Table 4.1 Characteristics and management of air bubble related complications following LASIK

Gas location	Description
Anterior chamber (AC) gas bubbles	**Incidence:** 0.14–1.6% [1, 2] **Physiology:** – Scattering of air bubbles may be a result of the femtosecond beam producing a direct photodissociation of the aqueous humor [3] – Bubbles enter through Schlemm's canal via the trabecular meshwork [4] **Risk factors**: Small cornea, large flap, and high applanation pressures [5] **Prevention:** Decreasing the flap diameter in small corneas, soft docking **Management:** Wait 2–4 h until the gas is reabsorbed and LASIK can be performed safely
Opaque bubble layer (OBL)	**Physiology:** Bubbles accumulate in the superficial layers of the stromal bed, creating diffuse opacity. Hard or soft bubble layer can form [6] **Risk factors:** Small flap, thick corneas, lower energy [7] **Prevention:** Larger flap diameter [8], using a pocket or a canal next to the hinge, creating the hinge at the edge of the cone so that the gas can dissipate outside cone [8], soft docking [9], high pulse repetition rate, higher energy, closer spots [10] **Management**: OBL may interfere with flap creation, measurement of residual stromal bed thickness, and the excimer laser tracking system and can delay the surgical procedure. Gentle corneal rubbing with the tip of instruments can resolve the issue
Vertical gas breakthrough (VGB)	**Physiology:** Bubbles dissect into the subepithelial space. Partial breaks will look gray/white and full breaks will look black. Lifting the flap may create a button hole or a strong adhesion may be located in the same area which may prevent flap lift **Risk factors:** Presence of corneal scars, abnormal stromal layers, epithelial defects or debris **Prevention**: Removal of surface debris on the cone or the cornea. PRK is recommended in case of corneal scars **Management:** Flap with central VGB should not be lifted, PRK can be performed. Flap with peripheral VGB can be lifted safely

J. Brenner (✉) · S. A. Melki
Boston Vision, Department of Ophthalmology, Harvard Medical School, Boston, MA, USA
e-mail: brenner@bostonvision.com; melki@bostonvision.com

W. Chanbour
Department of Ophthalmology and Visual Neurosciences, University of Minnesota, Minneapolis, MN, USA
e-mail: chanb013@umn.edu

S. A. Melki et al. (eds.), *Refractive Surgery Atlas*, https://doi.org/10.1007/978-3-031-60661-8_4

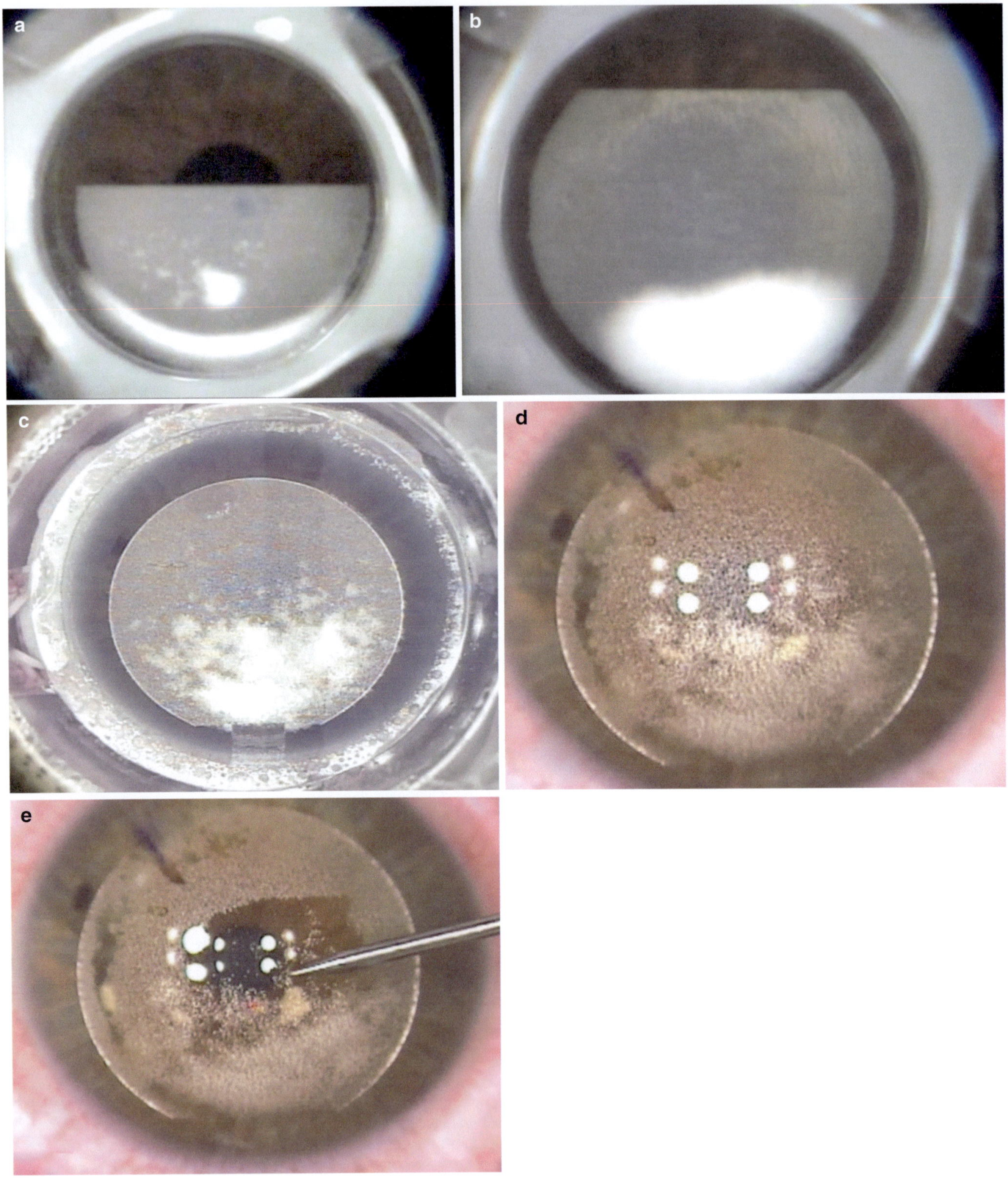

Fig. 4.1 Opaque bubble layer

Management: Flap should not be lifted as it may induce a buttonhole formation. Patient should be considered for PRK surgery.

Core message: The black appearance of VGB indicates that the air bubble may have dissected beyond Bowman's membrane. These cases are at high risk of inducing a buttonhole.

Case: A peripheral VGB formed at the hinge during flap creation; it has a whitish appearance (Fig. 4.4a). The bubble can be seen under the microscope (Fig. 4.4b). Strong adherence between the flap and the stroma was apparent at the location of the VGB during dissection (Fig. 4.4c).

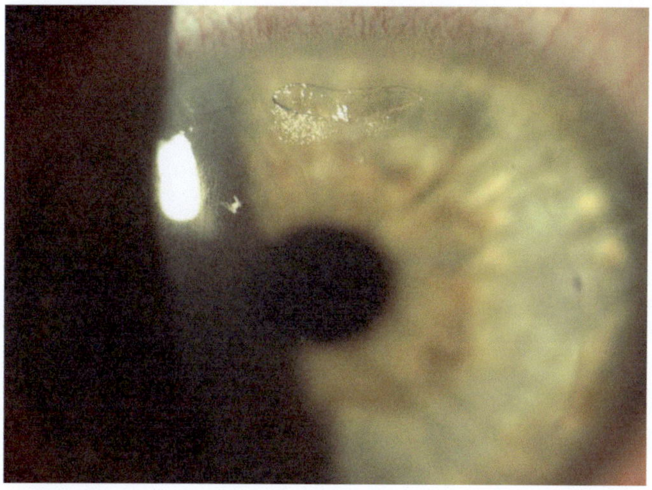

Fig. 4.2 Cataract incision

Management: Laser ablation can be performed as the adhesions between the flap and stroma is outside the visual axis, blade can be used to dissect the adherent area.

Core message: When the VGB is noted to have whitish appearance, the bubble may have stopped underneath the Bowman's layer. It is safer to lift the flap in these cases.

Case: A vertical gas breakthrough occurred during the creation of the superior air pocket with femtosecond laser. A large subepithelial gas bubble can be seen (*red arrow*) (Fig. 4.5a).

Management: Flap lift was performed, and the procedure was completed without complications. The Air bubble can be seen squeezed under the flap when it is lifted (*red arrowheads*) (Fig. 4.5b).

Case: Three small gas bubbles appeared during Femtosecond cut (*red arrow*) (Fig. 4.6a); bubbles appeared in the center of the pupil when the flap was lifted (Fig. 4.6b).

Management: When the gas bubble is large it will interfere with the pupillary tracker, the bubbles usually disappear within 3–4 h and the flap lift and excimer laser treatment can be performed. In this case, laser treatment was still possible as the pupil was still detectable.

Case: An irregular bubble pattern was noted at the interface during Femtosecond flap creation (Fig. 4.7a); compared with a normal pattern (Fig. 4.7b).

Management: There was no flap created on the patient's cornea. The pattern was caused by a cut through the contact lens that the patient forgot to remove. The contact lens was attached to the femtosecond LASIK cone. LASIK can still be performed safely later.

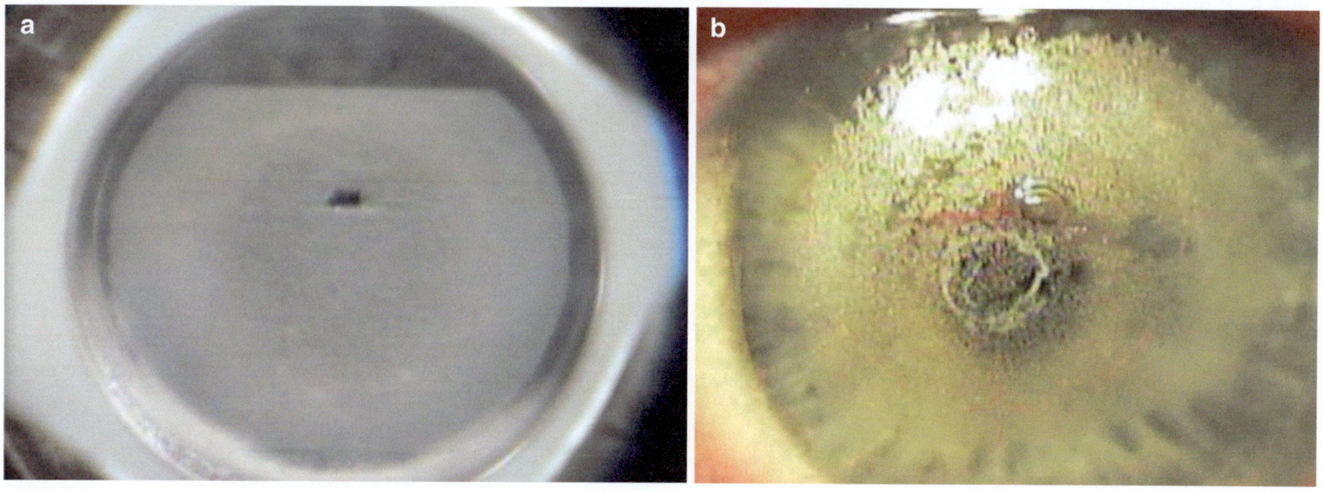

Fig. 4.3 Central vertical gas breakthrough

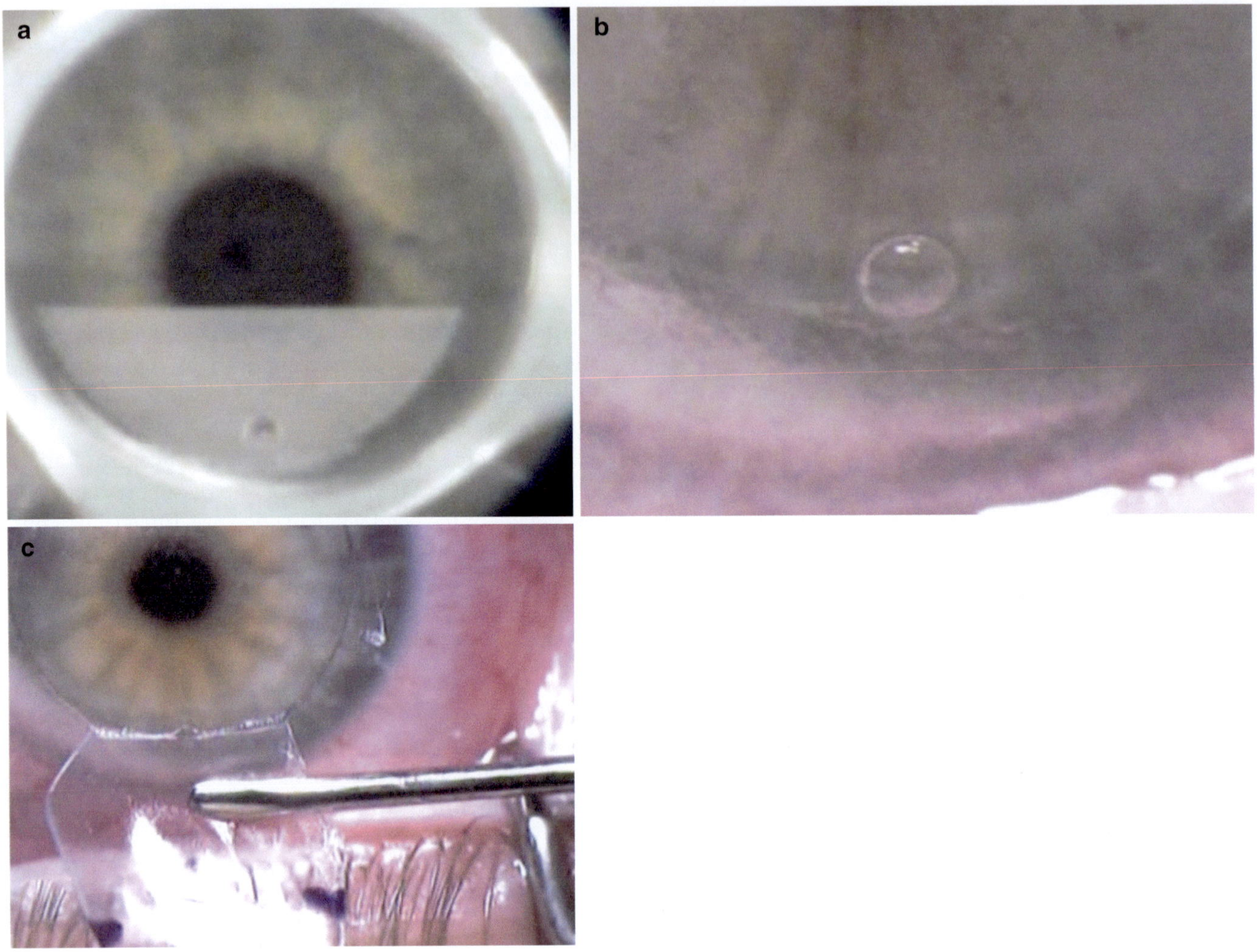

Fig. 4.4 Peripheral vertical gas breakthrough

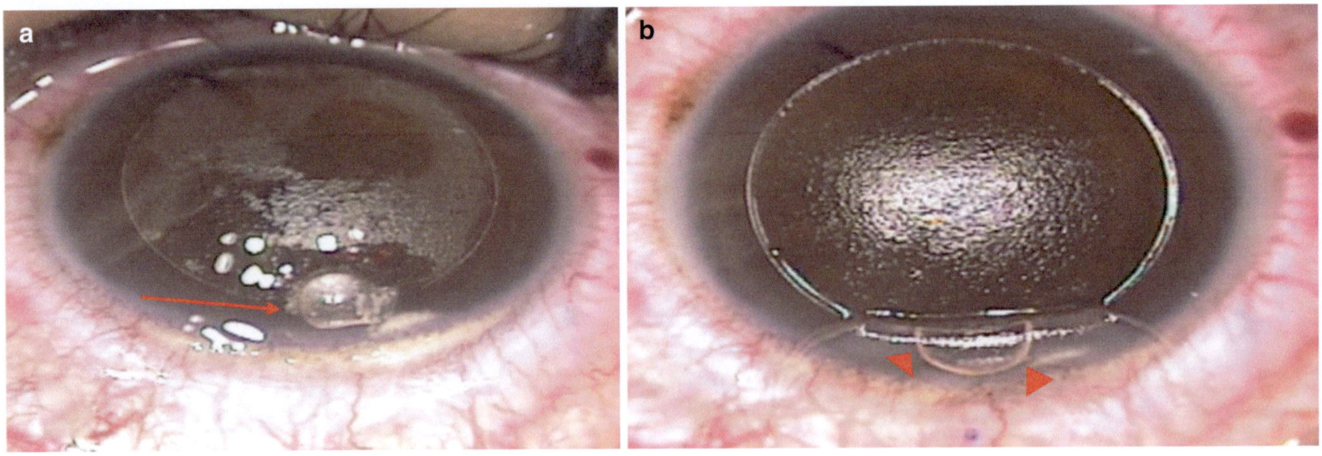

Fig. 4.5 Pocket air bubble

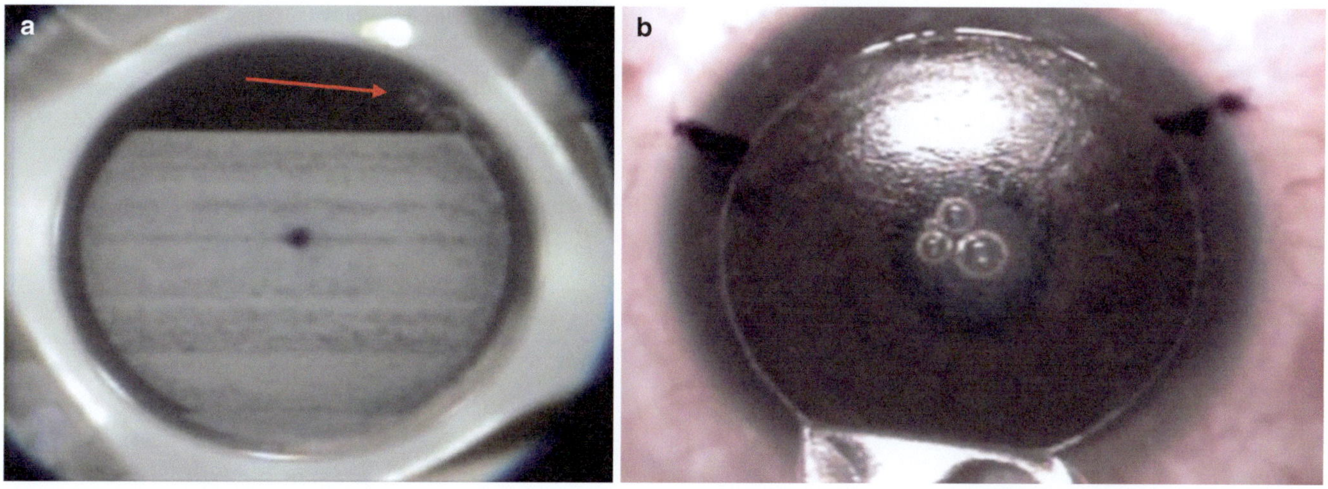

Fig. 4.6 Anterior chamber gas bubble

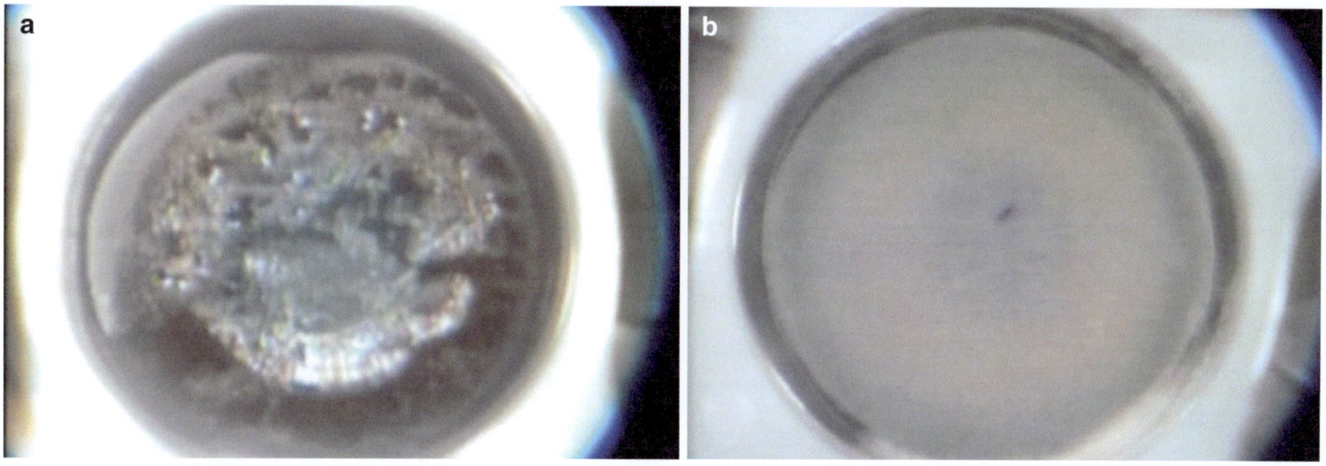

Fig. 4.7 Lasering a contact lens

Take-Home Message

- Air pocket is an optional setting that can help trap bubble during flap creation to prevent OBL formation.
- In small corneas, especially in Asian ethnicities, the flap diameter can be decreased to avoid AC gas bubbles.
- The flap can be lifted safely in the presence of a peripheral VGB.
- The flap should be left in place in case of central VGB and PRK can be performed later.
- PRK is a better option in patients with central superficial corneal scars to avoid VGB.
- Contact lens removal check should be added to the pre-op checklist.

References

1. Rush SW, Cofoid P, Rush RB. Incidence and outcomes of anterior chamber gas bubble during femtosecond flap creation for laser-assisted *in situ* keratomileusis. J Ophthalmol. 2015;2015:542127.
2. Niparugs M. Incidence and predisposing factors of anterior chamber gas bubbles during femtosecond laser flap creation. Int J Ophthalmol. 2020;13:1334–7.
3. Utine CA, Altunsoy M, Basar D. Visante® anterior segment OCT in a patient with gas bubbles in the anterior chamber after femtosecond laser corneal flap formation. Int Ophthalmol. 2010;30(1):81–4.
4. Wright JR. Gas bubbles after flap creation with femtosecond laser. J Cataract Refract Surg. 2006;32(7):1076.
5. Shah DN, Melki S. Complications of femtosecond-assisted laser *in situ* keratomileusis flaps. Semin Ophthalmol. 2014;29(5–6):363–75.
6. Liu CH, Sun CC, Hui-Kang Ma D, Chien-Chieh Huang J, Liu CF, Chen HF, Hsiao CH. Opaque bubble layer: incidence, risk factors, and clinical relevance. J Cataract Refract Surg. 2014;40(3):435–40.
7. Kaiserman I, Maresky HS, Bahar I, Rootman DS. Incidence, possible risk factors, and potential effects of an opaque bubble

layer created by a femtosecond laser. J Cataract Refract Surg. 2008;34:417–23.
8. Mastropasqua L, Calienno R, Lanzini M, et al. Opaque bubble layer incidence in femtosecond laser-assisted LASIK: comparison among different flap design parameters. Int Ophthalmol. 2016;37(3):635–41.
9. Jung H, Kim J, Lim T. Possible risk factors and clinical effects of an opaque bubble layer created with femtosecond laser–assisted laser in situ keratomileusis. J Cataract Refract Surg. 2015;41(7):1393–9.
10. Niparugs M. Incidence and predisposing factors of anterior chamber gas bubbles during femtosecond laser flap creation. Int J Ophthalmol. 2020;13(8):1334–7.

5 Flap Striae

Wassef Chanbour, Samir A. Melki, Jason Brenner, and Kevin G. Makhoul

See Table 5.1.

Case: Patient examined 20 min post LASIK procedure (Fig. 5.1).

Exam: Early slipping of the flap after LASIK and multiple vertical macrostriae (Fig. 5.1a).

Management: Partial refloating using an irrigation cannula was performed using a slit lamp (Fig. 5.1b). Slit lamp exam showing immediate resolution (Fig. 5.1c).

Core message: Flap check in the immediate post-operative period is necessary before the patient is discharge.

Case: One month following a LASIK procedure, a patient presented with halos and blurry vision with a BCVA 20/50 (Fig. 5.2).

Exam: Central macrostriae seen with slit lamp (Fig. 5.2a) and it showed negative linear staining with fluorescein stain (Fig. 5.2b).

Management: After de-epithelization the flap was sutured to stretch the folds. Day 1 following flap suturing (Fig. 5.2c) the central flap shows folds that eventually resolved.

Core message: Epithelium removal makes it easier to unfold the flap correctly.

Case: Multiple asymptomatic patients presenting for follow up, their UCVA is 20/20 (Fig. 5.3).

Exam: Patient 1: a temporal paracentral vertical microstriae (*red arrows*) (Fig. 5.3a). Patient 2: an inferior horizontal microstriae, not clearly visible with direct light (Fig. 5.3b), more evident on fluorescein exam with a negative staining (*red arrowhead*) (Fig. 5.3c). Patient 3: microstriae better identified using retro-illumination (*yellow arrowhead*) (Fig. 5.3d).

Management: Observation is recommended.

Case: One day following a LASIK procedure, an asymptomatic patient presented for follow up and his vision was 20/20 (Fig. 5.4a).

Case: A second patient having a 20/20 vision one day following LASIK (Fig. 5.4b).

Exam: Indirect illumination using the slit lamp shows peripheral microstriae formation (*red arrows*) (Fig. 5.4a, b).

Management: Observation is recommended.

Case: One day post LASIK procedure in two patients complaining of blurry vision, halos, and glare (Fig. 5.5).

Exam: Macrostriae with temporal gap shown on slit lamp (Fig. 5.5a) and on fluorescein staining (Fig. 5.5b, d).

Management: Refloating the flap should be performed. Alignment was corrected immediately following refloating (Fig. 5.5c, e).

Core message: On the first post-operative day, refloating using the slit lamp is a quick and safe method to adjust the flap. Any grown epithelium should be removed from the interface.

Case: Two weeks post LASIK procedure, a patient presented with decreased vision since the surgery. UCVA: 20/30 (Fig. 5.6).

Exam: Slit lamp exam showing macrostriae in the para central area (Fig. 5.6a).

Management: De-epithelization and ironing was performed (Fig. 5.6b) followed by BCL insertion. The Striae disappeared 1-week post-op (Fig. 5.6c).

Case: One month following a LASIK procedure a patient presented with blurry vision (Fig. 5.7).

Exam: Central macrostriae with inferior epithelial ingrowth (Fig. 5.7a, b).

Management: Flap lift with epithelial removal, ironing and epithelial ingrowth scraping should be performed.

W. Chanbour (✉)
Department of Ophthalmology and Visual Neurosciences, University of Minnesota, Minneapolis, MN, USA
e-mail: chanb013@umn.edu

S. A. Melki · J. Brenner
Boston Vision, Department of Ophthalmology, Harvard Medical School, Boston, MA, USA
e-mail: melki@bostonvision.com; brenner@bostonvision.com

K. G. Makhoul
KU Eye Center, University of Kansas Medical Center, Kansas City, KS, USA

S. A. Melki et al. (eds.), *Refractive Surgery Atlas*, https://doi.org/10.1007/978-3-031-60661-8_5

Table 5.1 Diagnosis, prevention, and management of flap striae

Onset	First few hours to days following LASIK surgery [1]
Rate	0.033%–12.8% clinically significant [2, 3]
Pathology	**Microstriae**: Almost universal in microkeratome created flaps, small, semi-random wrinkles, or irregularities in the LASIK flap [4] **Macrostriae**: Large wrinkles or folds with broad undulations of parallel or semi-parallel lines
Mechanism	Corneal flap misalignment, postoperative flap shifting, size differences between flap and stromal bed [5, 6]
Symptoms	Microstriae are mostly asymptomatic Symptomatic striae can cause: decrease in UCVA/BCVA, irregular astigmatism, loss of contrast sensitivity, halos, glare, ghosting, shadowing, and monocular diplopia [2, 7, 8]
Monitoring	Slit lamp, retro-illumination, ring light [8], fluorescein under cobalt blue filter [1]
Risk factors	**Preoperative**: higher manifest refraction sphere, cylinder, and/or spherical equivalence [2] **Perioperative**: flap misalignment, non-superior hinge [3], over-drying or excessive irrigation [8], thin or thick flaps [9], higher total ablation depth, and percentage of corneal tissue ablated [2] **Postoperative**: trauma
Prevention	• Use of a femtosecond laser rather than a microkeratome blade [3] • Proper flap construction, marking, and alignment [10] • Ensuring the flap is neatly positioned and not wrinkled when turned over [8] • Gentle stroking of the repositioned flap with a moistened surgical sponge [11] • Slade's striae test: gentle pressure applied just beyond the keratectomy to observe fine folds radiating into the flap [11] • Inspection of the flap with a slit lamp immediately after LASIK [11]
Indications for treatment	• Detection perioperatively or on slit lamp exam • Inducing refractive error or irregular astigmatism • Inducing halos, glare, shadowing, diplopia, or other undesirable visual effects
Treatment techniques	**Early Management**: • Flattening and stretching the flap in radial direction [11] • Refloating, hydrating, and repositioning the flap +/− de-epithelization [9] **Late Management**: • PTK [4, 7] • Suturing [7] • Donnenfeld method of hyperthermic ironing [12] • Application of a rigid contact lens [7] • Amputating the flap [7]

Core message: Any gap between the flap and the cornea should be fixed to prevent epithelial ingrowth in patients with striae.

Case: Patient examined day 1 following an uneventful LASIK. Patient is light sensitive and his vision is blurry (Fig. 5.8).

Exam: A peripheral folded flap is noted with a stage 1 DLK within and outside the folded area (*red arrows*).

Management: Flap lift, scraping of peripheral epithelium, unfolding the flap and irrigation should be performed.

Case: Two patients were examined few minutes post LASIK procedure (Fig. 5.9).

Exam: Macrostriae formation and flap slippage (Fig. 5.9a, c). Same folds visualized with negative fluorescein staining (Fig. 5.9b, d). Note that epithelium started growing on the stromal bed, which stains with fluorescein when exposed.

Management: Immediate flap refloating and alignment was performed.

Case 1: One day following a LASIK procedure, patient 1 presented with a complete peripheral flap folding with epithelization of the bare stroma and scattered epithelial cells under the flap (*red arrow*) (Fig. 5.10a). Fluorescein shows absence of staining in the epithelized area over the bare stroma (Fig. 5.10b).

Case 2: 4 days post LASIK, Patient 2 presented with macrostriae, a folded flap and a large epithelial ingrowth (Fig. 5.10c, d).

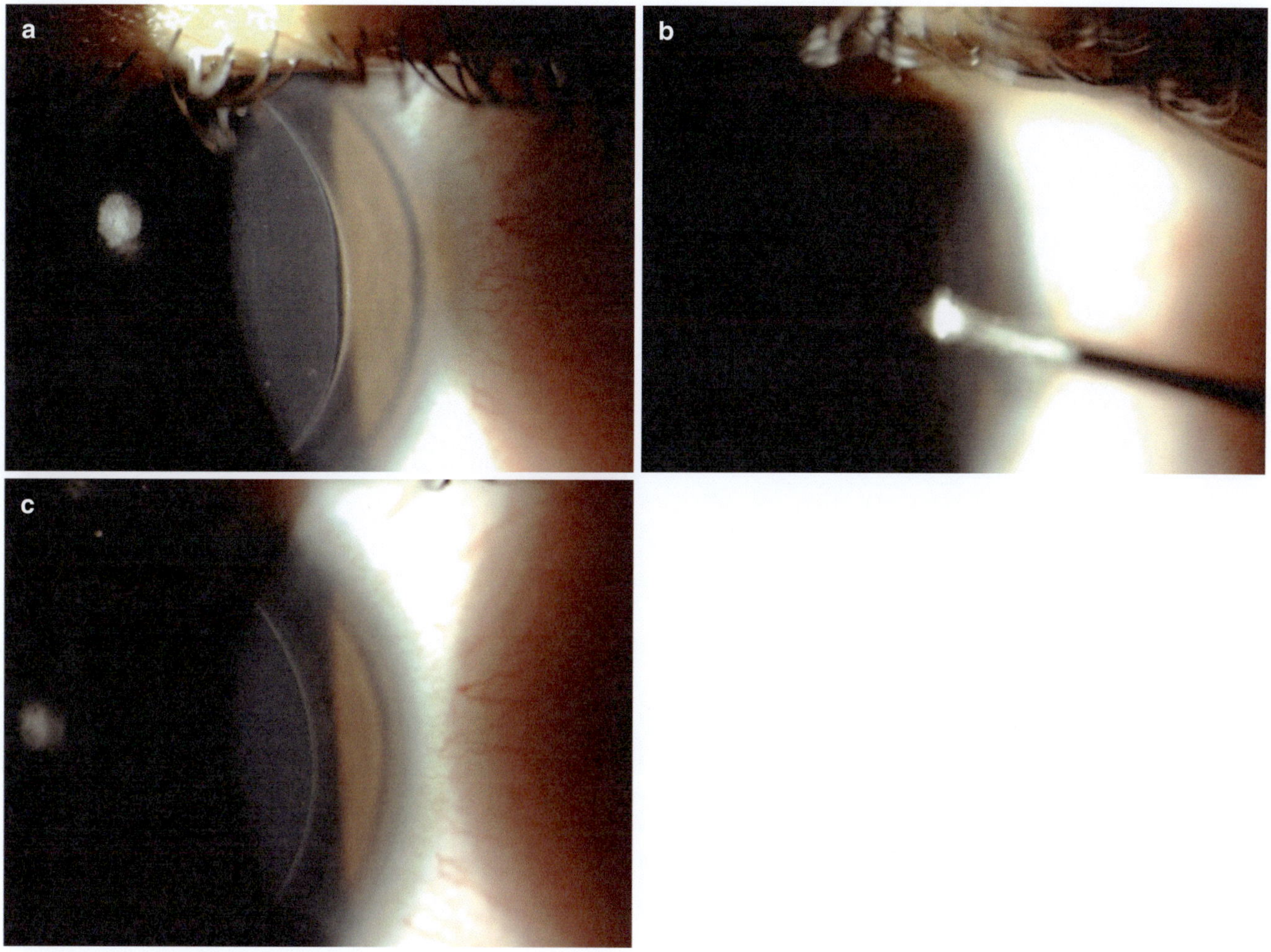

Fig. 5.1 Immediate peripheral macrostriae

Management: Flap lift, scraping of epithelial ingrowth, and unfolding should be performed.

Core message: Folding of the flap is an emergency that should be corrected surgically to prevent further complications.

Case: One year following a LASIK procedure, a patient was still complaining of severe glare and his BCVA was 20/30 (Fig. 5.11).

Exam: Slit lamp exam shows microstriae and negative fluorescein lines (Fig. 5.11a, b).

Management: Phototherapeutic keratectomy is recommended to smoothen the surface of the cornea.

Core message: Avoid late flap lift as the folds are less likely to resolve with ironing and epithelial removal.

Take-Home Message

- Corneal flap should be rechecked with slit lamp a few minutes following LASIK as striae may develop during speculum removal.
- De-epithelization followed by ironing is usually needed to remove microstriae persisting more than few days post-op.
- In case of longstanding visually significant striae, PTK is a well successful method that can be used to avoid flap lifting and the increased risks of post-operative epithelial ingrowth.
- Folded flap should be corrected urgently.

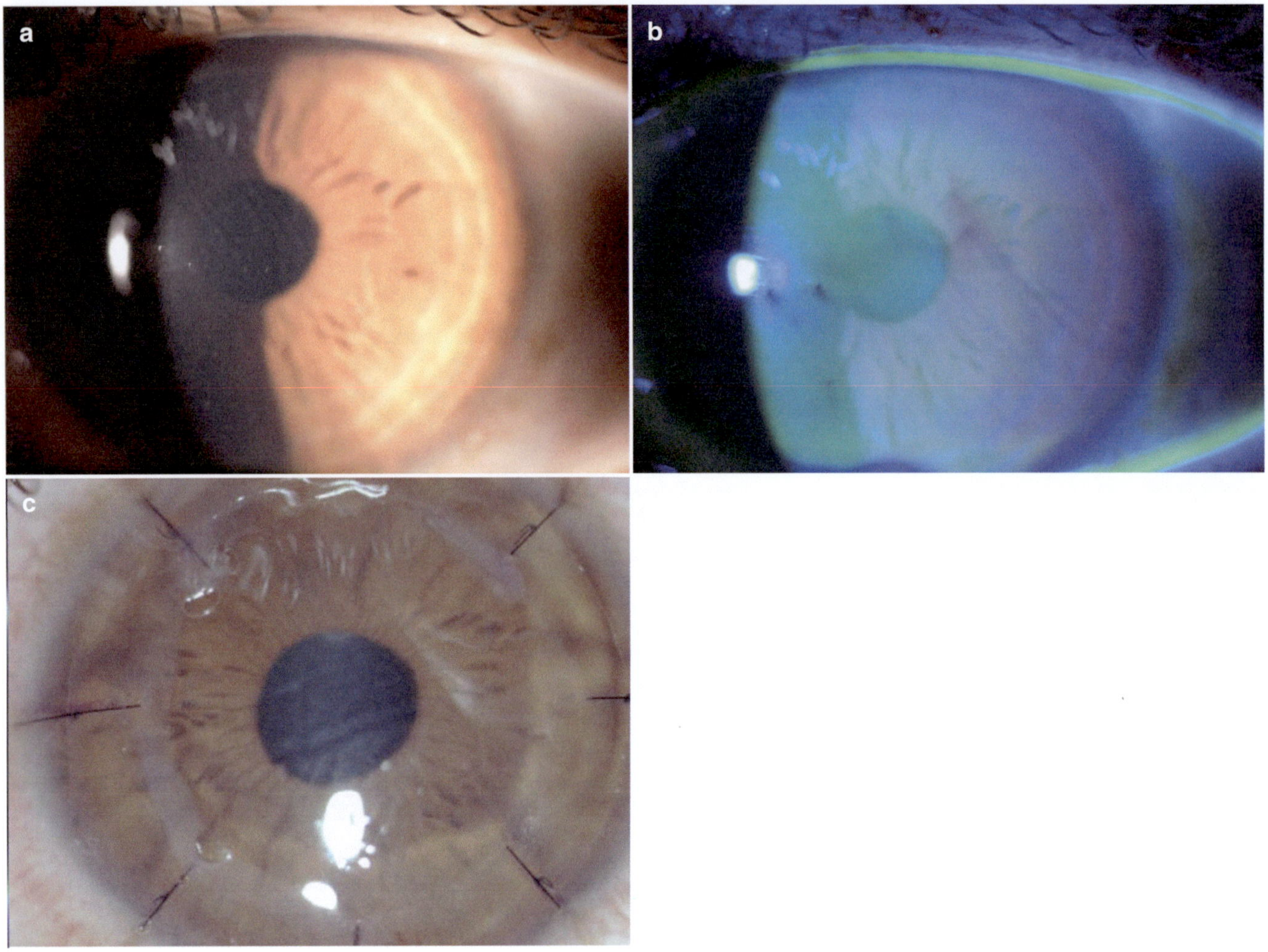

Fig. 5.2 Late presentation and sutures

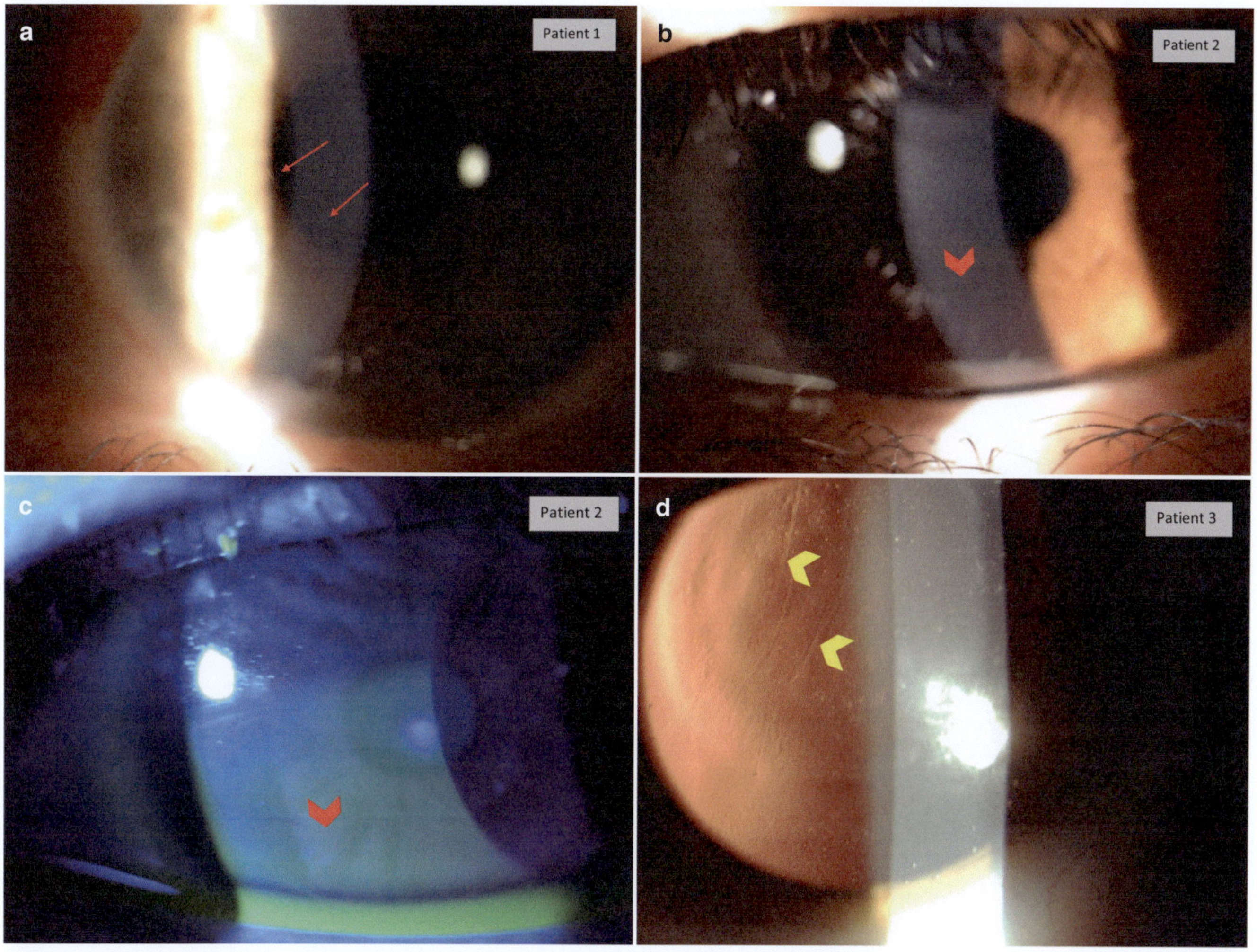

Fig. 5.3 Central microstriae

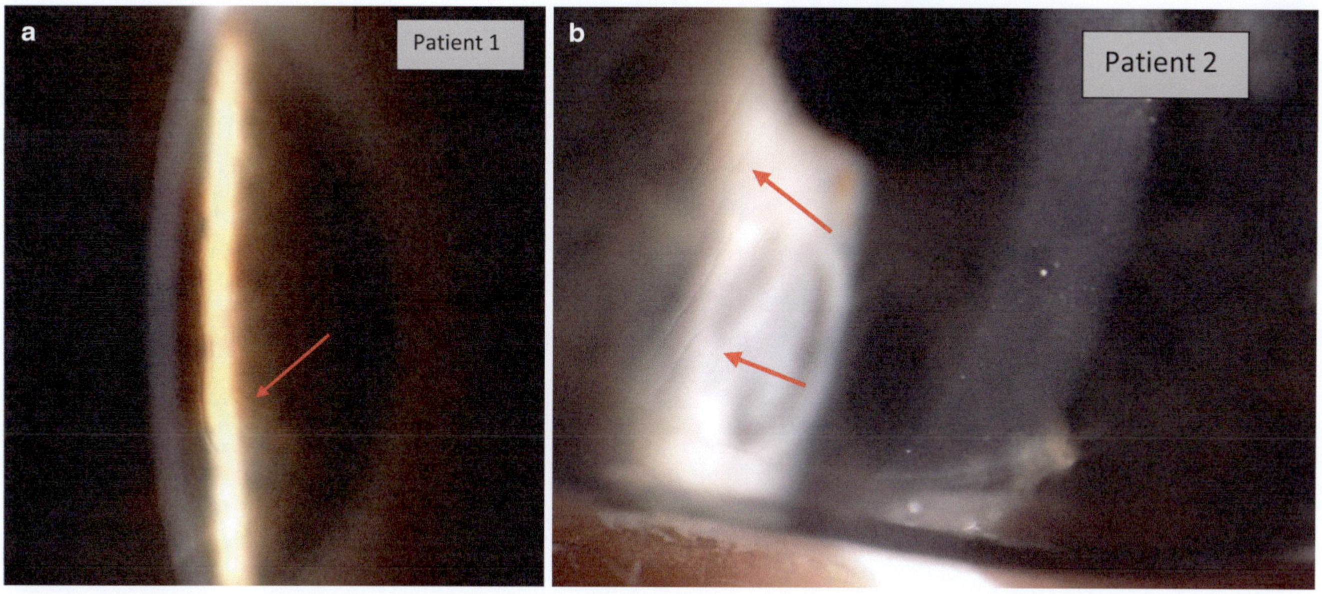

Fig. 5.4 Peripheral Folds. (Courtesy of Suphi Taneri, MD Augenzentrum am St. Franziskus Hospital Münste, Münster, Germany)

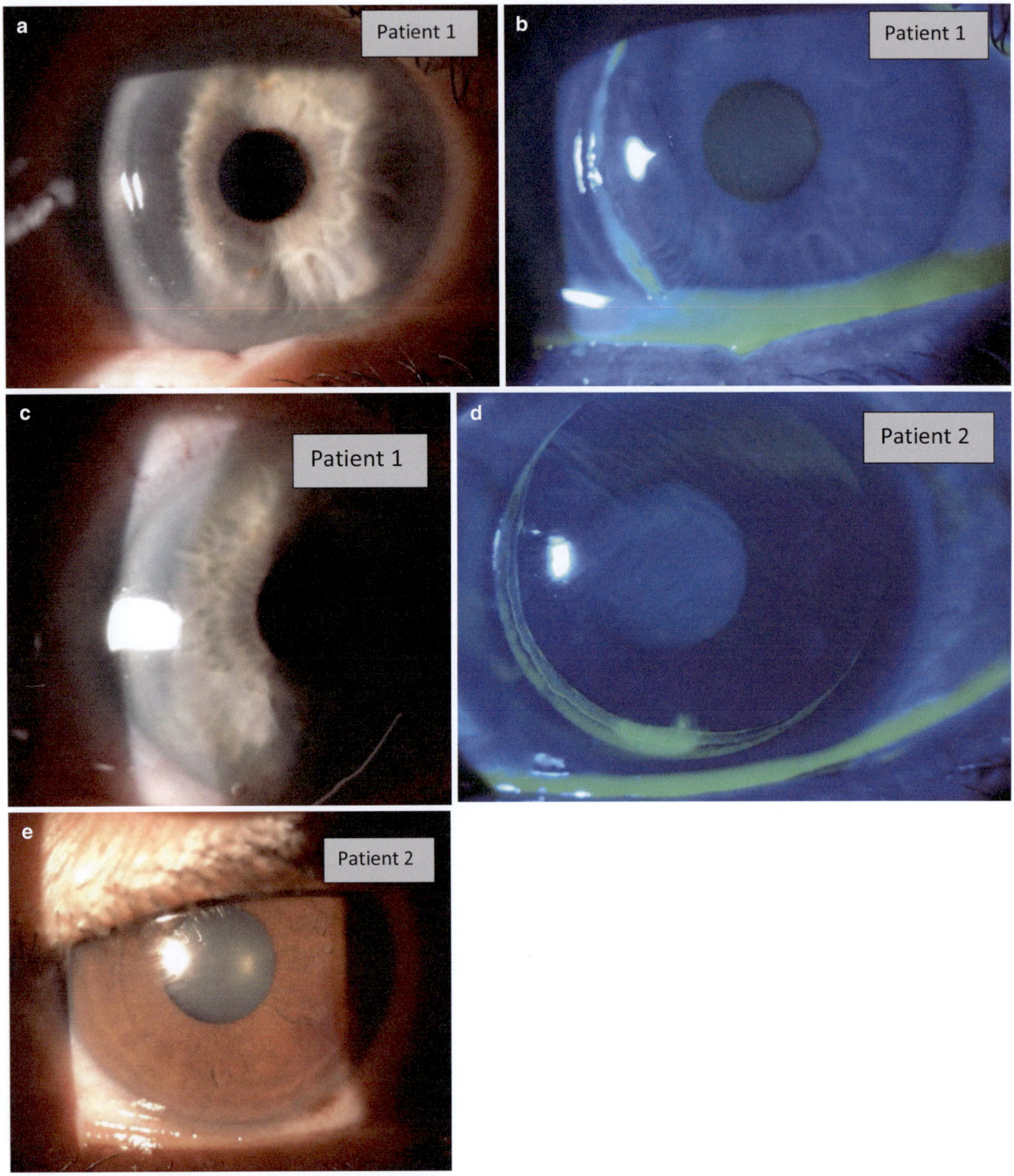

Fig. 5.5 Early macrostriae

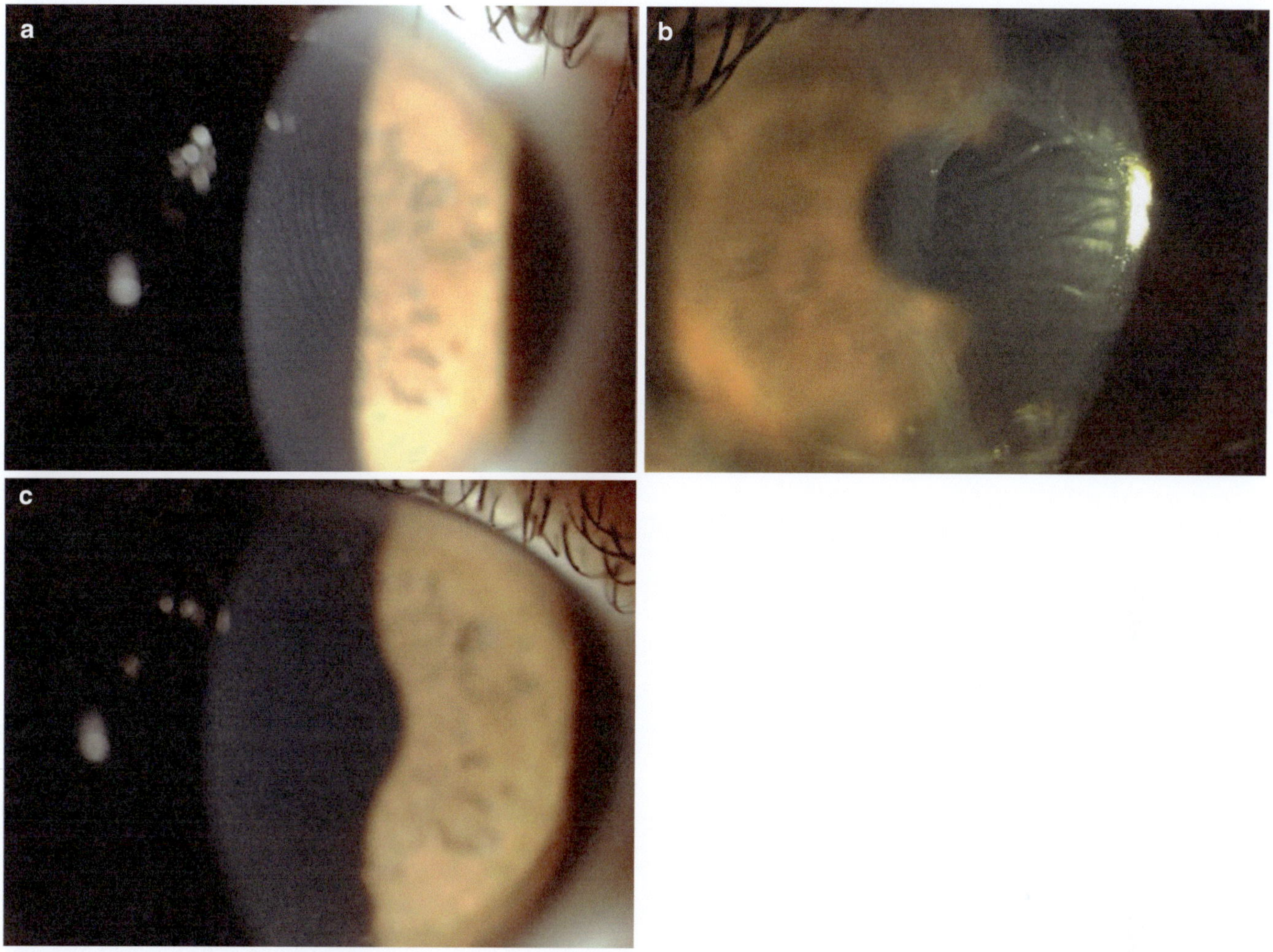

Fig. 5.6 Refloating after de-epithelization

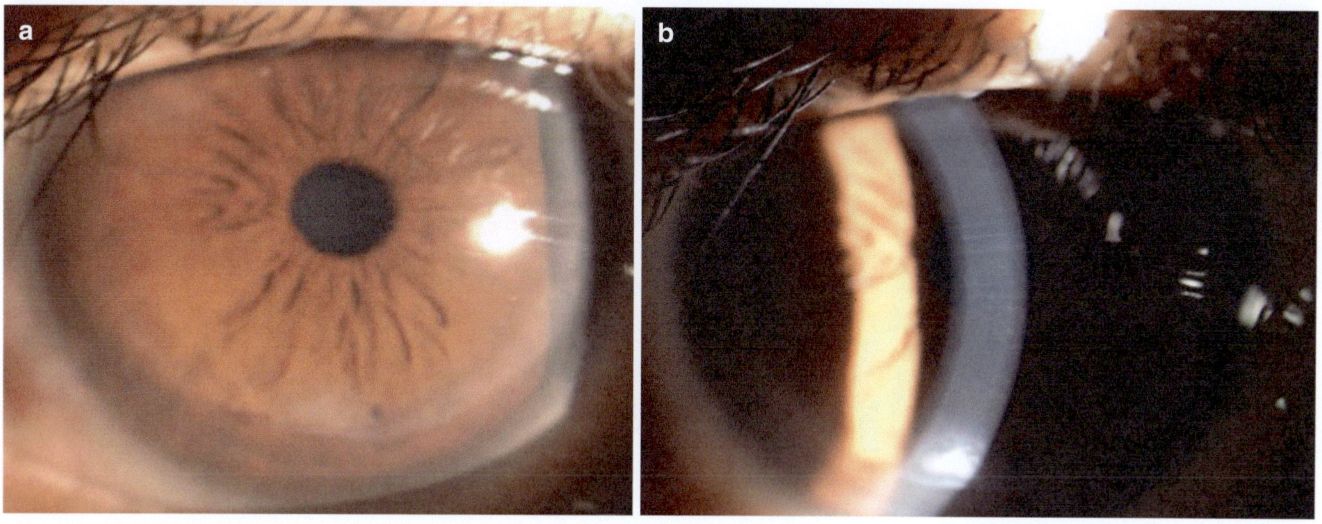

Fig. 5.7 Late macrostriae with epithelial ingrowth

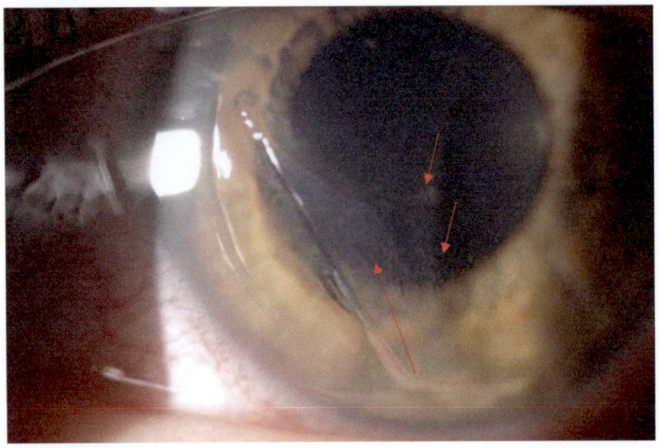

Fig. 5.8 Folded flap and DLK

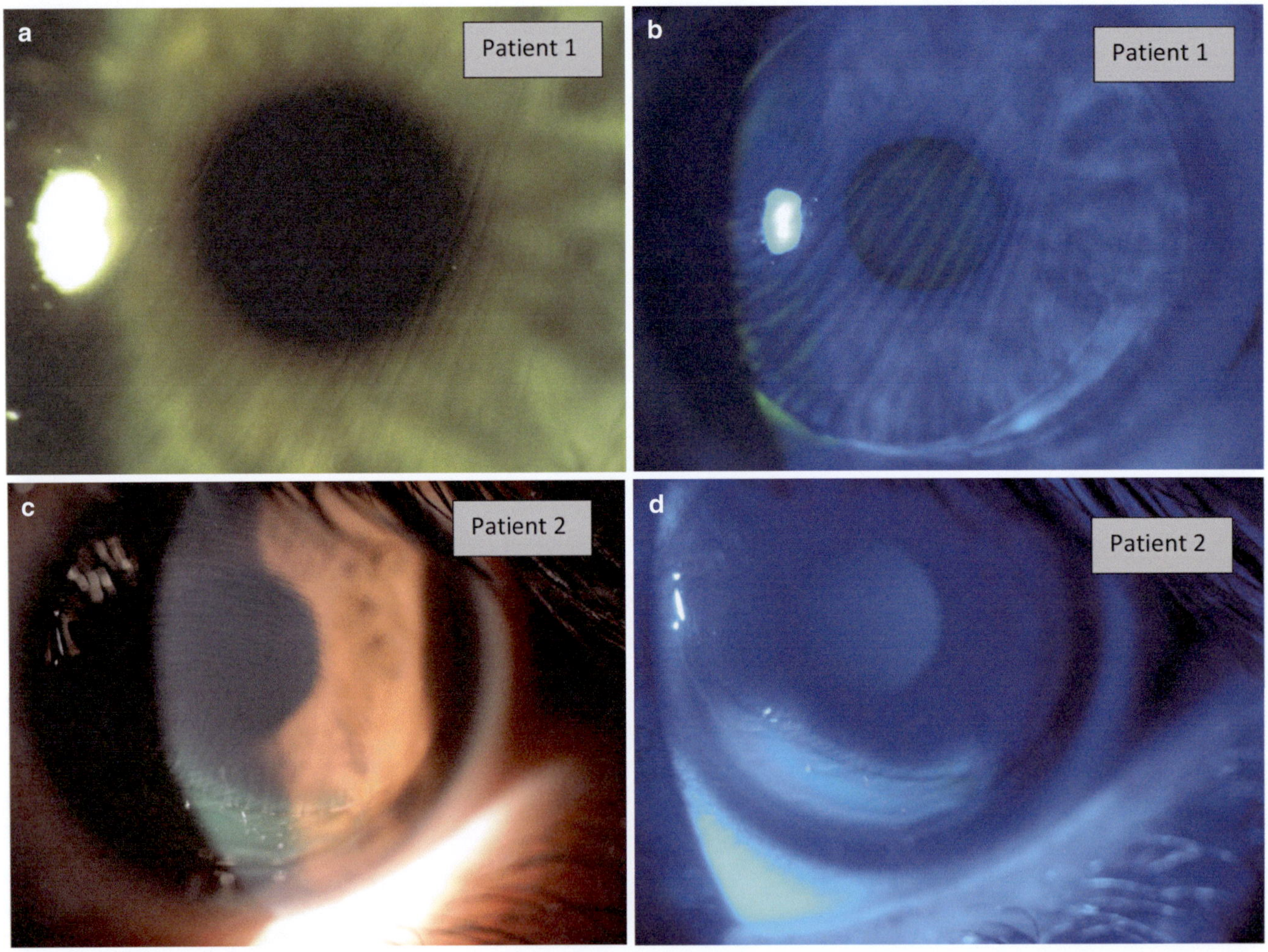

Fig. 5.9 Early macrostriae fluorescein staining

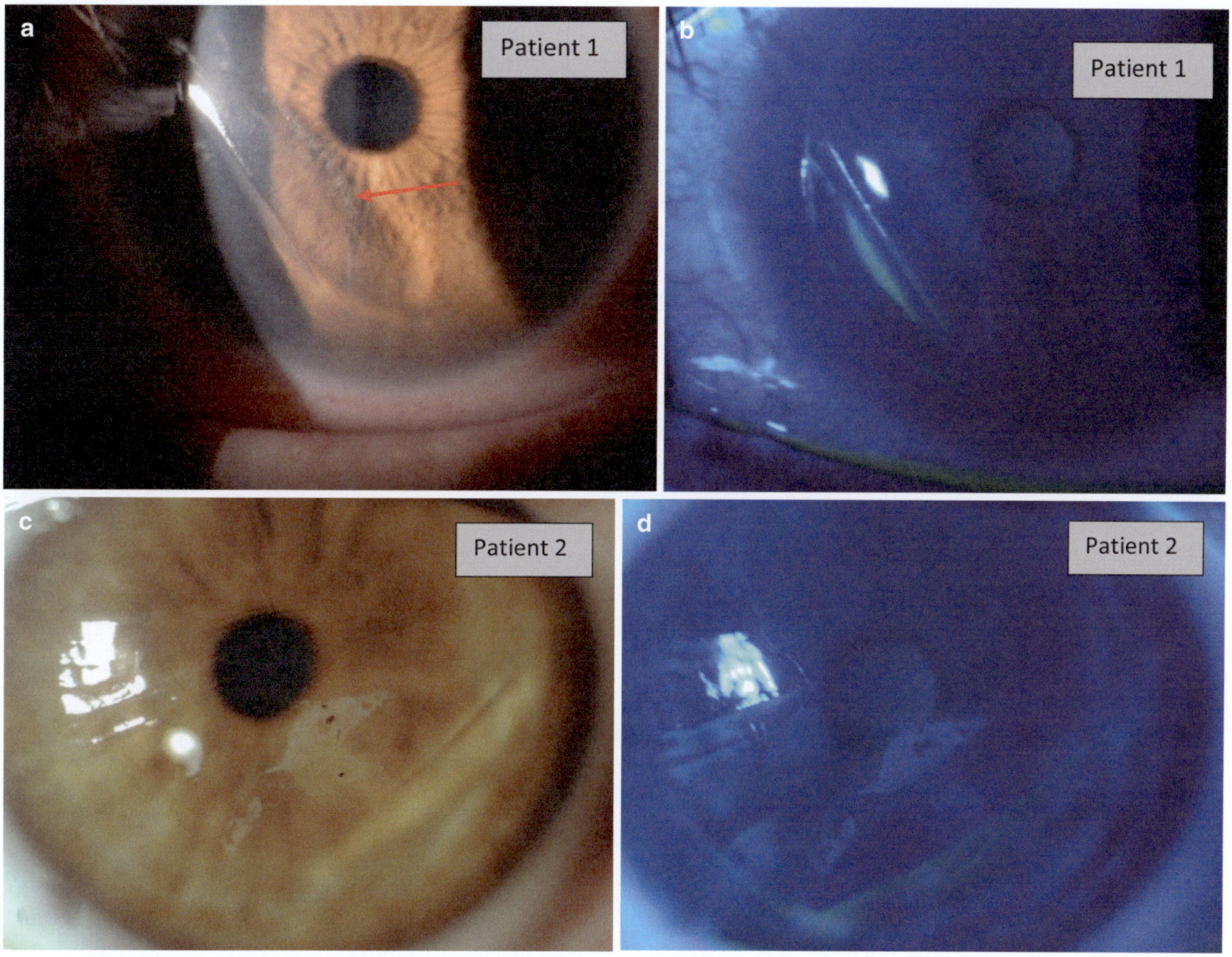

Fig. 5.10 Folded flaps

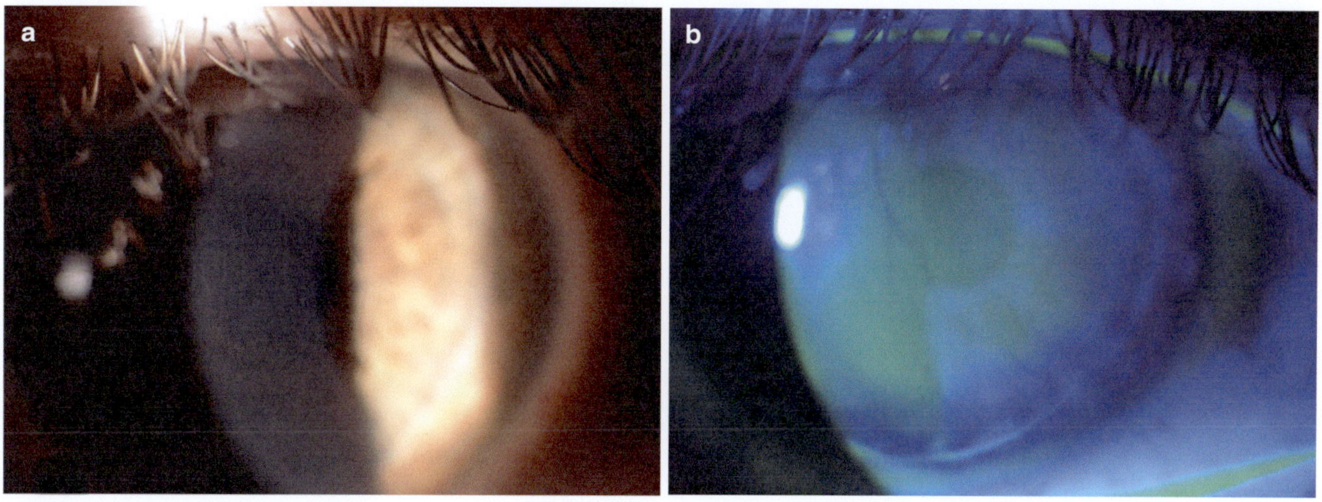

Fig. 5.11 PTK for chronic symptomatic microstriae

References

1. Sahay P, Bafna RK, Reddy JC, Vajpayee RB, Sharma N. Complications of laser-assisted *in situ* keratomileusis. Indian J Ophthalmol. 2021;69(7):1658–69.
2. Wallerstein A, Gauvin M, Adiguzel E, Singh H, Gupta V, Harissi-Dagher M, Cohen M. Clinically significant laser in situ keratomileusis flap striae. J Cataract Refract Surg. 2017;43(12):1523–33.
3. Galvis V, Tello A, Guerra AR, Rey JJ, Camacho PA. Risk factors and visual results in cases of LASIK flap repositioning due to folds or dislocation: case series and literature review. Int Ophthalmol. 2013;34(1):19–26.
4. Melki SA, Fava MA. Cornea and refractive atlas of clinical wisdom; 2011. p. 227.
5. Charman WN. Mismatch between flap and stromal areas after laser in situ keratomileusis as source of flap striae. J Cataract Refract Surg. 2002;28(12):2146–52.
6. Abdelazeem K, Nassr MA, Abdelmotaal H, Wasfi E, El-Sebaity DM. Flap sliding technique for managing flap striae following laser in situ Keratomileusis. J Ophthalmol. 2020;2020:5614327.
7. Ashrafzadeh A, Steinert RF. Results of phototherapeutic keratectomy in the management of flap striae after LASIK before and after developing a standardized protocol. Ophthalmology. 2007;114(6):1118–23.
8. Melki SA, Azar DT. 101 pearls in refractive, cataract, and corneal surgery. 2nd ed; 2006. p. 29–31.
9. Melki SA, Azar DT. LASIK complications. Surv Ophthalmol. 2001;46(2):95–116.
10. Shah DN, Melki SA. Complications of femtosecond-assisted laser in-situ keratomileusis flaps. Semin Ophthalmol. 2014;29(5–6):363–75.
11. Vajpayee RB, Sharma N, Melki SA, Sullivan L. Step by step lasik surgery, vol. 2; 2006. p. 173–7.
12. Donnenfeld ED, Perry HD, Doshi SJ, Biser SA, Solomon R. Hyperthermic treatment of post-LASIK corneal striae. J Cataract Refract Surg. 2004;30(3):620–5.

6 Epithelial Disease in Refractive Surgery

Samir A. Melki, Jason Brenner, Wassef Chanbour, and Perla Ibrahim

See Table 6.1.

Case: 30-year-old patient examined 7 days following a PRK surgery (Fig. 6.1).

Exam: Central epithelial star-like formation in the presence of a bandage contact lens.

Management: This presents normal healing following a PRK, and bandage contact lens can be safely removed at this stage.

Case: Patient presented for follow up 2 weeks post-PRK surgery (Fig. 6.2).

Exam: Following removal of the bandage contact lens, slit lamp exam (Fig. 6.2a) and fluorescein staining (Fig. 6.2b) show a central non-healing epithelial defect.

Management: Contact lens was reinserted, steroids and NSAIDS drops were discontinued, and more frequent use of lubricating drops was recommended. Epithelial defect resolved 1 week following treatment (Fig. 6.2c, d).

Core message: Delayed healing in PRK cannot be ignored as it's a source of difficult to manage haze.

Case: 25-year-old male presented for a follow up 2 weeks following a PRK surgery (Fig. 6.3).

Exam: A large epithelial defect was detected on slit lamp exam (Fig. 6.3a) and fluorescein staining (Fig. 6.3b).

Management: Bandage contact lens was reinserted and the steroid and NSAIDS drops were discontinued. One week later, the epithelial defect was smaller in size but persistent (Fig. 6.3c, d).

Amniotic membrane (Prokera® Bio-Tissue, Inc., Miami, FL) was applied over the cornea and the epithelial defect healed 1 week later.

Case: 52-year-old female patient presenting with progressive blurry vision 3 months following a non-complicated LASIK procedure. UDVA: 20/40. The patient was using artificial tears QID (Fig. 6.4).

Exam: Fluorescein staining showed diffuse superficial punctate keratitis. Corneal sensitivity was diminished and the patient was diagnosed with stage 1 neurotropic keratitis.

Management: Punctal plugs were inserted, more frequent application of artificial tear drops and ointment was recommended. 6 months following LASIK, symptoms and corneal sensitivity improved.

Case: 24-year-old female examined 1 day following a non-complicated LASIK procedure (Fig. 6.5).

Exam: Fluorescein staining of the right eye showed a cluster of small epithelial erosions occurring at 5 o'clock, at the same location where corneal was marked using a surgical skin marker.

Management: No additional treatment was given; same postoperative regiment of steroid/antibiotics combination and artificial tears was continued. The cornea healed completely within 3 days.

Case: Patient examined few minutes following a LASIK procedure (Fig. 6.6).

Exam: A small epithelial erosion noted next to the flap edge. Epithelial trauma occurred when attempting to lift the flap on the temporal aspect of the cornea.

Management: Continue the same postoperative regimen (steroid, antibiotics, and artificial tears).

Core Message: Small epithelial defects in the flap are usually painless and tend to heal spontaneously within 1 to 2 days.

Case: 42-year-old male presents with blurry vision 1 day following a LASIK procedure; during surgery the surgeon reported a loose surface epithelium (Fig. 6.7).

Exam: Central epithelial sloughing following flap manipulation (Fig. 6.7a). UDVA: 20/70.

S. A. Melki (✉) · J. Brenner
Boston Vision, Department of Ophthalmology, Harvard Medical School, Boston, MA, USA
e-mail: melki@bostonvision.com; brenner@bostonvision.com

W. Chanbour
Department of Ophthalmology and Visual Neurosciences, University of Minnesota, Minneapolis, MN, USA
e-mail: chanb013@umn.edu

P. Ibrahim
Cornea and Refractive Surgery Fellow, Boston Vision and Beth Israel Deaconess Medical Center, Boston, MA, USA
e-mail: perla.ibrahim@bostonvision.com

S. A. Melki et al. (eds.), *Refractive Surgery Atlas*, https://doi.org/10.1007/978-3-031-60661-8_6

Table 6.1 Common epithelial pathologies encountered during and following refractive surgeries

Disease	PRK	LASIK
Normal epithelial healing	• Epithelium regenerates in 3–5 days with contact lens • Regeneration of the basal membrane after PRK occurs within 6–8 weeks in rabbits [1] • At 6–8 months after the intervention of PRK, subepithelial nerve regeneration is almost complete [2] • Corneal sensitivity usually starts at 4–6 weeks, completing approximately within 6–12 months following PRK [3]	• No observed regenerated collagen between the corneal flap and the ablated stromal bed except in the wound margin • The number of sub-basal and stromal nerve fiber bundles in the flap decreases by 90% immediately after LASIK. It increases at 12 months but remains less than a half. Full recovery may take up to 5 years postoperatively [4, 5]
Dry eye syndrome	**Mechanism**: Iatrogenic corneal nerve damage caused by stromal ablation, changes in the corneal shape (ablation depth), increased tear film hyperosmolarity [6] **Incidence**: Variable; some studies reported lower incidence compared to LASIK; others reported higher incidence [6]	**Mechanism**: Iatrogenic corneal nerve damage caused by the flap creation, changes in the corneal shape (ablation depth), damage to goblet cells due to the suction, possibly a superior hinge [6] **Incidence:** Variable in studies. 50% of patients at 1 week, 40% at 1 month, 20% at 3 months, and 10–40% at 6 months [7]
	Possible risk factors: high myopia, high ablation depth, larger optical zone, preoperative dry eyes, previous intolerance to contact lens and female gender [8]	
	Treatment: Preoperatively: Treatment of preexisting dry eye with artificial tears or cyclosporine. Treatment of blepharitis and meibomian gland dysfunction with warm compresses, topical azithromycin, steroids or doxycycline Postoperatively: Preservative free artificial tears, punctal plugs, topical cyclosporine, lifitegrast. In severe cases, autologous serum eye drops and scleral contact lens may be considered	
Neurotrophic keratopathy	1 month following PRK, 9% of nerves regenerated; at 6 months, 50% had regenerated; and at 2 years, 92% of nerves had regenerated [9]	1 month following LASIK procedure, 11% of nerves regenerated; at 6 months, 27% had regenerated; at 2 years, 58% of nerves had regenerated; and at 5 years 79% had regenerated [9]
	Pathophysiology: Damage to corneal nerves leads to decreased tear production, reflex tearing, and decreased release of neuroprotective mediators. These factors lead to decrease in the quality and volume of the tear film. When severe, these same factors that pre-dispose patients to dry eye, can lead to neurotrophic keratitis **Incidence**: Unknown as the disease is rare, 1.7% of neurotrophic keratitis patient had refractive surgery [10] **Treatment**: In advanced stages serum tears, amniotic membrane, tarsorrhaphy and Cenegermin (Oxervate™) may be used	
Recurrent erosion syndrome	**Incidence**: 0.05% [11]–2.1% [12] of patients, close to general population incidence	**Incidence**: unknown, 6 cases reported in one study [13]
	Treatment: Dry eye management, contact lens may be placed for a prolonged period, stromal puncture, epithelial debridement, PTK	
Epithelial basement membrane dystrophy (EBMD)	PRK is indicated	• Relative contraindication to do LASIK • Diagnosis can occur intra/postoperatively leading to epithelial sloughing, recurrent erosions and map-dot-fingerprints on the cornea • PTK it therapeutic

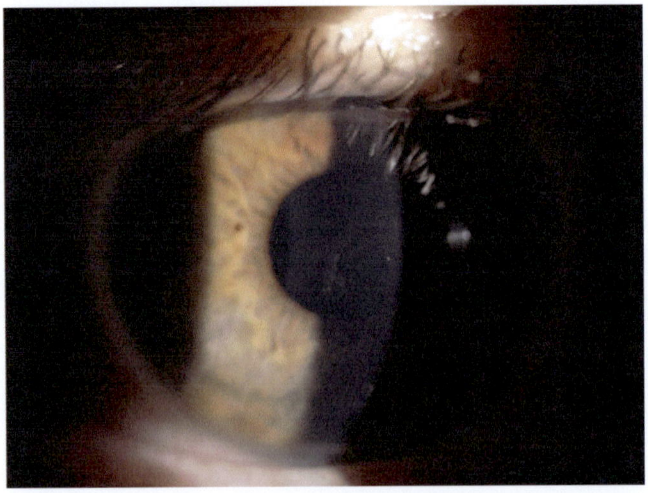

Fig. 6.1 Normal epithelial healing following PRK

Management: Bandage contact lens application may be considered. Patient should be reassured that the visual recovery is expected to be slow. Change in eye drop regiment is not recommended. Exam at 1 week showed fine central epithelial irregularities (Fig. 6.7b) and UDVA reached 20/20 after 2 weeks.

Core message: Pre-operative evaluation is important to detect epithelial membrane dystrophy which may have increased risks of corneal erosion following LASIK procedure.

Case: 27-year-old patient examined 1 day following LASIK surgery; patient was complaining of foreign body sensation and light sensitivity (Fig. 6.8).

Exam: Slit lamp exam showed grade 1 DLK (*blue arrow*) next to a corneal erosion that was induced by surgical trauma while lifting the flap (Fig. 6.8a, b). UDVA was 20/30.

Management: More frequent application of topical steroids and artificial tears is recommended. Contact lens is not necessary as small defects heal quickly. The DLK and the

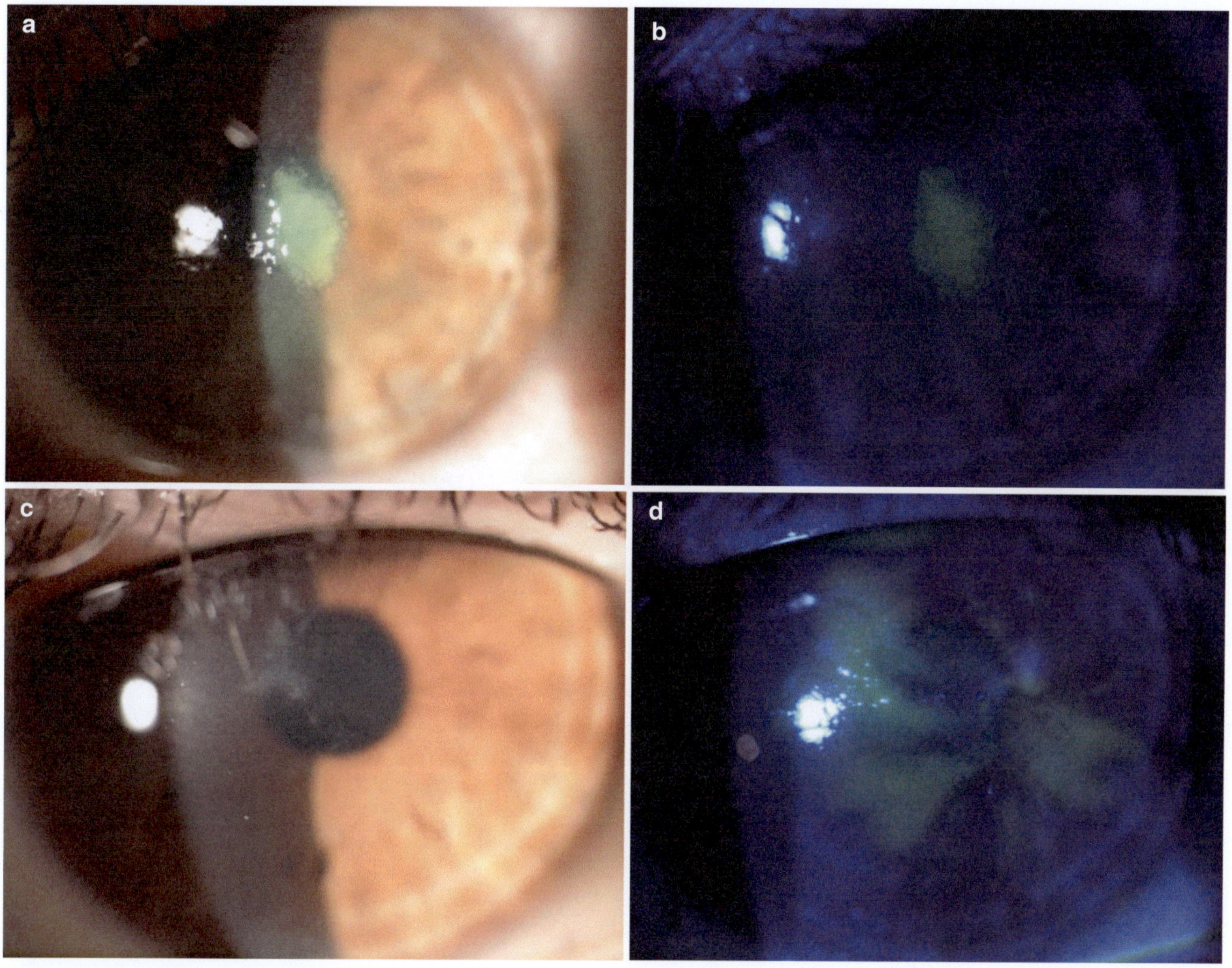

Fig. 6.2 Delayed epithelial healing following PRK. (**a**) Slit lamp exam following removal of bandage contact lens 2 weeks post PRK, (**b**) with fluorescein stain, (**c**) 1 week following treatment, (**d**) with fluorescein stain

erosion resolved completely after a week and the uncorrected visual acuity improved to 20/20.

Case: 25-year-old male patient presented for contact lens removal 1 week following a PRK procedure. Visual acuity was 20/50 (Fig. 6.9).

Exam: Central corneal epithelial clumping is detected.

Management: No additional treatment is recommended. Epithelial clumps disappeared 1 week later.

Case: 32-year-old female presenting to the emergency department with severe pain and light sensitivity since the morning. She had a non-complicated PRK procedure 3 months ago. Patient has been reporting dry eyes for the past month but she was not using any eye drops (Fig. 6.10).

Exam: Fluorescein staining shows an almost total corneal epithelial erosion with part of the epithelium attached inferiorly (Fig. 6.10a).

Management: Epithelial debridement was performed (Fig. 6.10b). Bandage contact lens was applied and the patient was started on topical antibiotics and artificial tears. 3 days following treatment, the size of the epithelial defect was smaller (Fig. 6.10c) and the cornea healed 10 days later (Fig. 6.10d).

Core Message: Dry eye should be detected and managed early following refractive surgeries.

Case: 28-year-old female presenting with pain upon waking up in the morning. She had a PRK procedure 3 weeks before (Fig. 6.11).

Exam: An area of epithelial defect with adjacent epithelial elevation.

Management: Epithelial debridement was performed. Bandage contact lens, topical antibiotics, and aggressive lubrication were used and symptoms resolved in 3 days.

Case: 35-year-old female presents with a delayed epithelial healing 14 days after a PRK procedure (Fig. 6.12).

Exam: Slit lamp exam following contact lens removal showed thick branch-like pattern of epithelial healing lines (Fig. 6.12a, b).

Management: No change needed in management; combined antibiotic/steroid eye drops should be continued.

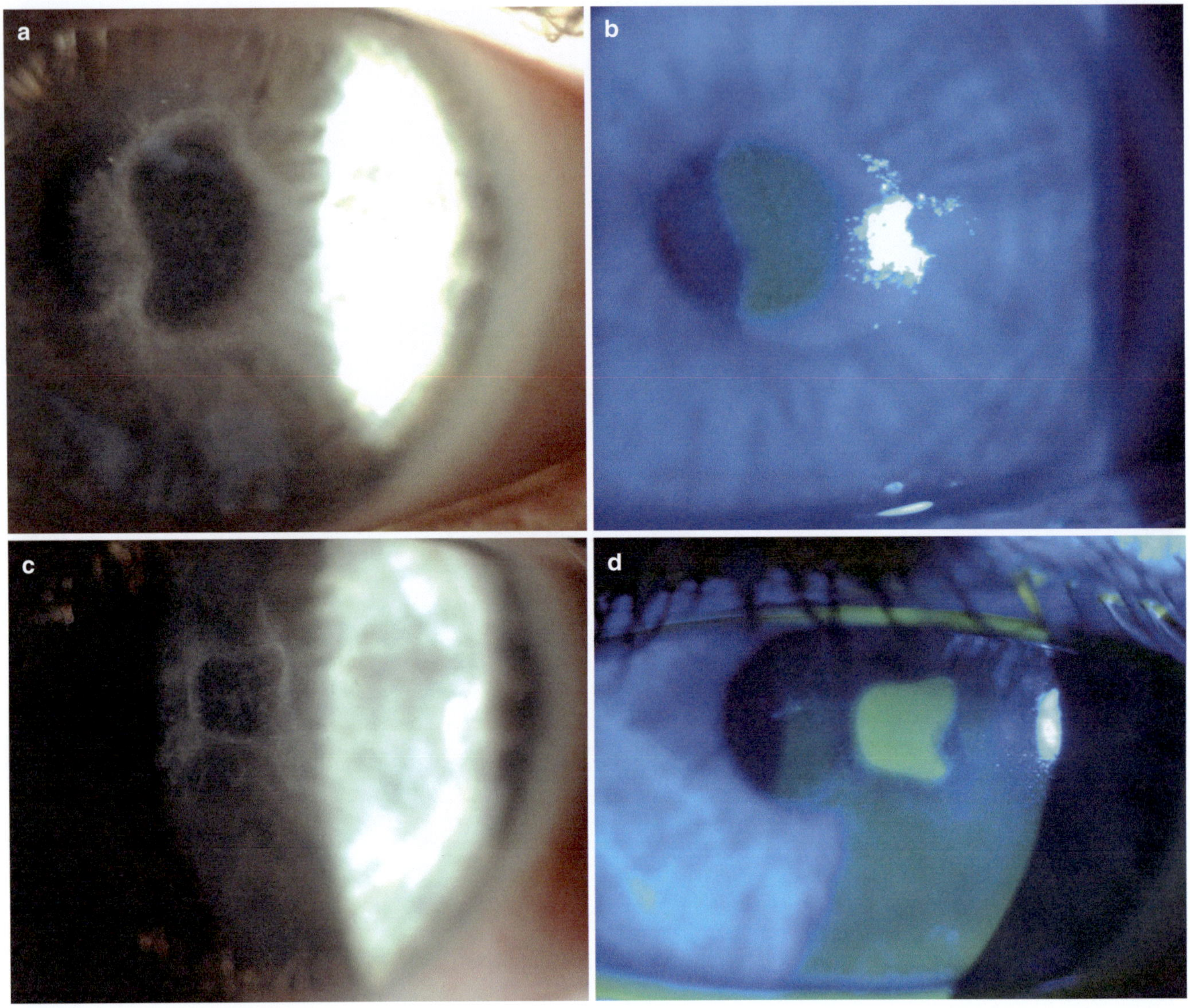

Fig. 6.3 Non-healing epithelial defect. (**a**) 2 weeks following PRK surgery, (**b**) with fluorescein stain). (**c**) 1 week after stopping steroids and NSAID drops, (**d**) with fluorescein stain

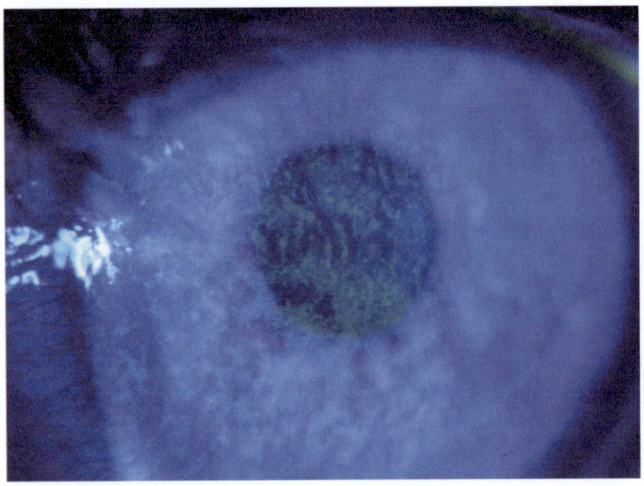

Fig. 6.4 Neurotophic cornea

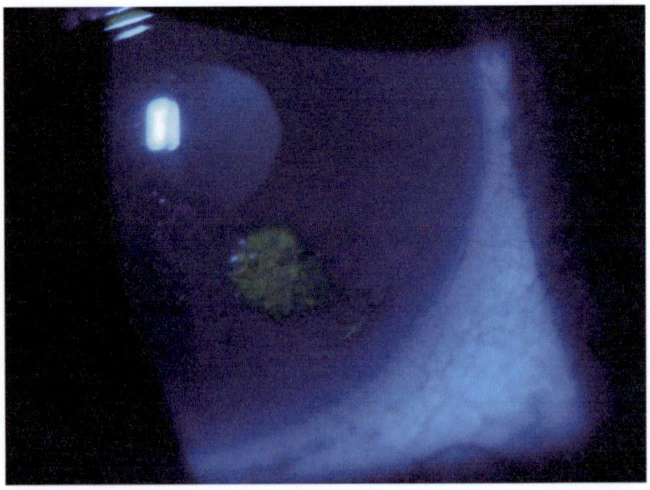

Fig. 6.5 Corneal marking

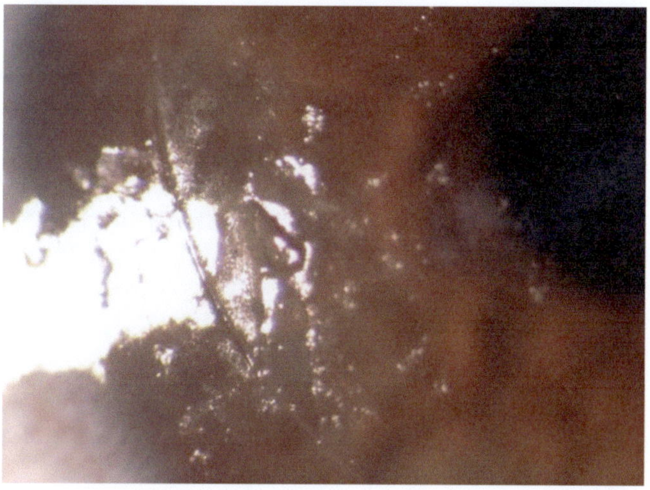

Fig. 6.6 Epithelial trauma in LASIK

Case: 45-year-old male examined 1 week following a PRK procedure (Fig. 6.13).

Exam: Central epithelial irregularities noted (Fig. 6.13a) and fluorescein staining shows a central dendritic like formation (Fig. 6.13b).

Management: Pseudo-dendrites can be managed by contact lens application or intensive lubrication in addition to the postoperative regiment.

Case: 38-year-old female presenting with dry eyes symptoms 5 months following a non-complicated PRK procedure (Fig. 6.14).

Exam: Slit lamp exam shows central superficial punctuate keratitis (Fig. 6.14a, b).

Management: Dry eye management involves increase in preservative free artificial tears and punctal plugs insertion. Patient symptoms improved partially; therefore, topical

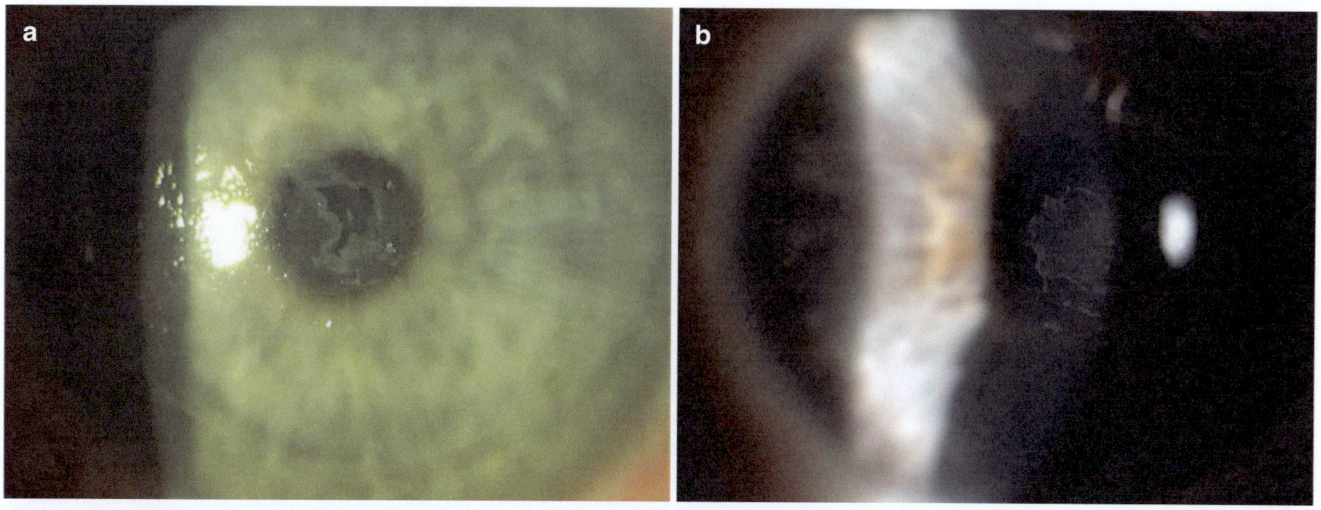

Fig. 6.7 Central epithelial sloughing following LASIK. (**a**) After flap manipulation, (**b**) 1 week later

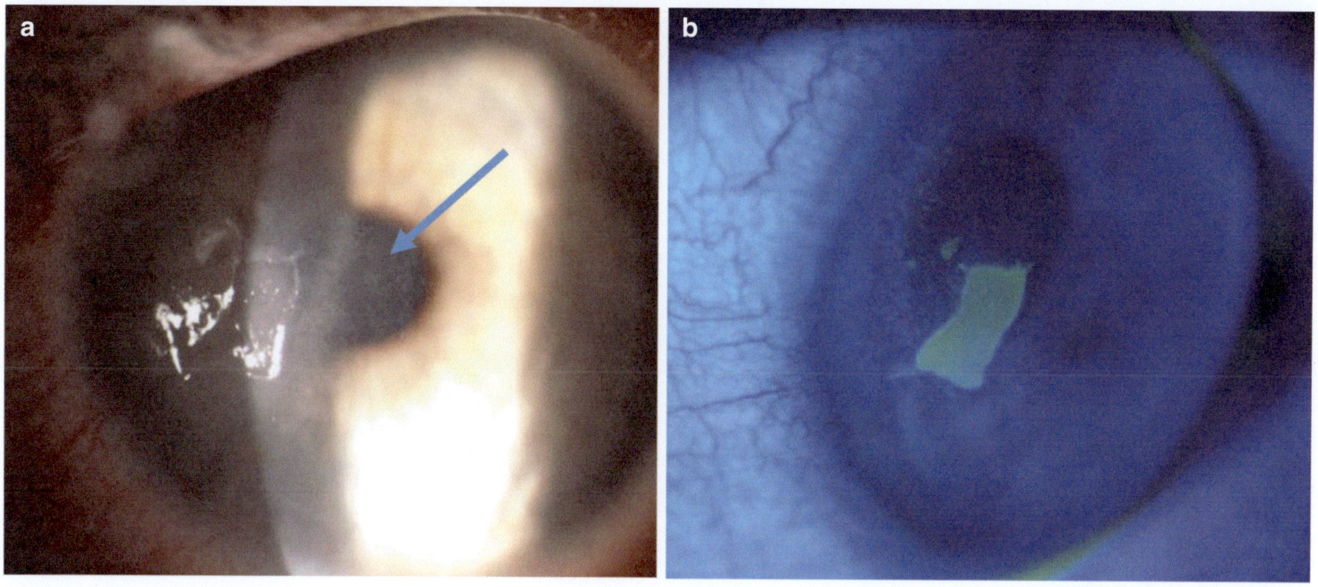

Fig. 6.8 Epithelial erosion inducing DLK. (**a**) 1 day following LASIK, (**b**) with fluorescein stain

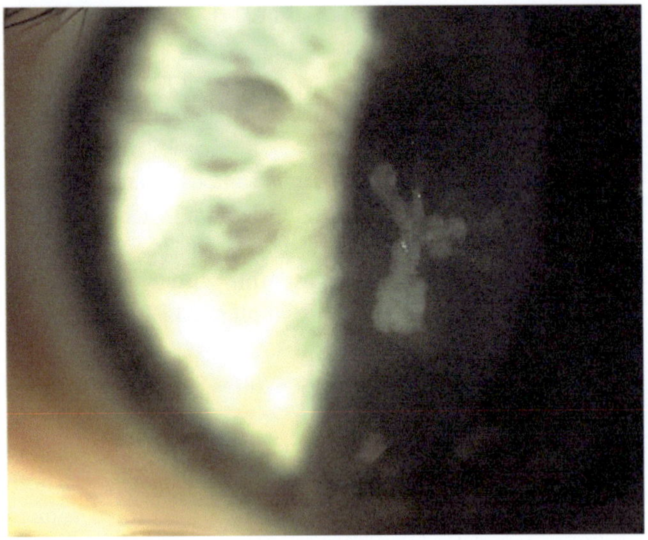

Fig. 6.9 Epithelial clumping

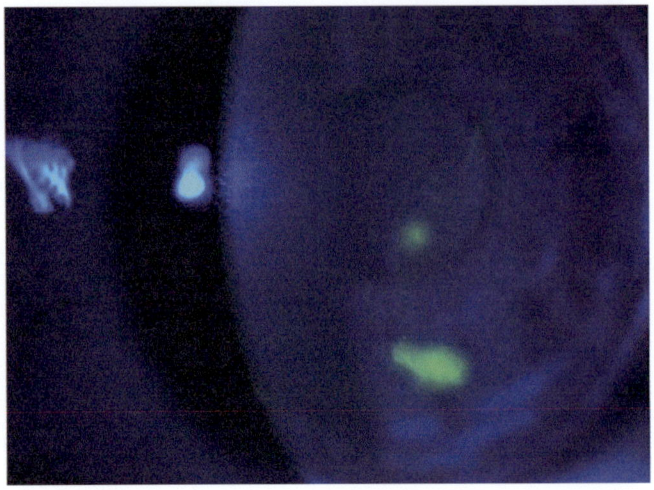

Fig. 6.11 Corneal erosion with epithelial hyperplasia

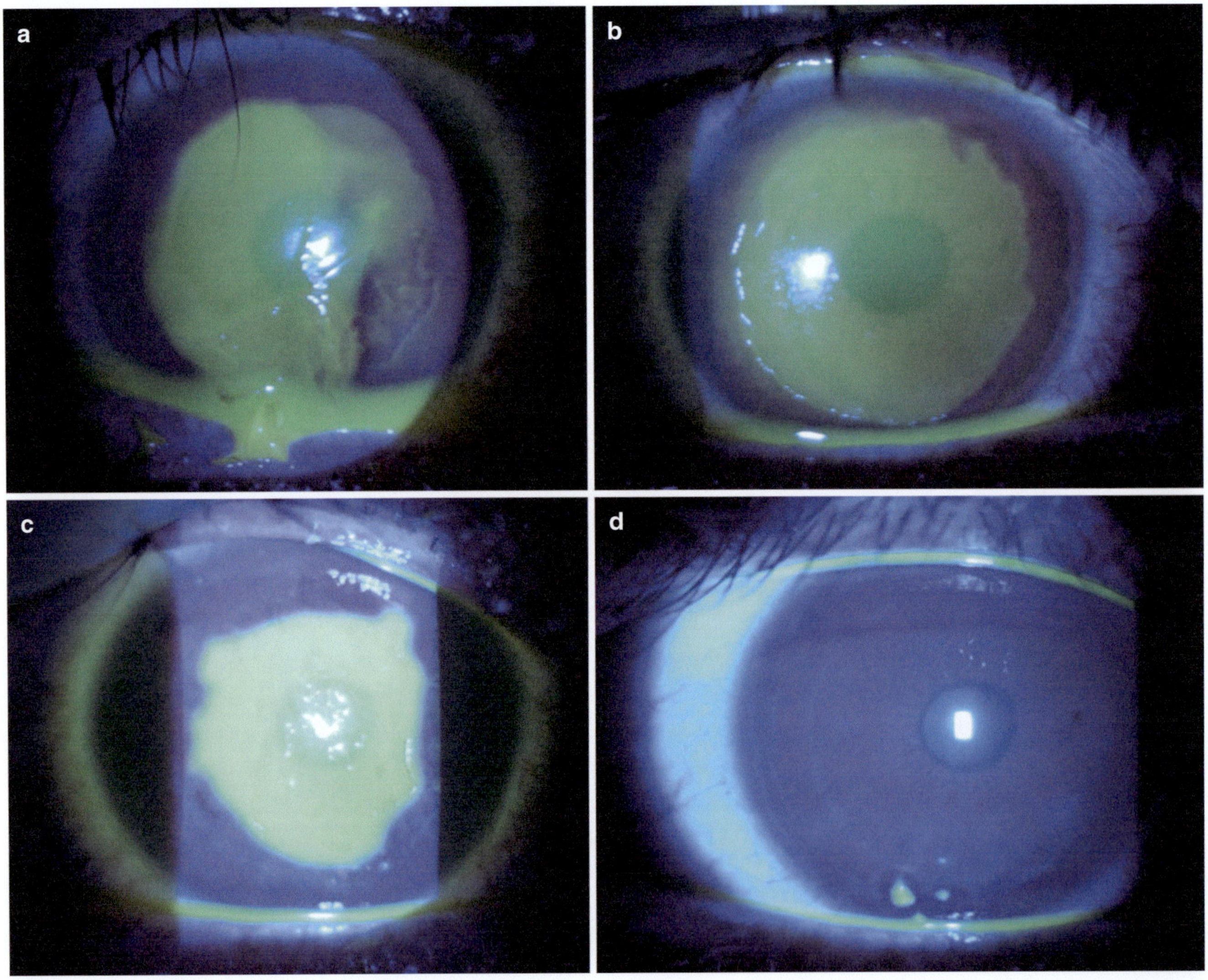

Fig. 6.10 Late epithelial erosion. (**a**) 3 months post PRK, with part of the epithelium attached inferiorly, (**b**) after epithelial debridement, (**c**) 3 days later, (**d**) 10 days later.

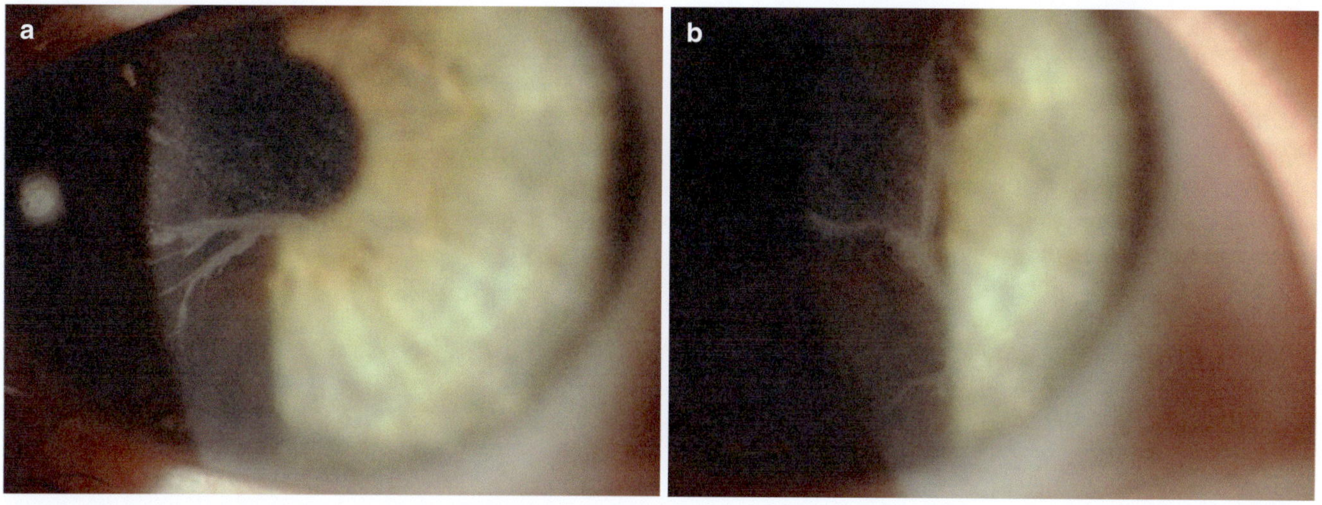

Fig. 6.12 Abnormal epithelial lines. (**a**, **b**) Branch-like pattern

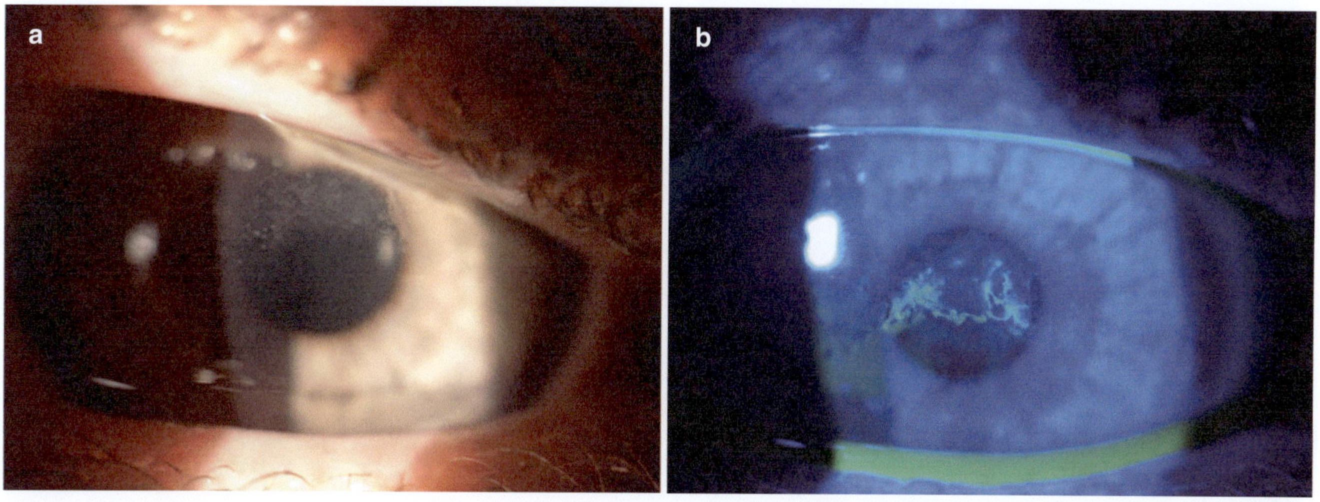

Fig. 6.13 Pseudo-dendritic formation. (**a**) Epithelial irregularities, (**b**) with fluorescein stain

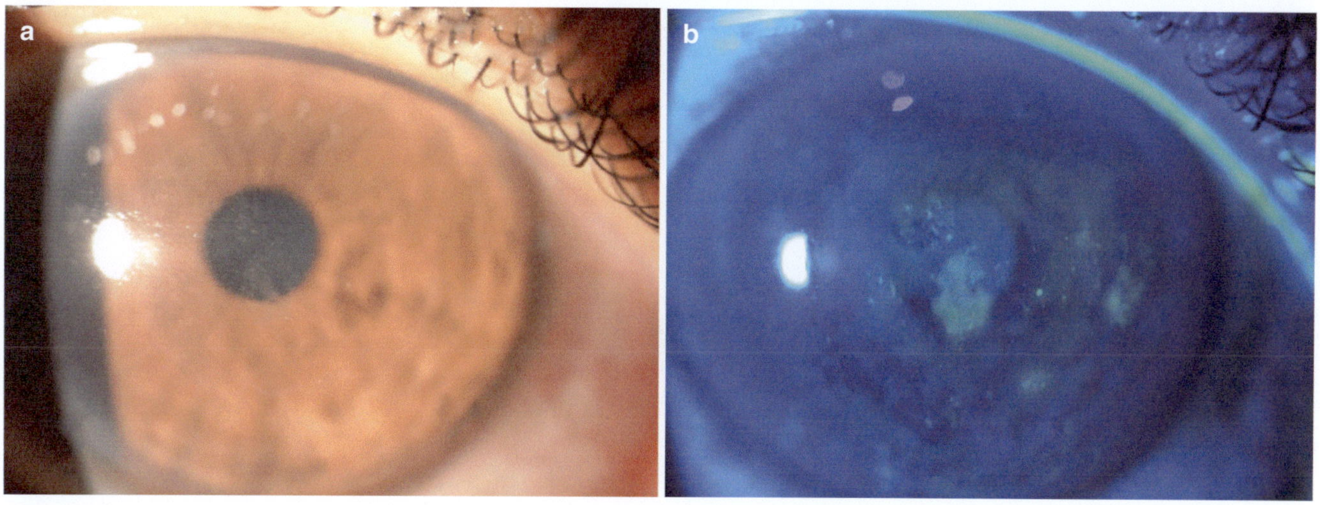

Fig. 6.14 Dry eyes. (**a**) Punctate keratitis, (**b**) with fluorescein stain

cyclosporine eye drops were prescribed and patient symptoms improved.

Case: Patient presented day one following an uneventful LASIK procedure with mild blurriness and irritation (Fig. 6.15).

Exam: A paracentral epithelial blister with circular border was noted with surrounding flap inflammation. A small linear crack occurred in the center of this blister (*red arrow*) (Fig. 6.15a, b). Topography showed corneal thickening in the area with the blister (Fig. 6.15d).

Management: Keep the same postoperative eye drop regiment (steroid and antibiotics). Patient healed completely within a week (Fig. 6.15c) and the topography normalized (Fig. 6.15e).

Core message: Even though the cause of this lesion is unknown, subclinical epithelial basement membrane dystrophy tends to cause epithelial sloughing or loosening during LASIK.

Take-Home Message

- Epithelial disease may occur following both LASIK and PRK.
- NSAIDs and steroids should be tapered in case of delayed healing following a PRK.
- Delayed epithelial healing may increase the risk of infection and corneal haze.
- A healing epithelium following PRK can simulate dendritic keratitis. Antivirals can be considered if epithelial defects persist beyond 2 weeks in patients with previously healthy corneas.
- LASIK and PRK may induce recurrent erosion syndrome.
- Traumatic corneal erosion is common during LASIK, especially in undiagnosed epithelial base-

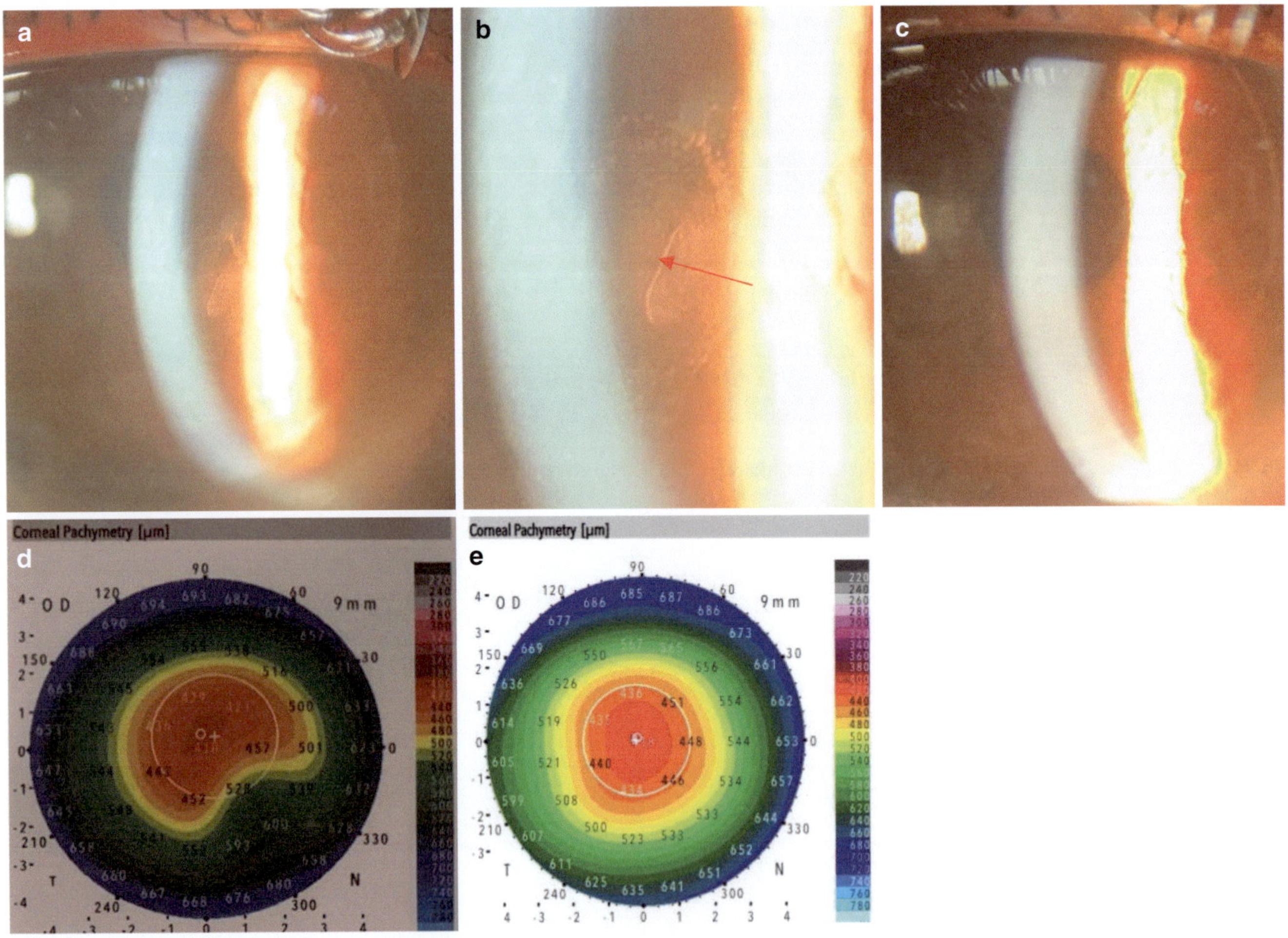

Fig. 6.15 Epithelial blister. (*Courtesy of Johnny Khoury, MD*)

ment membrane dystrophy; contact lens may be placed to decrease epithelial ingrowth.

- Corneal erosion over a flap may induce DLK.
- Evaluation of dry eye should be performed before surgery, on each postoperative visit, and when patients report decreased vision.
- Dry eye is common following refractive surgery and should be managed first with aggressive usage of artificial tears and punctal plugs.
- Severe dry eye syndrome may warrant the use of Cyclosporine, Lifitegrast, or serum tears.
- EBMD is a contraindication for microkeratome LASIK and a relative contraindication for femtosecond LASIK.
- Almost all corneal pathologies may still occur following refractive surgeries. However, their presentations may differ compared to non-operated corneas.

References

1. Javier JA, Lee JB, Oliveira HB, Chang JH, Azar DT. Basement membrane and collagen deposition after laser subepithelial keratomileusis and photorefractive keratectomy in the leghorn chick eye. Arch Ophthalmol. 2006;124:703–9.
2. Alio JL, Javaloy J. Corneal inflammation following corneal photoablative refractive surgery with excimer laser. Surv Ophthalmol. 2013;58:11–25.
3. Kauffmann T, Bodanowitz S, Hesse L, Kroll P. Corneal reinnervation after photorefractive keratectomy and laser in situ keratomileusis: an in vivo study with a confocal videomicroscope. Ger J Ophthalmol. 1996;5:508–12.
4. Lee BH, McLaren JW, Erie JC, Hodge DO, Bourne WM. Reinnervation in the cornea after LASIK. Invest Ophthalmol Vis Sci. 2002;43(12):3660–4.
5. Erie JC, McLaren JW, Hodge DO, Bourne WM. Recovery of corneal subbasal nerve density after PRK and LASIK. Am J Ophthalmol. 2005;140(6):1059–64.
6. Shehadeh-Mashor R, Mimouni M, Shapira Y, Sela T, Munzer G, Kaiserman I. Risk factors for dry eye after refractive surgery. Cornea. 2019;38(12):1495–9.
7. De Paiva CS, Chen Z, Koch DD, et al. The incidence and risk factors for developing dry eye after myopic LASIK. Am J Ophthalmol. 2006;141(3):438–45.
8. Schallhorn JM, Pelouskova M, Oldenburg C, Teenan D, Hannan SJ, Schallhorn SC. Effect of gender and procedure on patient-reported dry eye symptoms after laser vision correction. J Refract Surg. 2019;35(3):161–8.
9. Bilgihan K, Yesilirmak N, Yesim. Atlay. Evaluation of long-termcorneal morphology after photorefractive keratectomy by in vivo confocalmicroscopy and specular microscopy; 20-year follow-up. Eye Contact Lens Sci Clin Pract. 2019;45:360–4.
10. Saad S, Abdelmassih Y, Saad R, et al. Neurotrophic keratitis:frequency, etiologies, clinical outcomes, and management. Ocul Surf. 2020;18:231–6.
11. Seiler T. Photorefractive keratetcomy: European experience. In: Thompson FB, McDonnell PJ, editors. Color atlas/text of excimer laser surgery. The cornea. New York, NY: Igaku-Shoin; 1993. p. 53–62.
12. Maguen E. Results of laser photorefractive keratectomy for the correction of myopia. Ophthalmology. 1994;101:1548–56.
13. Ti SE, Tan DT. Recurrent corneal erosion after laser in situ keratomileusis. Cornea. 2001;20(2):156–8.

7 Epithelial Ingrowth

Alexander Melki, Jason Brenner, Wassef Chanbour, and Samir A. Melki

See Tables 7.1 and 7.2.

Case: Two weeks post LASIK enhancement procedure in a 40-year-old patient, which was performed 1 year after his primary treatment. UDVA is 20/20 (Fig. 7.1).

Exam: Paracentral epithelial island; discrete cells evident within nest, distant from the edge of the flap without connection to the surface epithelium (Fig. 7.1a).

Management: Spontaneous resolution of ingrowth after 2 months and residual scarring at the flap-stroma interface (Fig. 7.1b).

Core message: Observation is advised when the island is not visually significant and there is no identified fistulous tract with the corneal epithelium.

Case: Patient examined 1 week after a non-complicated primary LASIK procedure with no improvement in her UCVA of 20/40 (Fig. 7.2).

Exam: Isolated epithelial cell clumps noted under the flap (Fig. 7.2a). There was an increase in the anterior axial curvature on the topography causing irregular astigmatism (Fig. 7.2b).

Management: Flap lift was performed. The epithelial clump can be seen isolated in the center of the cornea, and it was scraped with a Weck-Cel (Fig. 7.2d–f). Topography normalized 1 month following the procedure (Fig. 7.2c).

Case: 30-year-old female presented 1 week after her LASIK enhancement procedure. Her primary surgery, 1 year ago, was complicated with a large epithelial defect and micro-striae (Fig. 7.3).

A. Melki
UCLA, Los Angeles, CA, USA

J. Brenner (✉) · S. A. Melki
Boston Vision, Department of Ophthalmology, Harvard Medical School, Boston, MA, USA
e-mail: brenner@bostonvision.com; melki@bostonvision.com

W. Chanbour
Department of Ophthalmology and Visual Neurosciences, University of Minnesota, Minneapolis, MN, USA
e-mail: chanb013@umn.edu

Exam: Progression from Grade 1 (Fig. 7.3a) to Grade 2 (Fig. 7.3b) epithelial ingrowth after 2 months. A thicker ingrowth is noted containing discrete cells evident within nest, at least 2 mm from flap edge without melting or erosion (Fig. 7.3b).

Management: Monthly observation.

Core message: Mild progression outside the visual axis must be followed closely, without intervention as spontaneous resolution is still possible.

Case: 8 months following a LASIK enhancement procedure, a patient presented with decreased UDVA from 20/20 in the early post-operative period to 20/30 (Fig. 7.4).

Exam: Grade 2 epithelial ingrowth with a dense nest of white epithelial cells surrounded by a translucent area of advancing cells towards the visual axis (Fig. 7.4a). Multiple fistulas, stained with fluorescein, provide an entry point for more cells (Fig. 7.4b).

Management: Surgical removal of epithelial ingrowth was performed.

Core message: Epithelial ingrowth that threatens the visual axis or causes a decrease in the visual acuity should be treated aggressively.

Case: An asymptomatic patient presented 1 year after a non-complicated LASIK procedure, the UDVA was 20/20 (Fig. 7.5).

Exam: Grade 2 epithelial ingrowth (Fig. 7.5a), fluorescein staining shows one open epithelial fistula (Fig. 7.5b), corneal flap edge is gray, indicating a possible progression to melting (Fig. 7.5c).

Management: Patient was followed monthly. One year later the epithelial cells aggregated and became scar tissue, ingrowth shrunk in size and the flap edge healed completely (Fig. 7.5d).

Case: Asymptomatic patient presenting for a 1-month follow-up after LASIK enhancement procedure, UDVA was 20/20 (Fig. 7.6).

Exam: A grade 2 epithelial ingrowth consistent of multiple small epithelial islands advancing in the cornea (*red arrowheads*) (Fig. 7.6a). Fluorescein staining highlighted a

S. A. Melki et al. (eds.), *Refractive Surgery Atlas*, https://doi.org/10.1007/978-3-031-60661-8_7

Table 7.1 Diagnosis, prevention, and management of epithelial ingrowth

Onset	2–3 months after LASIK
Rate	1% after primary treatment with microkeratome [1] 0.03% after primary treatment with femtosecond laser [2] 1.8–20% after enhancement treatment [1, 3]
Pathology	Islands of epithelial cells trapped in the flap-stromal interface [4]
Mechanism	• Invasion through the flap edge or stromal laceration (buttonhole) • Implantation during dissection of the flap or irritation under the flap [4]
Symptoms	Asymptomatic, becomes symptomatic with decreased visual acuity [5] if: • Ingrowth migrates onto the visual axis • Irregular astigmatism • Melting
Monitoring	Photograph, topography [5], fluorescein staining (shows an epithelial fistula)
Risk factors	Preoperative: age, diabetes mellitus, RK, basement membrane dystrophy, recurrent erosion syndrome Perioperative: enhancement surgery, epithelial defect, thin flap, buttonholes, free cap, DLK, flap misalignment, ablation zone larger than the flap diameter [6, 7]
Prevention	• Use of femtosecond laser instead of microkeratome • Bandage contact lens in case of flap lift (enhancement surgery) or in case of intraoperative epithelial defect • Push peripheral corneal epithelium away during enhancement procedure • Use vertical side cuts in femtosecond laser
Indication for observation	• Isolated epithelial cells at the interface without connection to the surface • Localized non-progressive peripheral melting leading to a scar
Indications for treatment	• Invades the visual axis • Induces refractive error or irregular astigmatism • Stromal melting • Nighttime glare • Induces foreign body sensation
Surgical technique	• Lifting the flap and scraping the epithelial cells from the stromal bed and undersurface of the flap with a scalpel blade • Additional proposed treatments of recurrent ingrowth: sutures [8], ethanol [9], mitomycin [10], phototherapeutic keratectomy [11], Nd:YAG laser [12], glue [13], and if everything fails with progressive melting, then the flap should be amputated

Table 7.2 Grades of epithelial ingrowth

Grades	Probst/Machat epithelial ingrowth classification [3]	Treatment
Grade 1	Thin ingrowth, 1–2 cells thick, limited to within 2 mm of flap edge, transparent, difficult to detect, well-delineated white line along advancing edge, no associated flap changes, and non-progressive	Monthly observation
Grade 2	Thicker ingrowth, discrete cells evident within nest, at least 2 mm from flap edge, individual cells translucent, easily seen on slit lamp, no demarcation line along nest, corneal flap edge rolled or gray, no flap edge melting or erosion, and usually progressive	Non-urgent treatment within 2–3 weeks
Grade 3	Pronounced ingrowth, several cells thick, greater than 2 mm from flap edge, ingrowth areas appear opaque, obvious on slit lamp, white geographic areas of necrotic epithelial cells without a demarcation line, and corneal flap margins rolled with thickened white-grayish appearance	Urgent treatment required with close follow-up
Grade 4	Large areas of flap melting from collagenase release from necrotic epithelium. Confluent haze develops peripheral to the flap edge as flap pulls away, leaving exposed stromal bed in contact with surface epithelium	Urgent treatment required with close follow-up

rolled corneal flap edge and area of pooling between the flap edge and the corneal bed (*red arrow*) (Fig. 7.6b).

Management: Non-urgent epithelial ingrowth scraping is considered due to high risk of progression.

Core message: A non-healed flap edge increases the risk of ingrowth progression; early surgery may be considered.

Case: Following a LASIK enhancement procedure. UDVA: 20/20 (Fig. 7.7).

Exam: Grade 1 epithelial ingrowth detected 6 weeks post enhancement, composed of thin layer, 1–2 cells thick, limited to within 2 mm of flap edge, transparent, and difficult to visualize (Fig. 7.7a). Ingrowth progressed to Grade 2 and moved closer to the visual axis 1 month later (Fig. 7.7b).

Management: Close monitoring and early surgical intervention is advised.

Case: 39-year-old patient followed for 1 year after a non-complicated LASIK procedure (Fig. 7.8).

Exam: Progression from Grade 1 (Fig. 7.8a, b) epithelial ingrowth starting 1 month after the procedure, into Grade 2 epithelial ingrowth. Diffuse nests of epithelial cells are scattered through the cornea (Fig. 7.8c). Patient was lost to follow up and presented 2 months later with Grade 4 epithelial

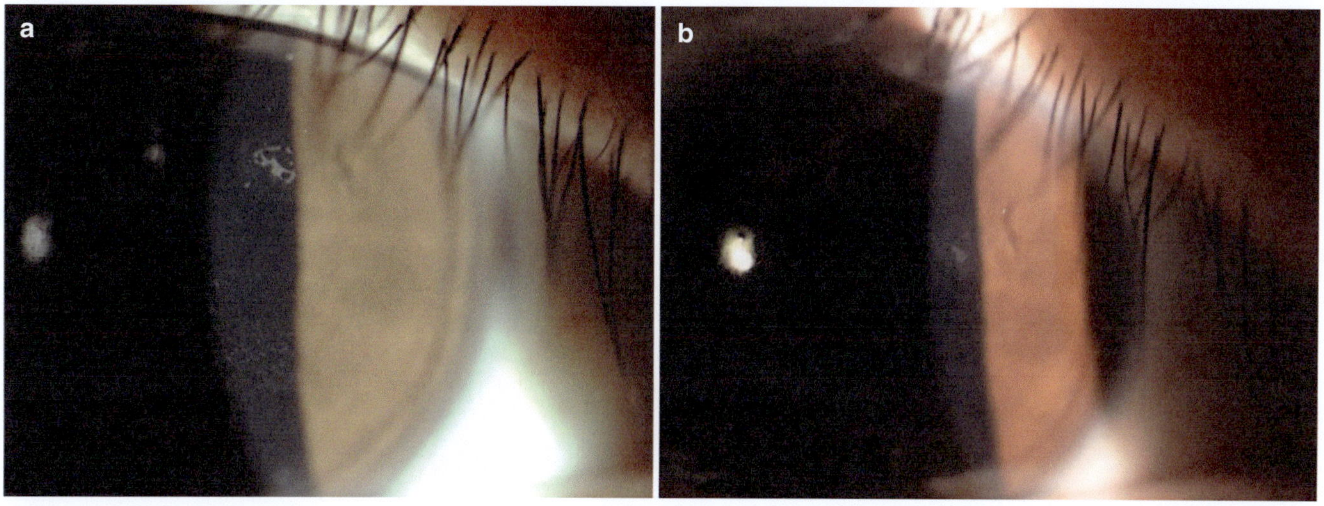

Fig. 7.1 Paracentral island

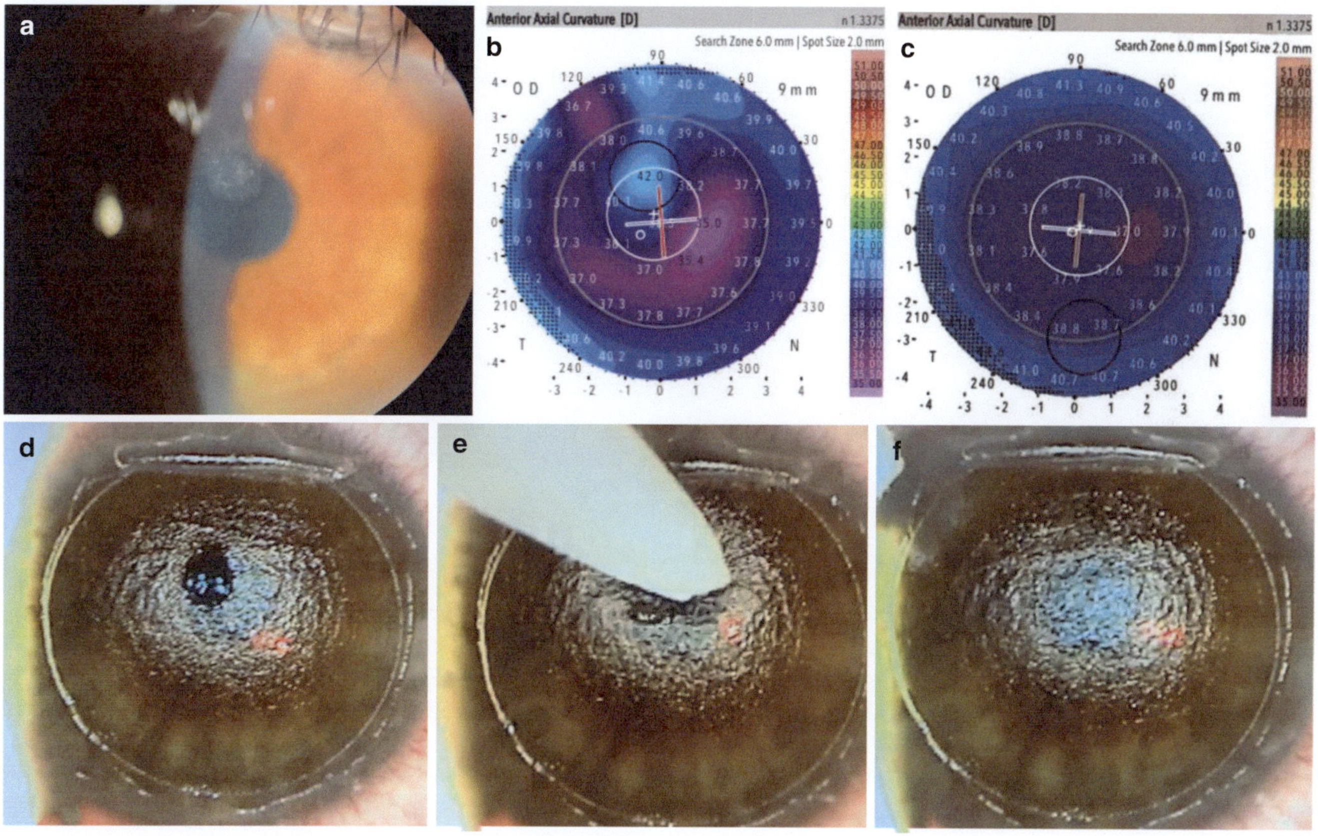

Fig. 7.2 Isolated epithelial island. (*Courtesy of Johnny Khoury, MD*)

ingrowth, large area of flap melting with central areas of translucent sheet of epithelial cells including multiple islands of epithelial cells (Fig. 7.8d).

Management: Urgent surgical intervention is recommended.

Core message: In cases of fast epithelial ingrowth progression, early treatment may have prevented flap melting.

Case: 35-year-old female was followed after a LASIK enhancement procedure. UDVA was 20/20 (Fig. 7.9).

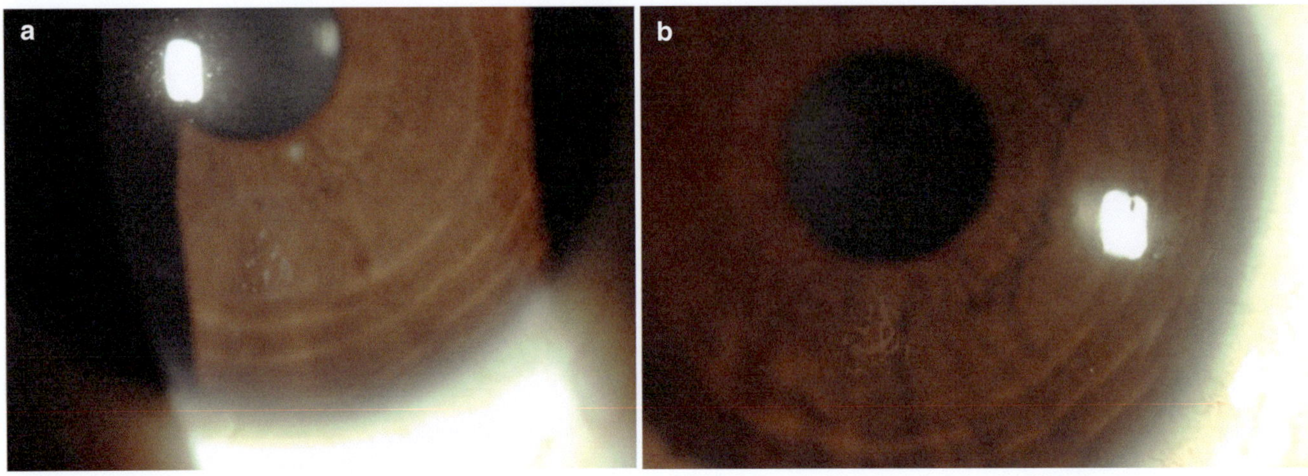

Fig. 7.3 Progressing epithelial ingrowth

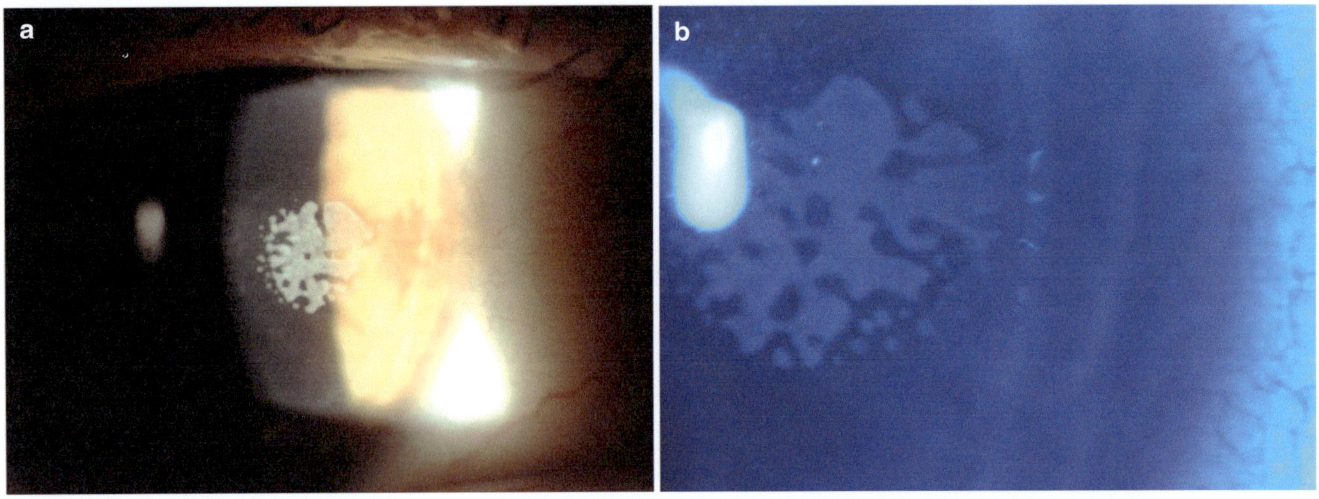

Fig. 7.4 Epithelial fistula

Exam: Progressive increase in epithelial ingrowth from Grade 1 (Fig. 7.9a) at 6 months' post Enhancement to Grade 2 (Fig. 7.9b) at 1 year, followed by spontaneous regression, leading to shrinking in the size of the ingrowth (Fig. 7.9c) into one white isolated island (Fig. 7.9d) at 2 years post enhancement.

Management: Patient was observed, and 3 years after the enhancement, a visually non-significant sup-epithelial haze persisted (Fig. 7.9e).

Core message: In slowly progressing epithelial ingrowth, observation is advised as late spontaneous resolution is common.

Case: Patient presented with blurry vision 1 week following a LASIK surgery complicated with a superior interface hemorrhage (Fig. 7.10).

Exam: Grade 3 epithelial ingrowth affecting the visual axis. Additionally, there was a hemorrhage at the edge of the ingrowth, which was an unrelated incident (Fig. 7.10a).

Management: Urgent surgical management with flap lift and scraping was performed and the cornea recovered completely after 1 week (Fig. 7.10b).

Core message: Early post-operative follow-up and yearly screening is imperative to detect and treat epithelial ingrowth before progression into melting.

Case A: 3 months after a non-complicated enhancement procedure, UDVA: 20/20 (Fig. 7.11a).

Case B: 1 year after a non-complicated enhancement procedure, UDVA: 20/30 (Fig. 7.11b).

Exam: Grade 3, advanced opaque ingrowth with a thickened corneal flap margin, white and rolled with minimal melting (Fig. 7.11a, b).

Management: Corneal debridement with or without suturing is advised to prevent melting.

Case: Patient had a central flap laceration following a trauma years after a LASIK surgery. Flap was lifted cleaned and realigned (Fig. 7.12).

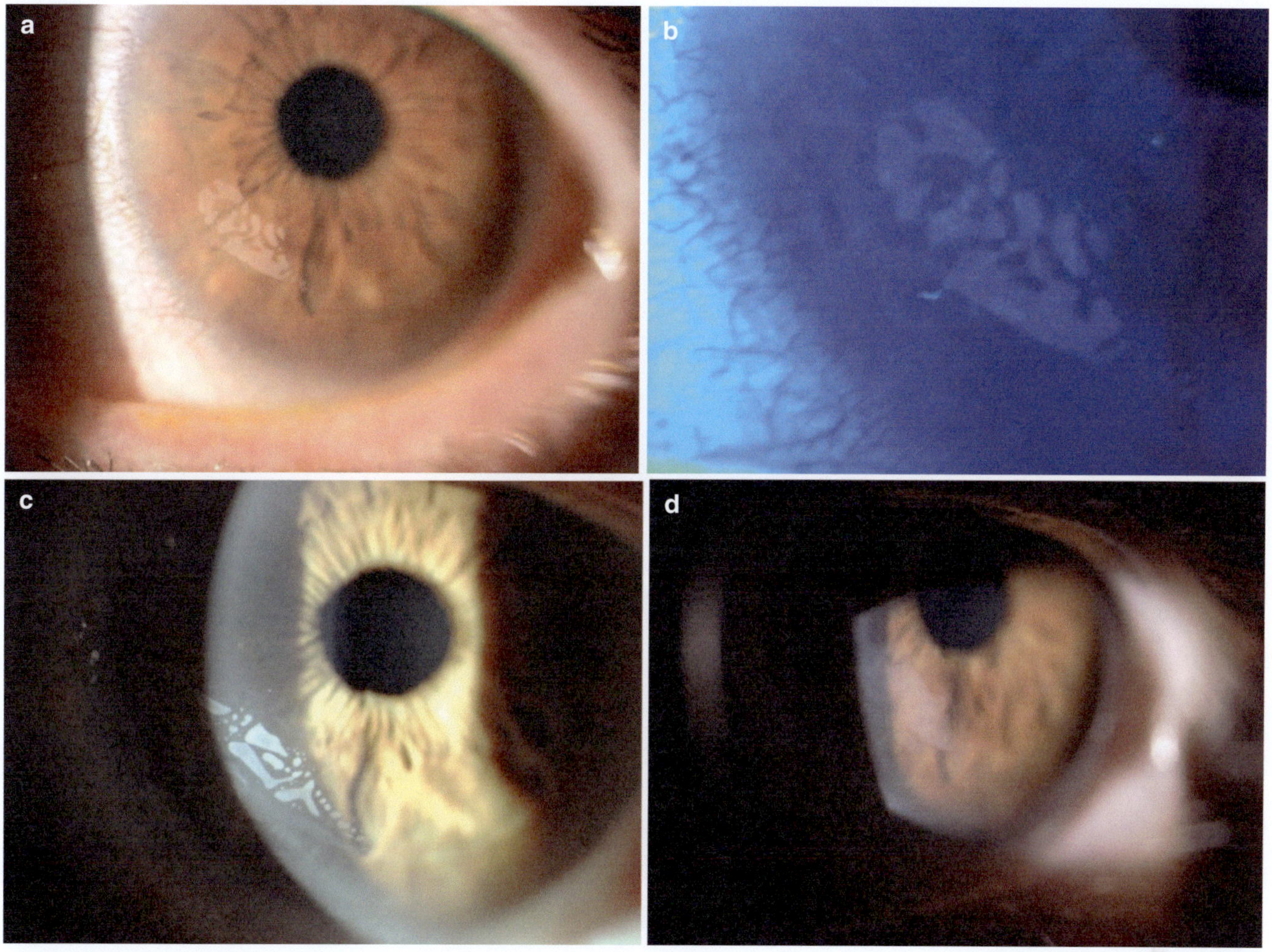

Fig. 7.5 Late epitelial ingrowth resolution

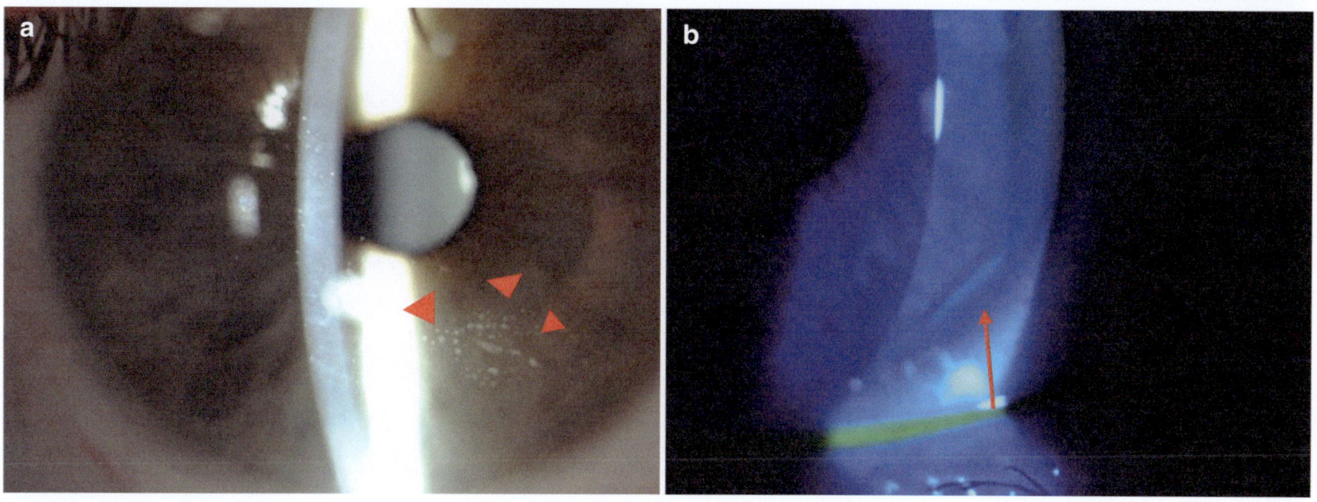

Fig. 7.6 Flap-stroma gap

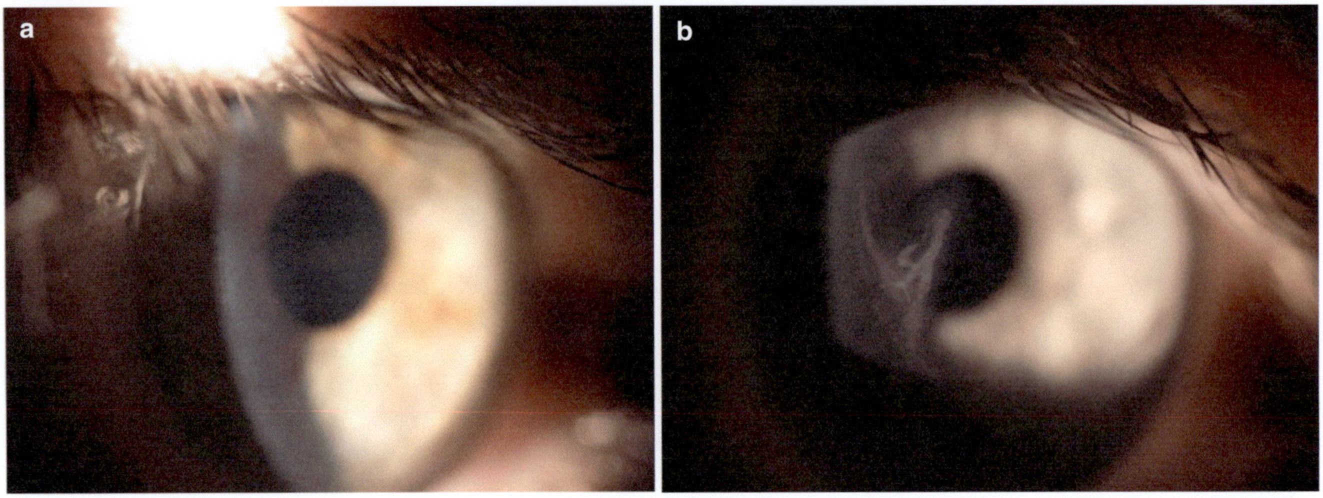

Fig. 7.7 Progression from Grade 1 to 2

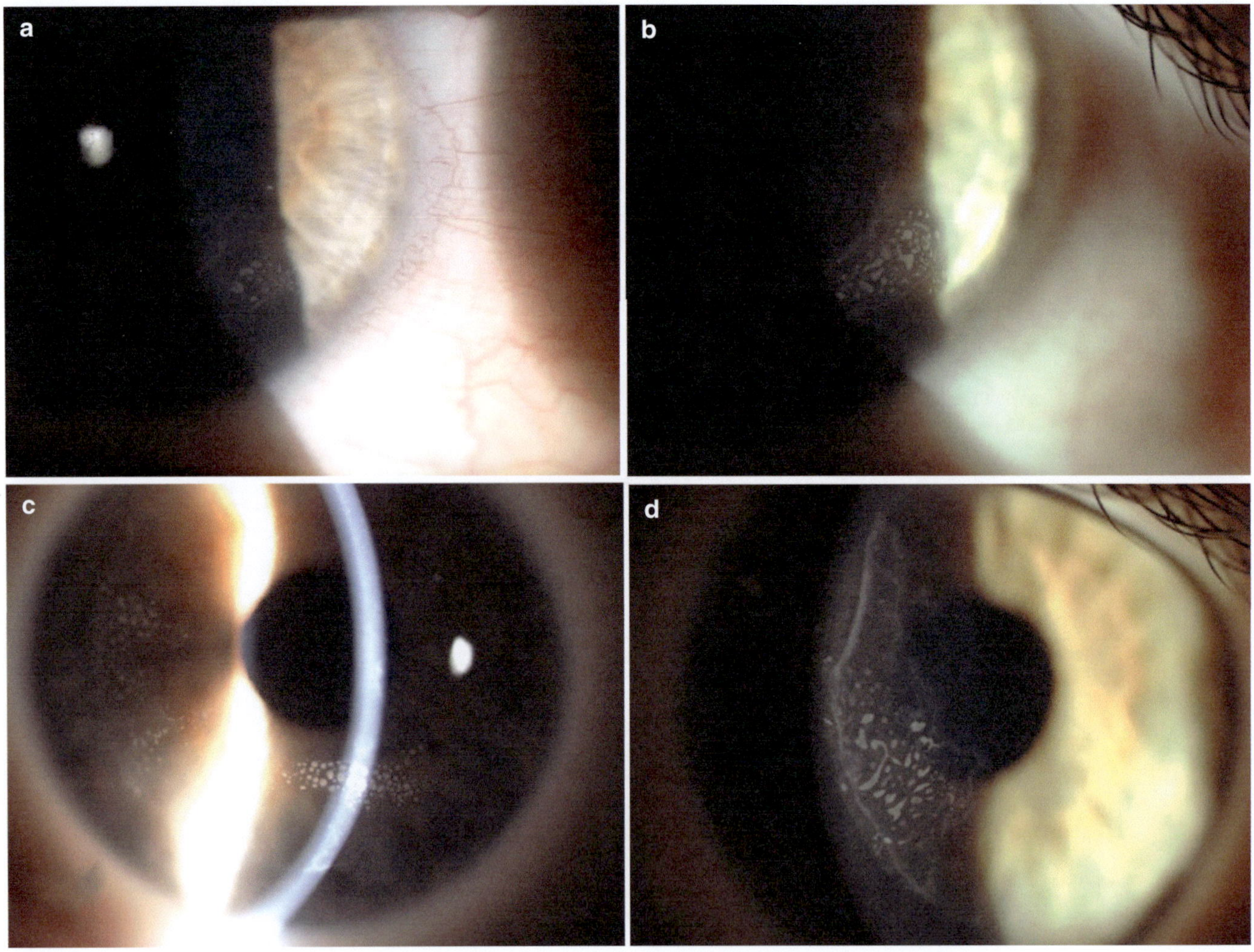

Fig. 7.8 Rapid progression to melting

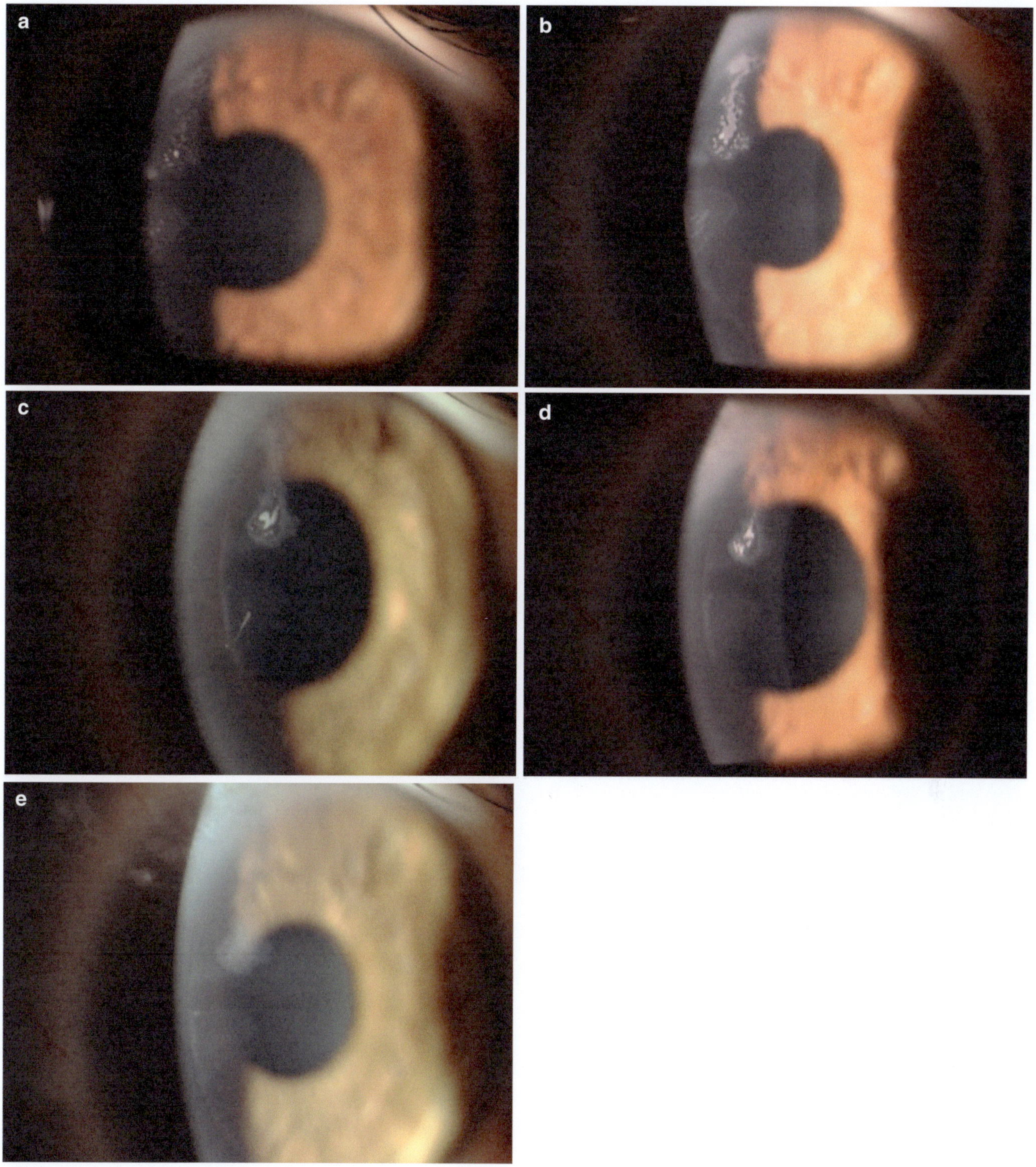

Fig. 7.9 Spontaneous resolution

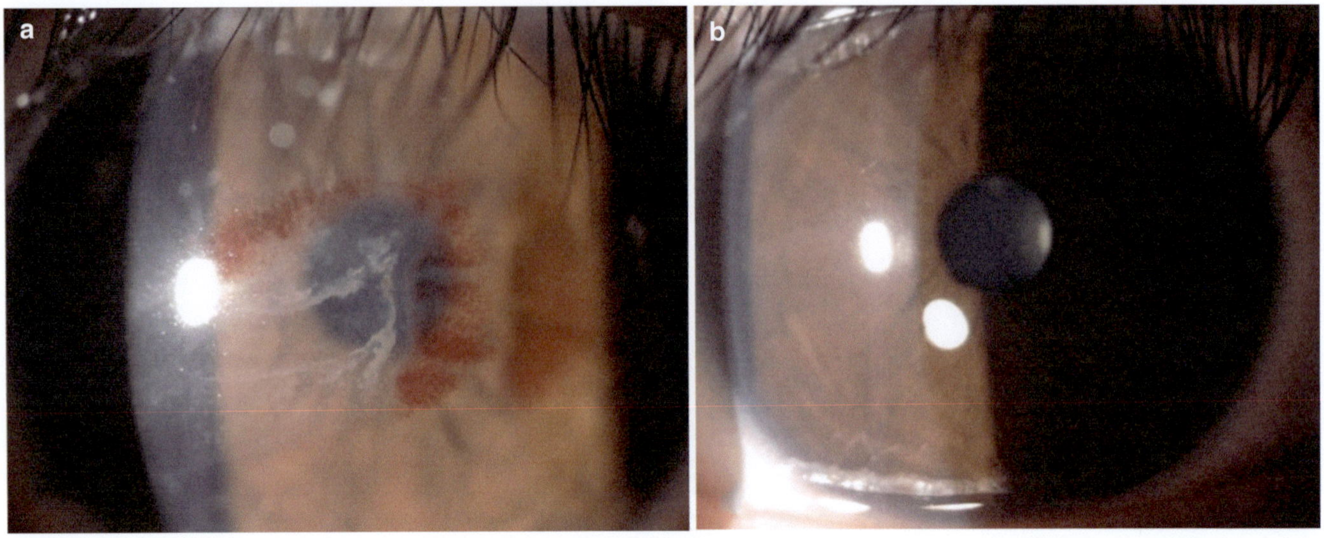

Fig. 7.10 Urgent treatment

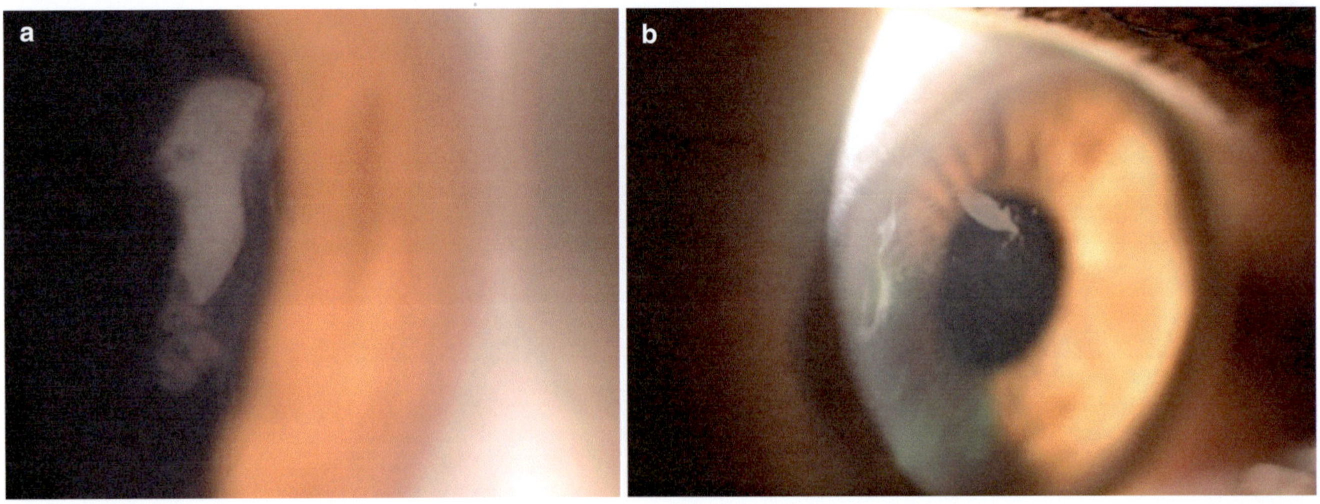

Fig. 7.11 Rolled flap edge

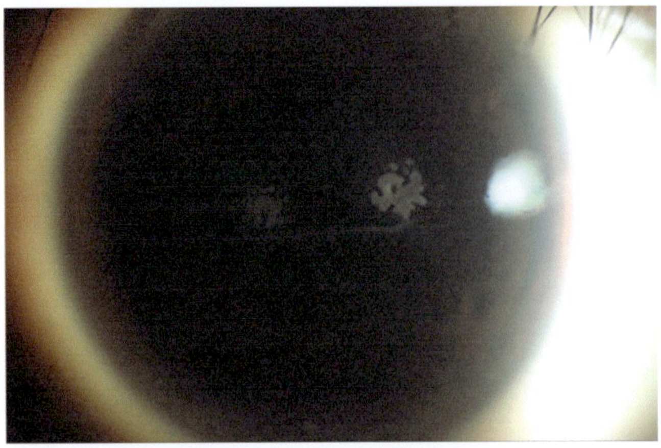

Fig. 7.12 Traumatic epithelial ingrowth. (*Courtesy of Joshua H. Hou, MD. University of Minnesota, Minnesota, USA*)

Exam: Two Grade 2 central epithelial ingrowth extending from the laceration area.

Management: Flap lift and debridement is recommended if the ingrowth is affecting the visual axis. Para central sutures can be placed to prevent recurrence.

Case: 75-year-old male presented 8 months following an enhancement following LASIK 15 years before. Vision worsened and the patient was photophobic. MRx OS: +2.50–3.50 × 068 (20/40) (Fig. 7.13).

Exam: Slit lamp exam showed grade 3 epithelial ingrowth (Fig. 7.13a); topography showed increased steepness over the area of the ingrowth (Fig. 7.13b). Corneal OCT showed hyperreflective material under the flap (Fig. 7.13c).

Management: Flap lift and debridement is recommended.

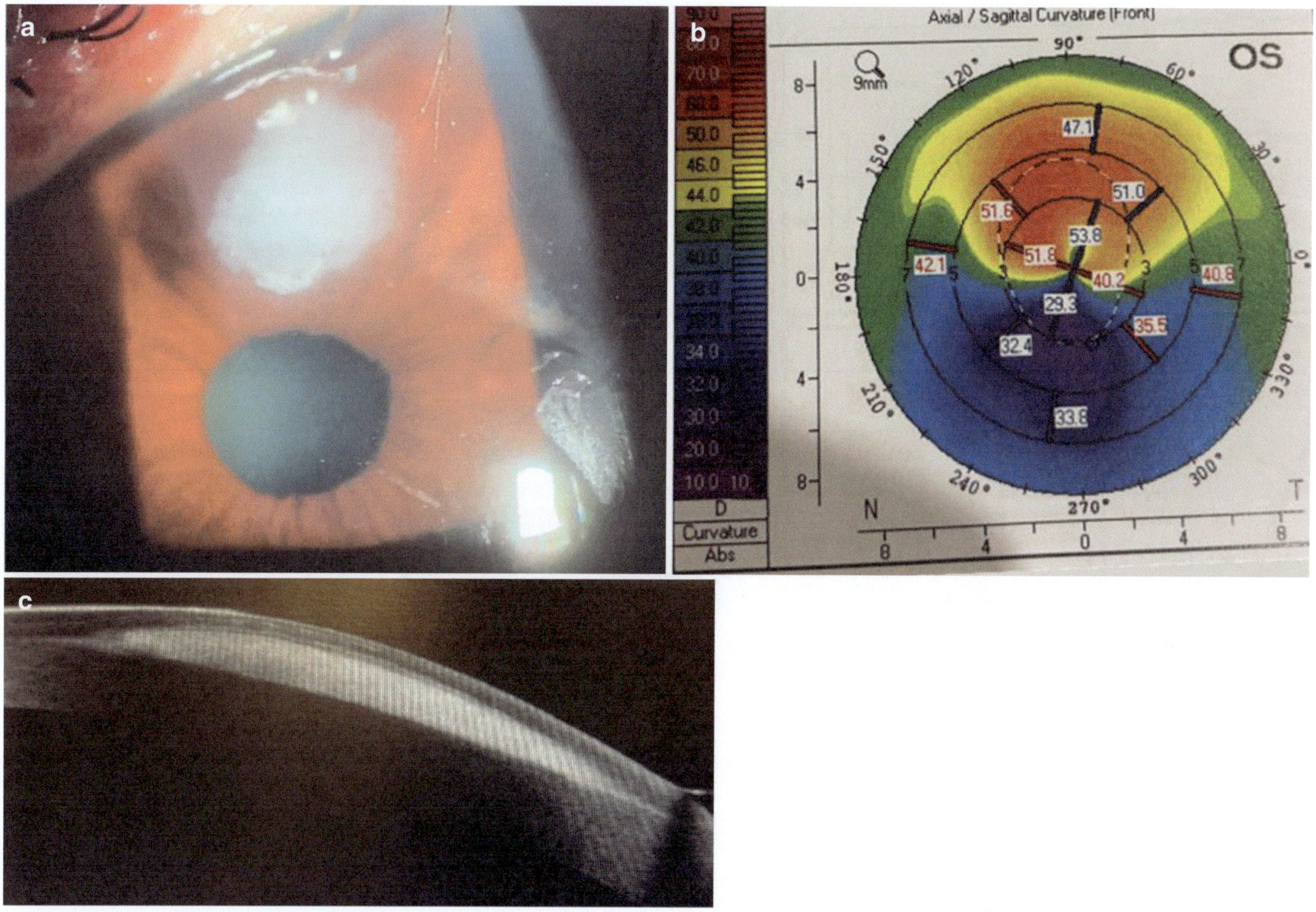

Fig. 7.13 Elevated flap. (*Courtesy of Matthew McCauley, MD, Berkeley Eye Center, Texas, USA*)

Core Message: Topography and Corneal OCT can be used to assess the severity and monitor progression of the epithelial ingrowth.

Case: 39-year-old patient presented 2 years after a non-complicated LASIK procedure; she is asymptomatic and her UDVA is 20/20 (Fig. 7.14).

Exam: Grade 2 dense and large epithelial ingrowth is easily seen on slit lamp. A gray flap border indicates a possible progression to melting (Fig. 7.14a, b).

Management: Flap lift, scraping, and 10-0 nylon suturing were performed. Two weeks post-operative appearance showed a compete disappearance of the ingrowth without recurrence, but the flap edge retained the gray color (Fig. 7.14c, d).

Case: 4 months following a primary LASIK procedure, a patient was followed closely; UDVA was 20/20. (Fig. 7.15).

Exam: Grade 2 epithelial ingrowth >2 mm in size with no melting (Fig. 7.15a) was first noticed 4 months after the LASIK. It increased its density and threatened the visual axis at 1 year postoperatively (Fig. 7.15b); fluorescein staining showed an inferior fistula (Fig. 7.15c).

Management: Ingrowth was threatening the visual axis even though the visual acuity was preserved. The patient underwent flap lift, scraping, and flap suturing. Post-scraping picture shows inferior recurrence 1 mm from the edge of the flap (Fig. 7.15d). Post-operative fluorescein staining shows multiple fistulous tracts between two sutures (Fig. 7.15e).

Core message: Epithelial ingrowth can still occur with the presence of sutures.

Case: 70-year-old female patient s/p LASIK 20 years ago, presented with progressive blurry vision. UCVA: 20/80 (Fig. 7.16).

Exam: Large stage 4 epithelial ingrowth noted inferiorly (*red arrowheads*) (Fig. 7.16a), extending into the visual axis. Anterior segment OCT shows a paracentral area of flap melting (*red arrow*) (Fig. 7.16b).

Management: A complete flap lift, scraping, and suturing was performed. One month following the procedure, a new ingrowth was noted inferotemporally (yellow arrowheads) (Fig. 7.16c). Another flap lift and suturing was performed (Fig. 7.16d). One month later, a third recurrence of ingrowth was noted inferonasally (*yellow arrow*) (Fig. 7.16e).

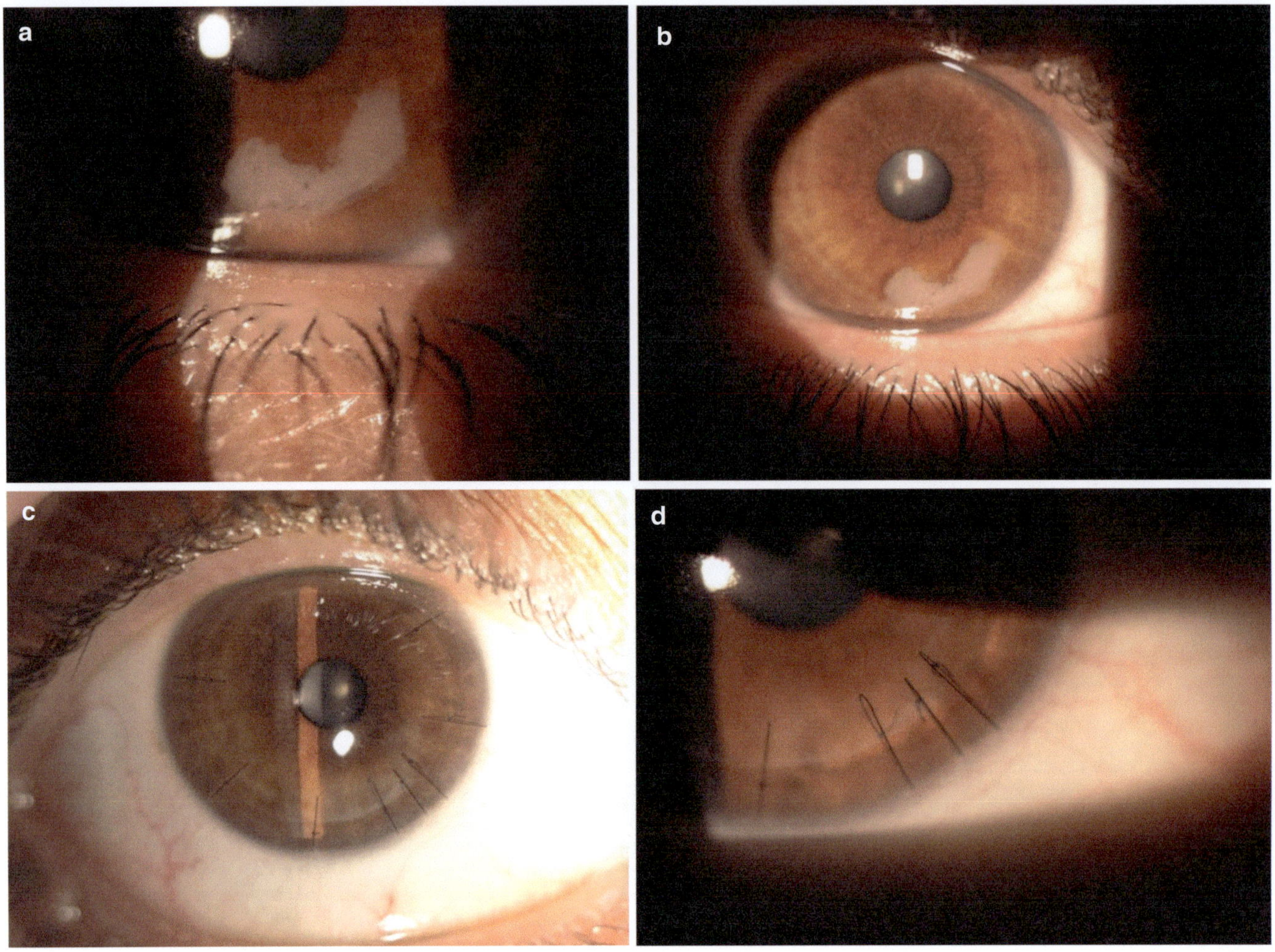

Fig. 7.14 Preventive measures

Disruption of epithelial ingrowth with Nd:YAG laser (1 mJ) was performed and there was no recurrence following complete suture removal (Fig. 7.16f).

Core Message: With good management and follow up, the flap can still be preserved in cases of peripheral melting due to stage 4 epithelial ingrowth.

Epithelial ingrowth patterns (Fig. 7.17a–c) and method of removal thorough scraping of both the stromal bed and the underside of the flap (Fig. 7.17d).

The Melki LASIK FLAP suction stabilizer, an instrument used as a support for scraping the underside of a flap for epithelial ingrowth (Fig. 7.18a) and also used for straightening flap folds by applying the Pineda Iron to smoothen the surface (Fig. 7.18b).

Extra Illustrations

See Figs. 7.19, 7.20, 7.21, 7.22, 7.23, 7.24, 7.25, 7.26, 7.27, 7.28, 7.29, 7.30, 7.31 and 7.32.

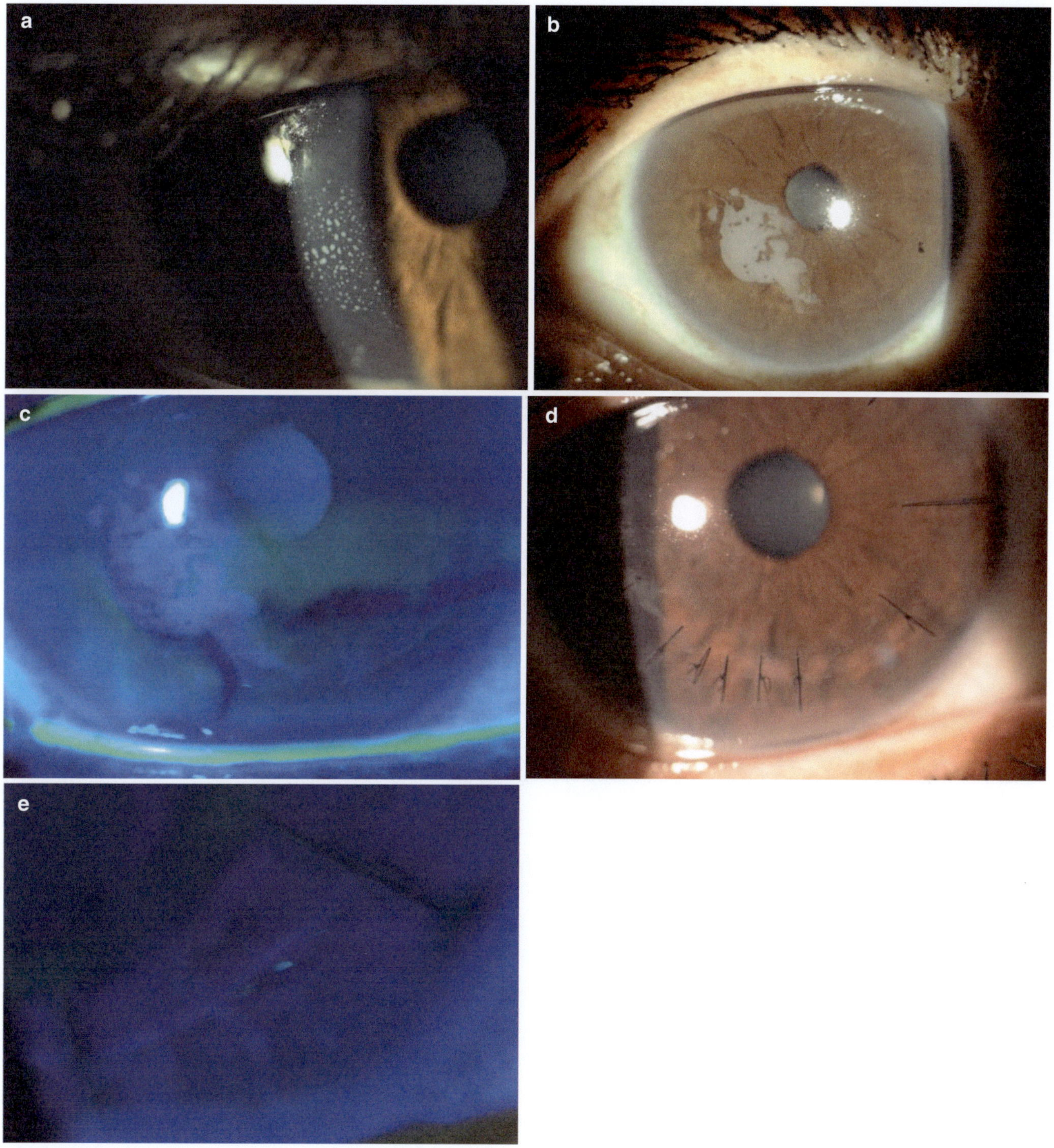

Fig. 7.15 Recurrent ingrowth following flap suturing

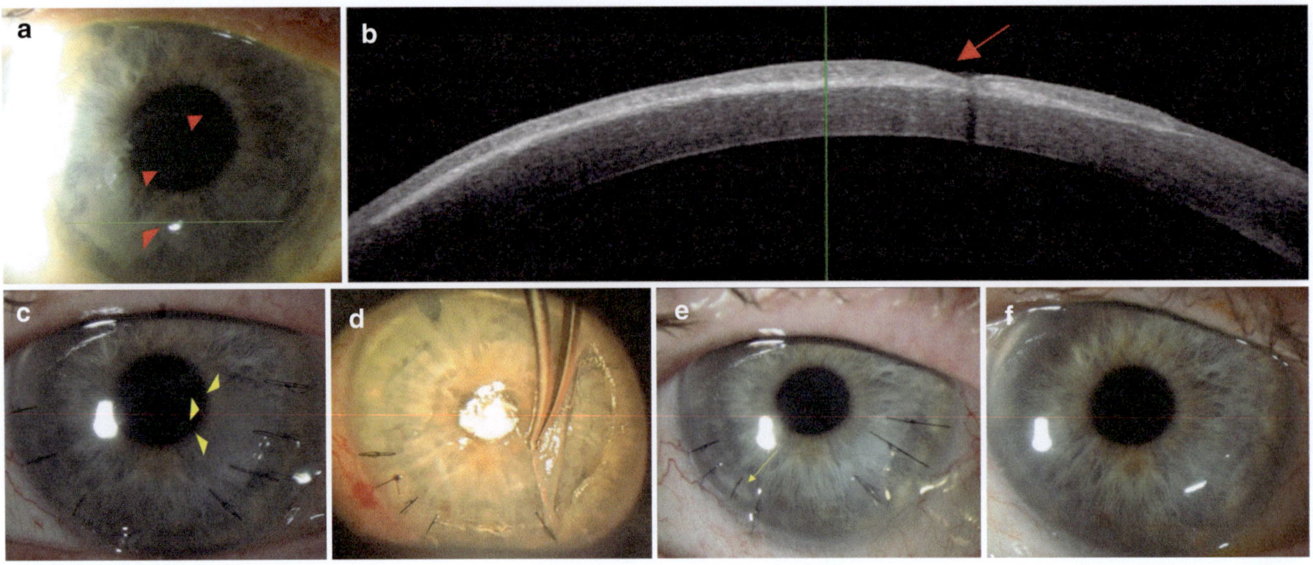

Fig. 7.16 YAG epithelial disruption

Fig. 7.17 Surgical debredement technique

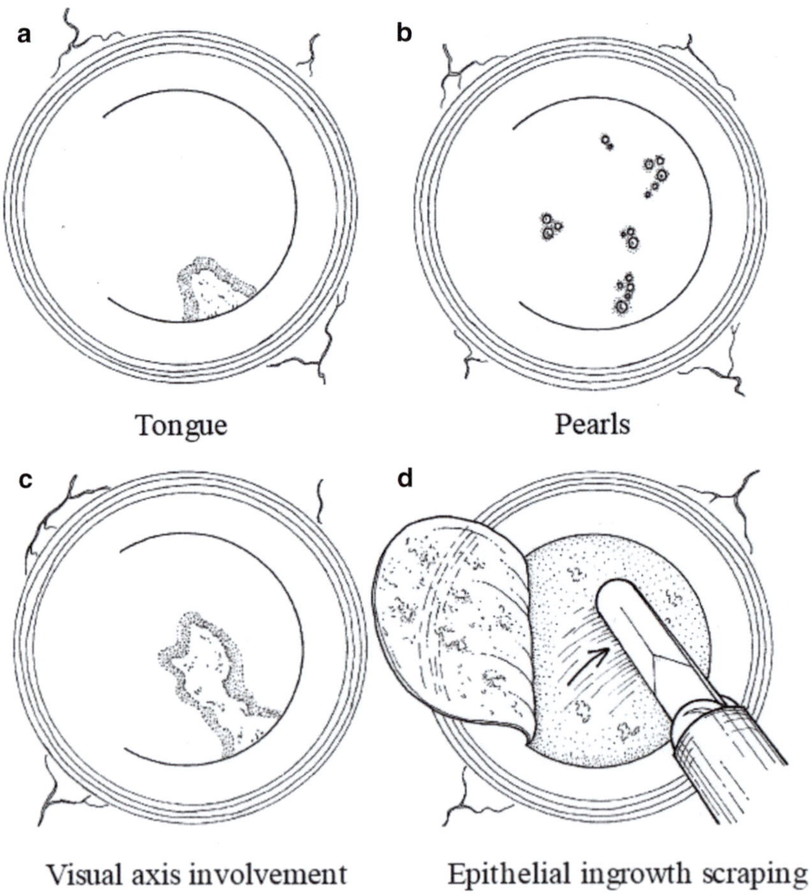

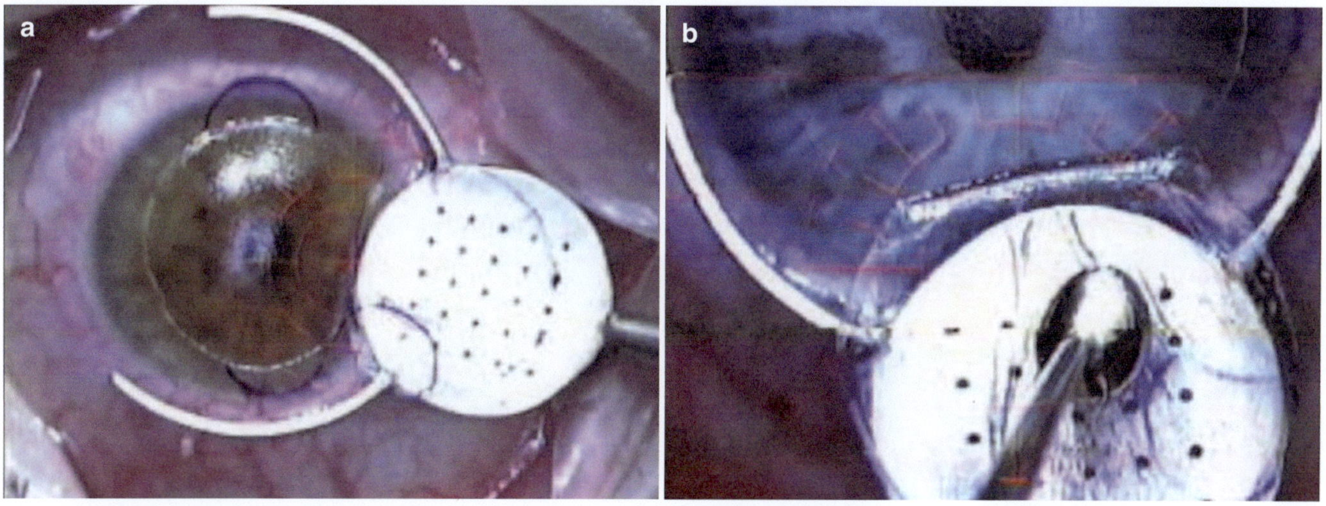

Fig. 7.18 Flap stabilizer

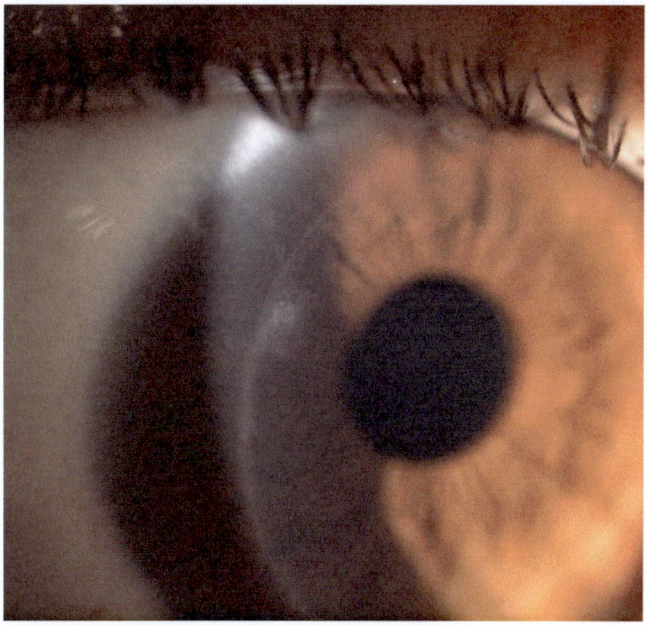

Fig. 7.19 Grade 1 epithelial ingrowth: thin ingrowth, within 2 mm of flap edge

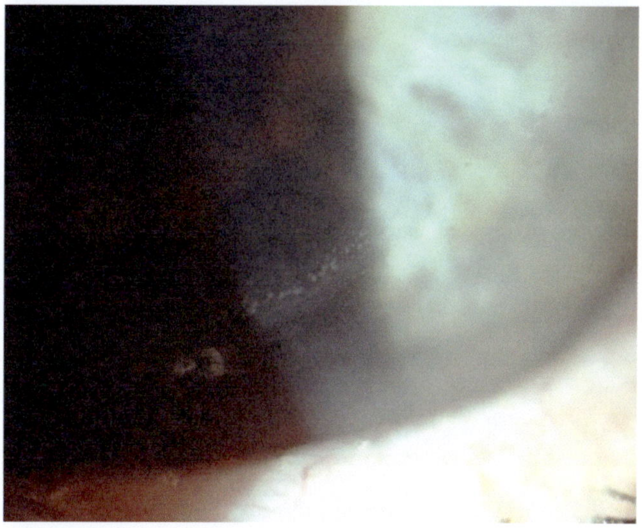

Fig. 7.20 Thin grade 1 epithelial ingrowth layers, limited to within 2 mm of the flap edge, transparent and difficult to detect

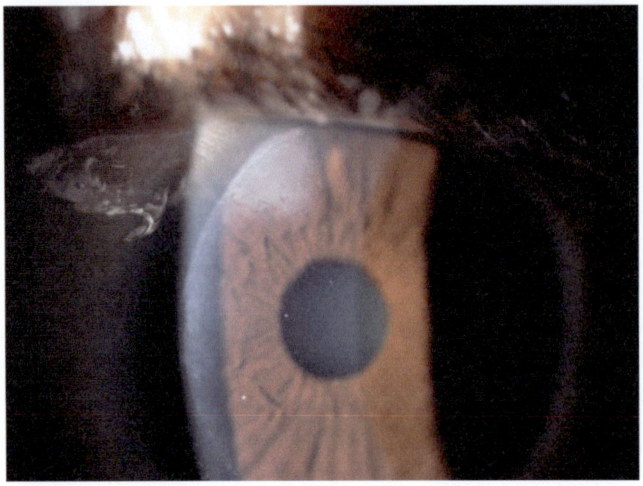

Fig. 7.21 Grade 2 thick ingrowth

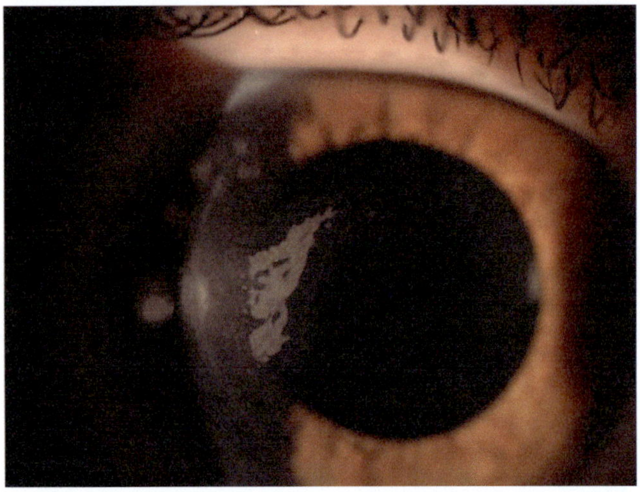

Fig. 7.22 Grade 2 thick ingrowth, advancing more than 2 mm from the flap edge

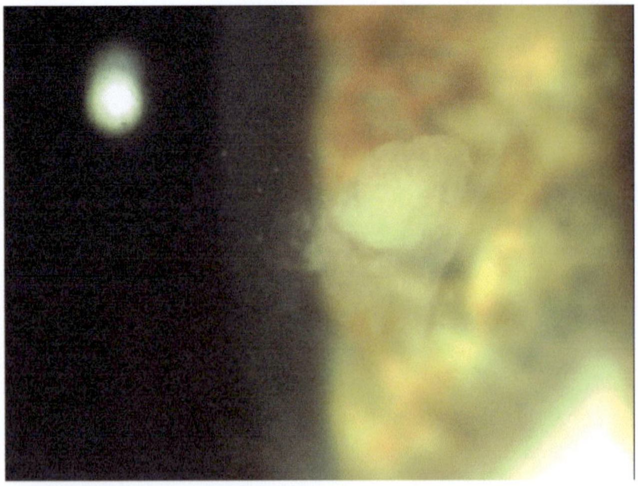

Fig. 7.23 Grade 2 epithelial ingrowth, the flap edges are rolled and gray in appearance without flap melting

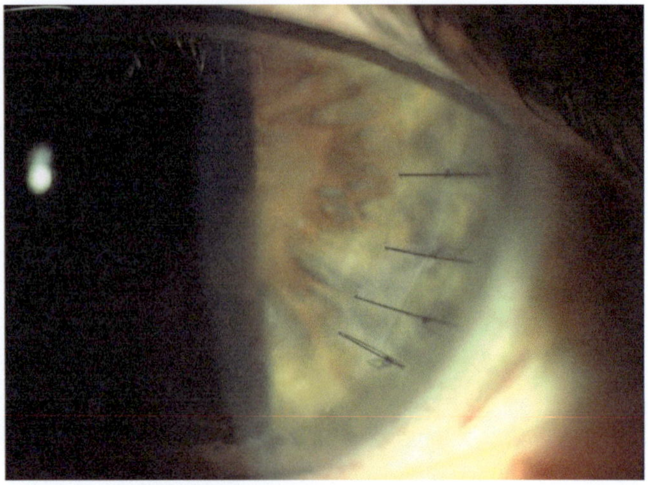

Fig. 7.24 Following flap suturing of the patient in Fig. 7.23

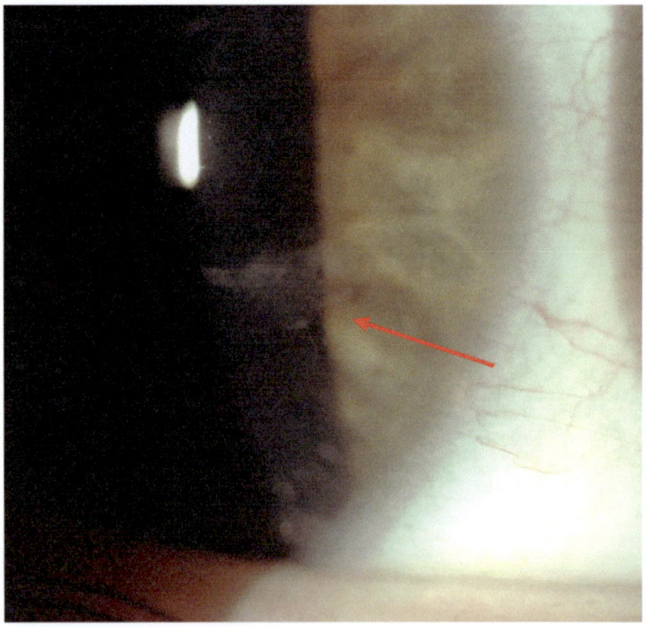

Fig. 7.25 Grade 3 epithelial ingrowth with a small area of melting detected at the flap edge (*red arrow*), 5 months after the enhancement procedure

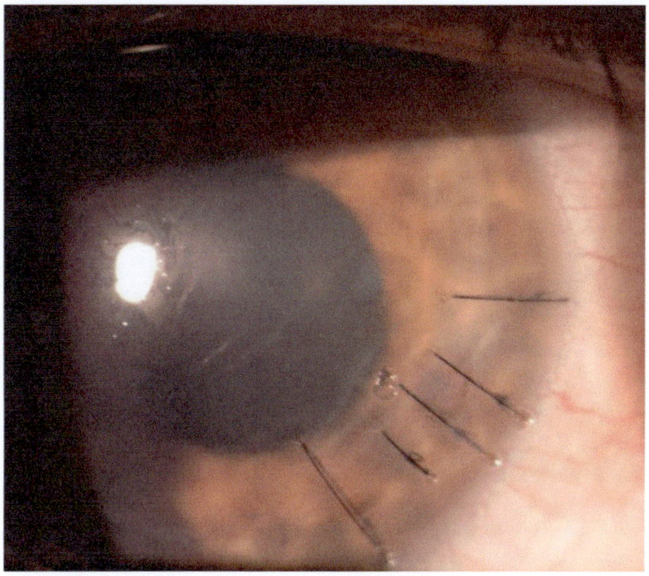

Fig. 7.26 Macro-striae, epithelial defect, and flap edema were noted following a flap lift and scraping of the patient in Fig. 7.25. Sutures are asymmetric and have different lengths

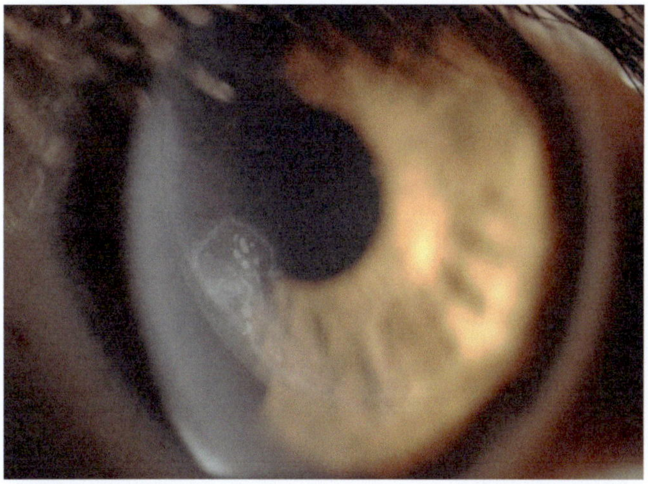

Fig. 7.27 Grade 4 ingrowth with melting

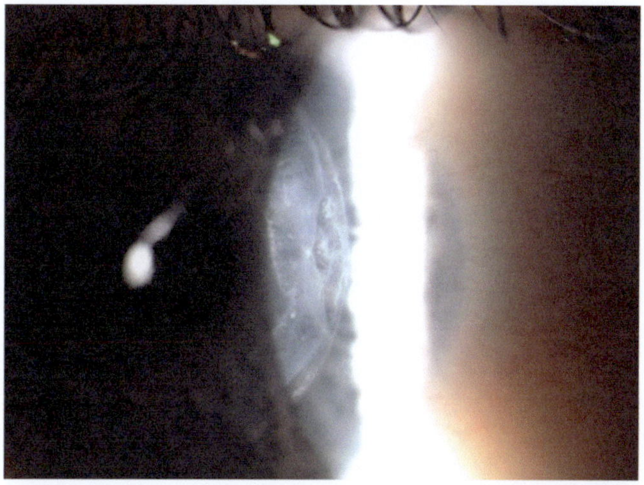

Fig. 7.28 Grade 4 epithelial ingrowth leading to melting of the flap with a wide area of exposed stroma 3 years following LASIK surgery

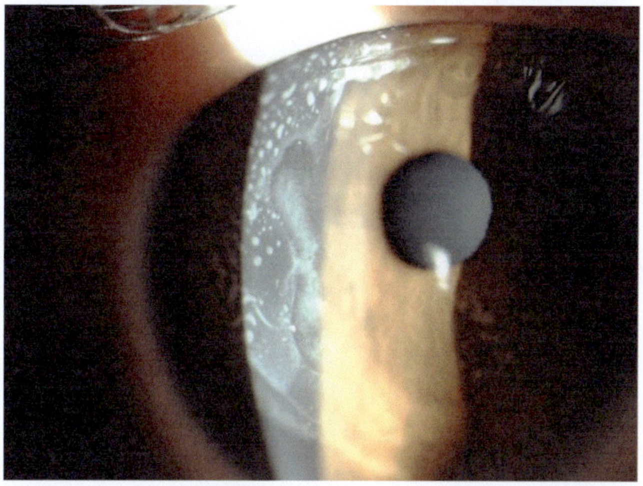

Fig. 7.29 Grade 4 epithelial ingrowth, greater than 2 mm from flap edge associated with a with a large geographic area of necrotic flap

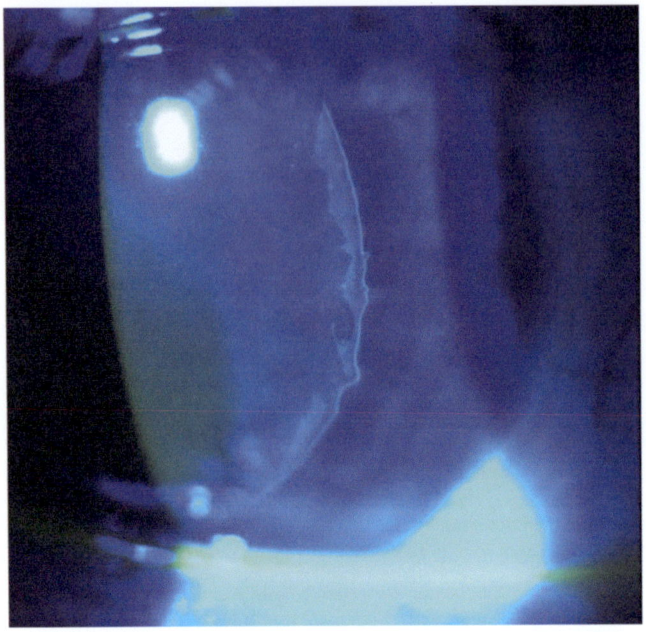

Fig. 7.30 Fluorescein staining showing an extensive area of connection between the epithelium and the interface inducing an epithelial ingrowth

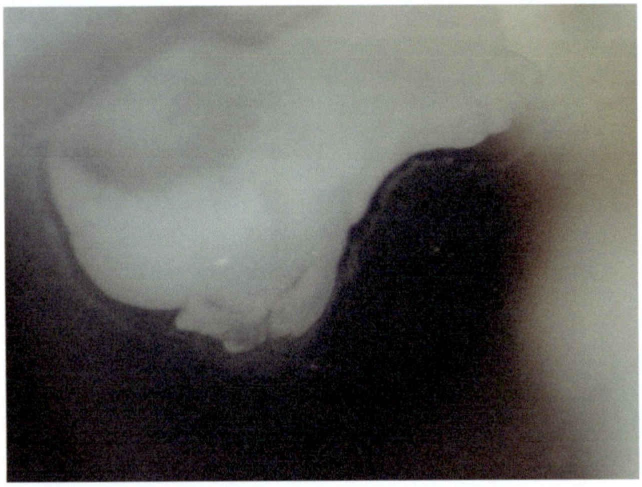

Fig. 7.31 A grade 2 epithelial ingrowth with a central white area of multilayer epithelial cells surrounded by a thin transparent monolayer of cells indicating an active progression

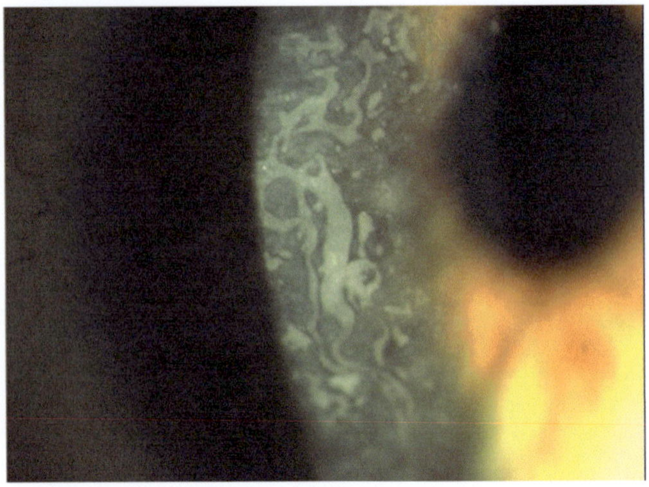

Fig. 7.32 A extensive geographic area of grade 3 epithelial ingrowth

Take-Home Message

- Epithelial ingrowth is most commonly encountered following LASIK enhancement procedures.
- Early post-operative follow-up and close observation is necessary to identify and treat epithelial ingrowth.
- Fluorescein staining must be performed to identify fistulous tract.
- Most of the grade 1 to grade 2 epithelial ingrowth will resolve spontaneously.
- Abnormal flap border (gap, rolled, melted...) should be managed surgically to stop epithelial ingrowth progression.
- Flap melting may be more extensive than recognized at the slit lamp.
- During enhancement surgery, epithelial scraping with weck-cel or a blade at the border of the flap followed by BCL application may prevent epithelial ingrowth.
- Flap suturing should be considered in case of flap melting or recurrence of ingrowth.
- The disruption of the epithelial tract using Nd:YAG laser is an effective method to avoid flap lift. The laser creates a local inflammation, resulting in the formation of a scar and a denser attachment between the flap and the stroma. More than one treatment may be necessary to achieve complete resolution.

References

1. Wang MY, Maloney RK. Epithelial ingrowth after laser in situ keratomileusis. Am J Ophthalmol. 2000;129(6):746–51.
2. Kamburoğlu G, Ertan A. Epithelial ingrowth after femtosecond laser-assisted in situ keratomileusis. Cornea. 2008;27:1122–5.
3. Ting DS, Srinivasan S, Danjoux J-P. Epithelial ingrowth following laser in situ keratomileusis (LASIK): Prevalence, risk factors, management and visual outcomes. BMJ Open Ophthalmol. 2018;3(1):e000133.
4. Danjo S, Friend J, Thoft RA. Conjuctival epithelium in healing of corneal epithelial wounds. Invest Ophthalmol Vis Sci. 1987;28:1445–9.
5. Helena MC, Meisler D, Wilson SE. Epithelial growth within the lamellar interface after in situ keratomileusis (LASIK). Cornea. 1997;16(3):300–5.
6. Stulting RD, Carr JD, Thompson KP, et al. Complications of laser in situ keratomileusis for the correction of myopia. Ophthalmology. 1999;106:13–20.
7. Carr JD, Nardone R Jr, Sulting RD, et al. Risk factors for epithelial ingrowth after LASIK. Invest Ophthalmol Vis Sci. 1997;38(4):S232.
8. Rowsey J. Suture laser-assisted in situ keratomileusis flaps after epithelial ingrowth removal. Arch Ophthalmol. 2002;120(11):1601.
9. Haw WW, Manche EE. Treatment of progressive or recurrent epithelial ingrowth with ethanol following laser in situ keratomileusis. J Refract Surg. 2001;17(1):63–8.
10. Taneri S, Koch JM, Melki SA, Azar DT. Mitomycin-C assisted photo refractive keratectomy in the treatment of buttonholed laser in situ keratomileusis flaps associated with epithelial ingrowth. J Cataract Refract Surg. 2005;31:2026–30.
11. Domniz Y, Comaish IF, Lawless MA, et al. Epithelial ingrowth: causes, prevention, and treatment in 5 cases. J Cataract Refract Surg. 2001;27(11):1803–11.
12. Ayala MJ, Alio JL, Mulet ME, et al. Treatment of laser in situ keratomileusis interface epithelial ingrowth with neodymium:yttrium-aluminum-garnet laser. Am J Ophthalmol. 2008;145:630–4.
13. Anderson NJ, Hardten DR. Fibrin glue for prevention of epithelial ingrowth after laser in situ keratomileusis. J Cataract Refract Surg. 2003;29(7):1425–9.

Corneal Haze

8

Wassef Chanbour, Samir A. Melki, and Jason Brenner

See Tables 8.1 and 8.2.

Case A: 3 weeks following an uncomplicated PRK (Fig. 8.1a).

Case B: 1 month following a PRK procedure (Fig. 8.1b).

Exam: Diffuse Grade 1 early corneal haze (Fig. 8.1).

Management: Observation is recommended as long as the patients are asymptomatic and the visual acuity is not affected.

Core message: Early Grade 1 corneal haze usually disappears within a few months without treatment.

Cases: (Fig. 8.2) Late central Grade 2 corneal haze occurring >3 months following PRK in 3 different patients (Fig. 8.2a–c).

Management: Short course of topical steroid treatment is recommended for 1–2 months.

Case: 4 months following a noncomplicated PRK, patient presented with blurry vision, UDVA: 20/40 (Fig. 8.3).

Exam: Central Grade 2 late corneal haze (Fig. 8.3a).

Management: Steroid eye drops were given. Haze decreased to Grade 1 after 1 month (Fig. 8.3b) and UDVA increased to 20/25. Patient was satisfied and did not require further treatments.

Core message: A trial of topical steroid should always be considered even in late presentations.

Case: Two patients previously diagnosed with corneal haze 5 months post-PRK procedures presented for follow up. They were previously given steroid eye drops for 1 month without improvement (Fig. 8.4).

Exam: Grade 3 central corneal haze with a circular (Fig. 8.4a) and star shape superficial scars (Fig. 8.4b).

Management: PTK + Mitomycin-C was performed. Figure 8.4c, d shows almost complete resolution of Grade 2 haze weeks following PTK.

Core message: Mitomycin-C should be always considered with PTK to decrease the recurrence rates of haze.

Case: A patient presented for follow up 3 months following a complicated PRK with a delayed epithelial healing. His corneal surface healed but the vision is still blurry (Fig. 8.5).

Exam: Grade 4 corneal haze with dense scar completely covering the pupillary axis (Fig. 8.5a).

Management: PTK with Mitomycin-C was performed, vision improved, and corneal haze decreased to Grade 1 (Fig. 8.5b).

Cases: Multiple nummular sub epithelial opacities (Fig. 8.6) occurring more than 3 months following noncomplicated PRK in patient 1 (Fig. 8.6a, b) and in patient 2 (Fig. 8.6c, d).

Management: Topical steroid eye drops can be considered if the patient is complaining of blurry vision or glare.

Case: 6 months following PRK, patient presented with blurry vision. UDVA: 20/60 (Fig. 8.7).

Exam: Grade 3 late central corneal haze (Fig. 8.7a). The opacity is located in the superficial stroma (Fig. 8.7b).

Management: Patient did not improve with steroids. PTK was then performed; haze decreased to grade 2 (Fig. 8.7c) and the opacities can be seen decreased in the superficial stoma (Fig. 8.7d).

Case: 4 months following a noncomplicated PRK a patient presented with progressive blurry vision (Fig. 8.8).

Exam: Central scar with a pseudo-dendritic pattern (Fig. 8.8a); fluorescein shows a negative staining cause by elevated stomal lesions (Fig. 8.8b).

Management: PTK was performed since the steroids were not effective. Slit lamp exam shows disappearance of the lesions (Fig. 8.8c).

Exam: Corneal scars can take different forms (Fig. 8.9). Central grade 2 corneal pinpoint corneal scar (Fig. 8.9a). Paracentral Grade 3 plaque-like corneal haze covering partially the pupil (Fig. 8.9b–d). Arcuate shape grade 3 corneal

W. Chanbour (✉)
Department of Ophthalmology and Visual Neurosciences, University of Minnesota, Minneapolis, MN, USA
e-mail: chanb013@umn.edu

S. A. Melki · J. Brenner
Boston Vision, Department of Ophthalmology, Harvard Medical School, Boston, MA, USA
e-mail: melki@bostonvision.com; brenner@bostonvision.com

S. A. Melki et al. (eds.), *Refractive Surgery Atlas*, https://doi.org/10.1007/978-3-031-60661-8_8

Table 8.1 Diagnosis and management of corneal haze following PRK

Onset	• Early: 1 week or less than 3 months postoperative [1] • Late: more than 3 months postoperative [2] • Greatest intensity between 3 and 6 months postoperative
Rate	In low myopia: 1.4% had trace haze in the Mitomycin treated group versus 11.8% without Mitomycin at 6 months postoperatively [3] In high myopia: 7.5% had stage 1 haze with Mitomycin, while 12.9% had a stage 1 haze, and 11.3% stage 2 haze [4]
Patho-physiology	• Early haze: activation of keratocytes to corneal fibroblasts [3] • Late haze: increased corneal myofibroblasts formation [3] • Deposition of collagen fibers [5] • Decreased corneal crystallin production (less common) [5]
Symptoms	Low contrast, glare, and decreased visual acuity
Monitoring	**Subjective**: Slit lamp **Objective:** Opacity lensometer, OCT, Scheimpflug anterior eye segment analysis, confocal microscopy, forward-scattered light
Risk factors	**Preoperative**: high myopia, hyperopia, or astigmatism [6], age, male sex, and UV-B exposure [2] **Perioperative**: epithelial defects, use of alcohol>transepithelial [7]
Prevention	• Preoperative control of periocular inflammation and dryness with Cyclosporine • Intraoperative use of pharmacological agents (e.g., Mitomycin-C) to minimize myofibroblast activation • Oral Ascorbate (Vitamin C) [8] • Usage of steroidal drops to reduce risk of short-term corneal haze [9] • Usage of UV-protective eyewear, since UV-B radiation can prolong stromal healing response [10]
Indication for observation	Asymptomatic Grade 1 to Grade 2 corneal haze that is non-progressive
Indications for treatment	• Invading the visual axis • Inducing refractive error or irregular astigmatism • Elevated scar, causing foreign body sensation • Obscuring details of iris or intraocular structures
Medical treatment	• Topical corticosteroid eye drops for 1-3 months • Treatment is less effective in late corneal haze
Surgical treatment	• Indication: Failed steroid treatment • Techniques – Scraping or burr – Manual superficial keratectomy – Phototherapeutic keratectomy – Mitomycin-C 0.02% should be used following the scar removal

Table 8.2 Grades of corneal haze following PRK

Grade	Corneal haze grading scale [11]	Treatment
Grade 0	No haze, completely clear cornea	None
Grade 0.5[a]	Trace of faint haze seen only by indirect, broad tangential illumination	Observation
Grade 1	Haze of minimal density seen with difficulty with direct or diffuse examination	Mostly observation; topical steroids if patient is symptomatic
Grade 2	Mild haze easily visible with direct focal slit lamp illumination	Non-urgent treatment starting with topical steroid followed by surgical treatment if there is no improvement
Grade 3	Moderate opacity that partially obscure the details of iris	Urgent treatment required with close follow-up; usage of mechanical debridement or PTK if no improvement with steroid
Grade 4	Severe opacity that completely obscures the details of intraocular structures	Urgent treatment required with close follow-up; anterior lamellar keratoplasty may be required if no improvement with superficial keratectomy or PTK

[a]G 0.5 is considered clear

haze; these occur usually following hyperopic treatments (Fig. 8.9e, f).

Management: A trial of topical steroid is the first line of therapy, PTK would be considered in case of no improvement in a symptomatic patient.

Core Message: Corneal haze and scarring following PRK can have different shapes but the management is the same.

Case: 23-year-old patient presenting 1 month following a PRK procedure. Patient had stopped steroid eye drops at 2 weeks post operatively (Fig. 8.10).

Exam: Grade 2 sub-epithelial scar was noted on slit lamp exam (Fig. 8.10a); Ant. segment OCT showing hyper-reflective sub-epithelial/superficial stromal haze (Fig. 8.10b).

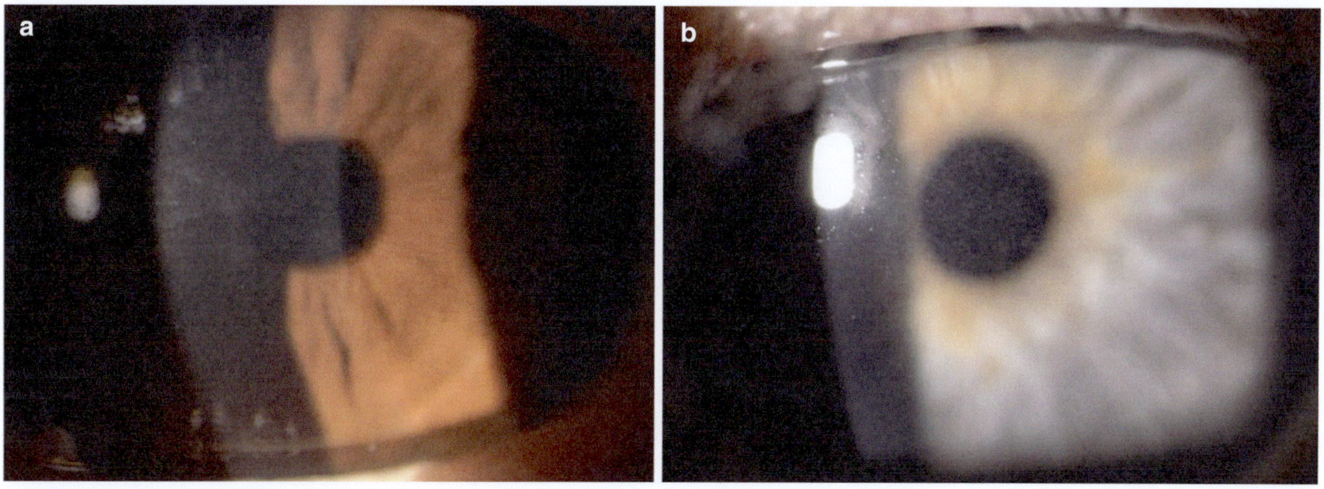

Fig. 8.1 Early Grade 1 corneal haze

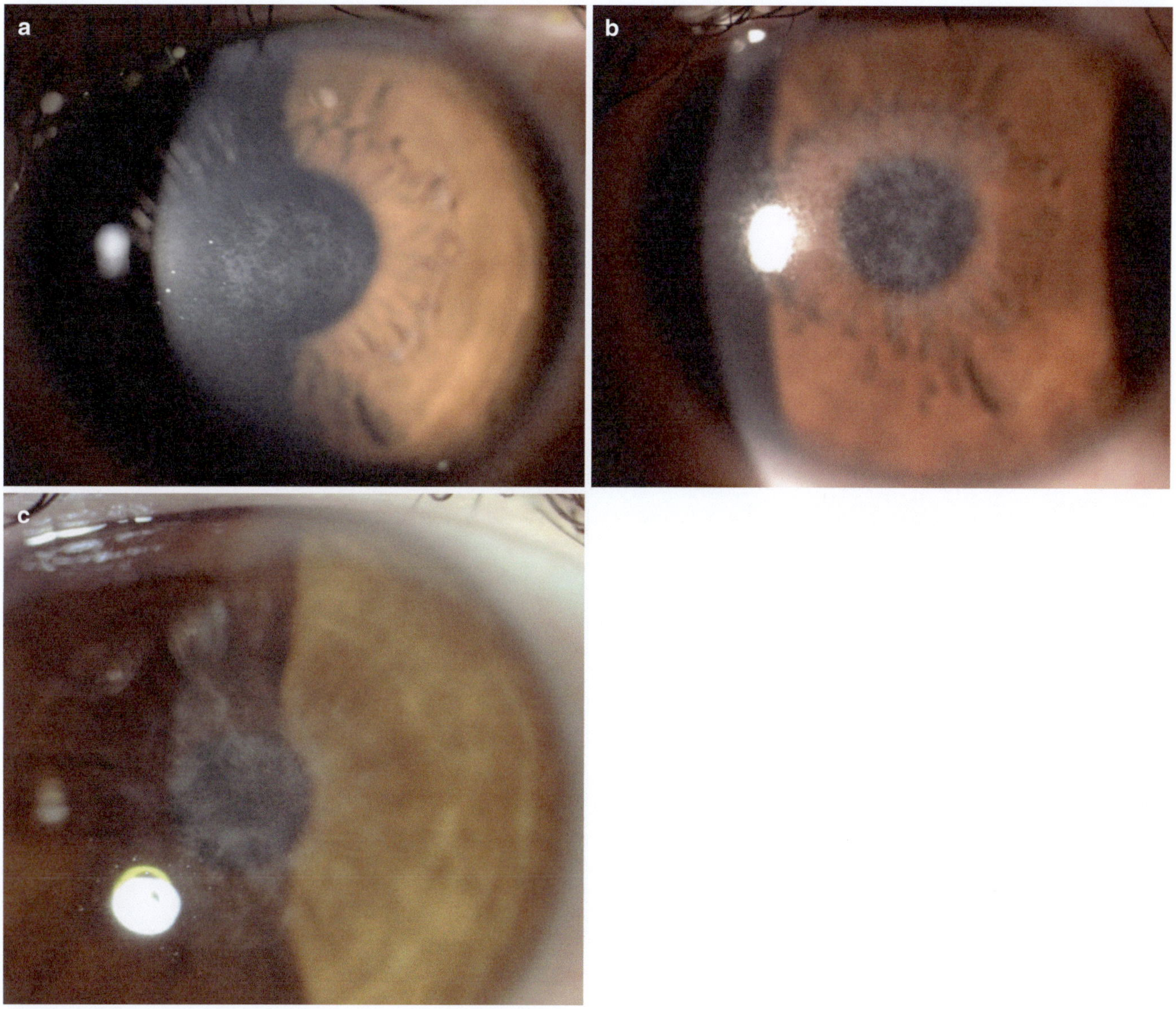

Fig. 8.2 Grade 2 corneal haze

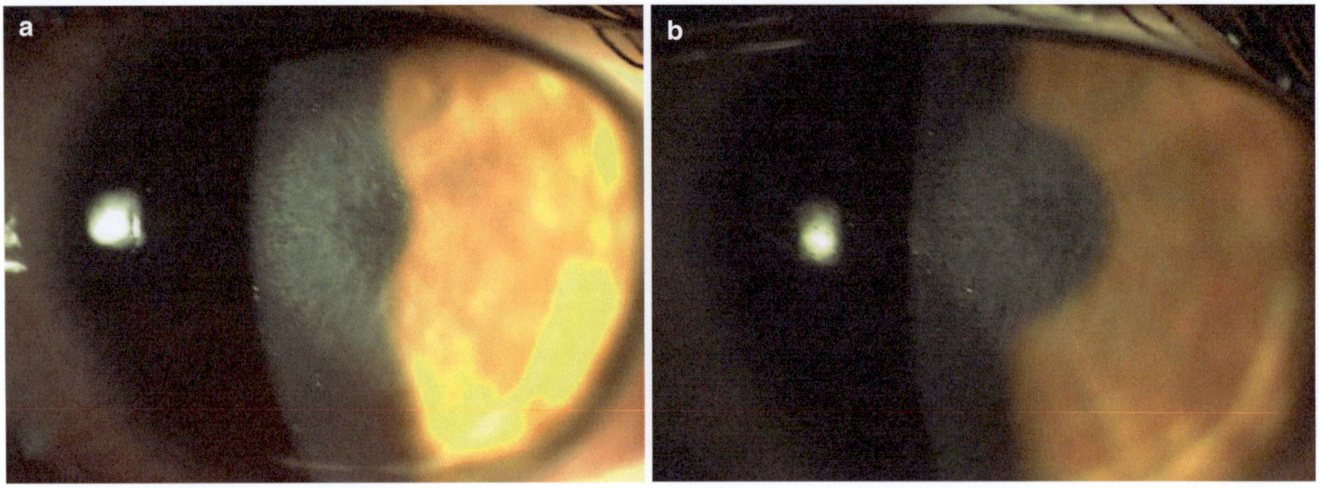

Fig. 8.3 Partial resolution

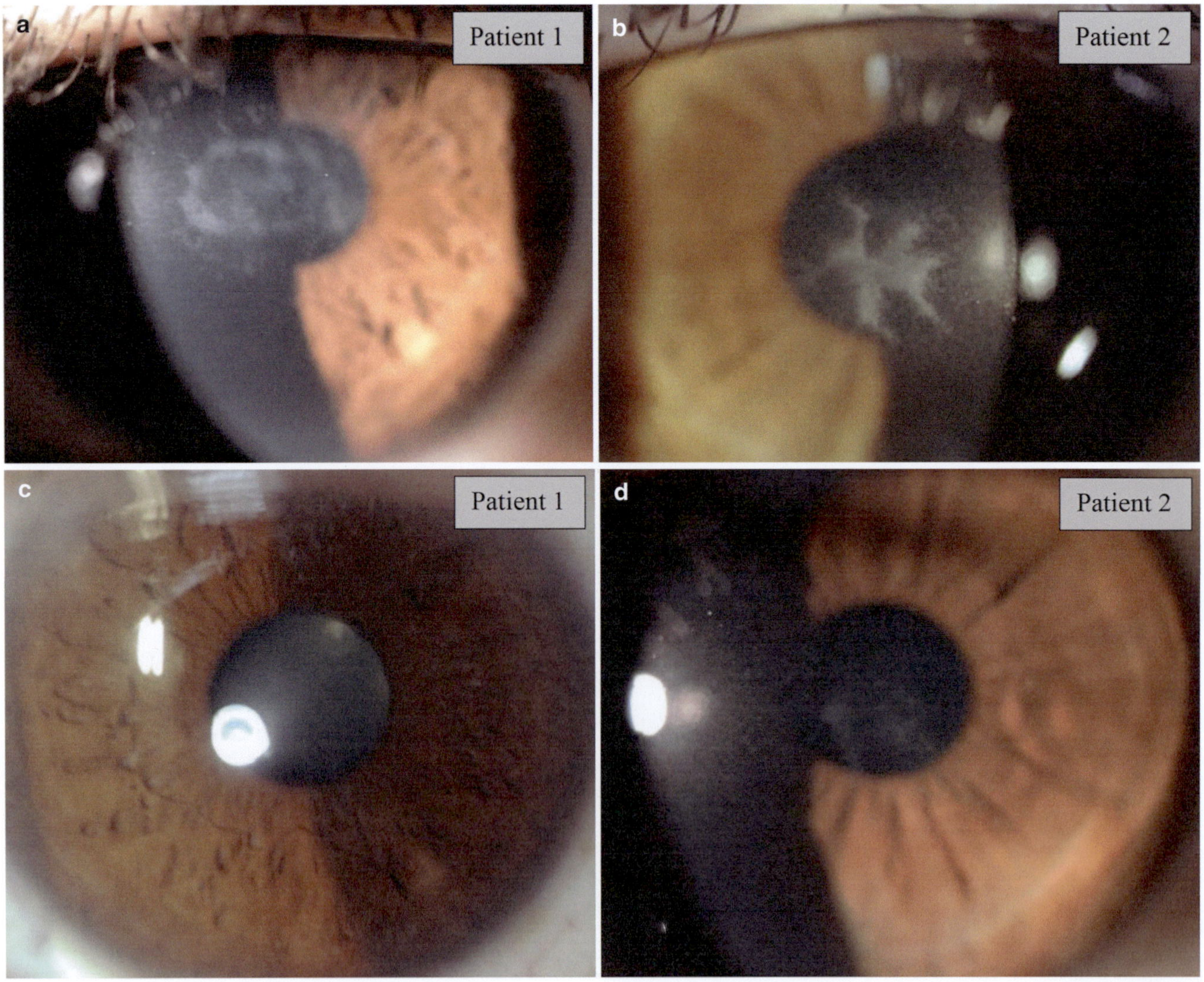

Fig. 8.4 Central dense opacities

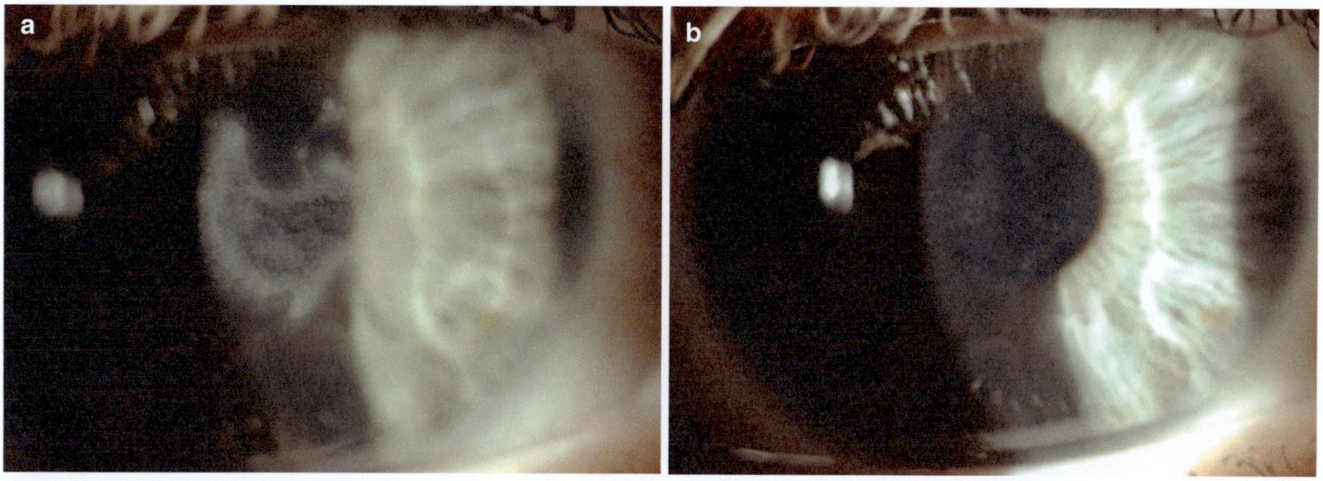

Fig. 8.5 Grade 4 haze

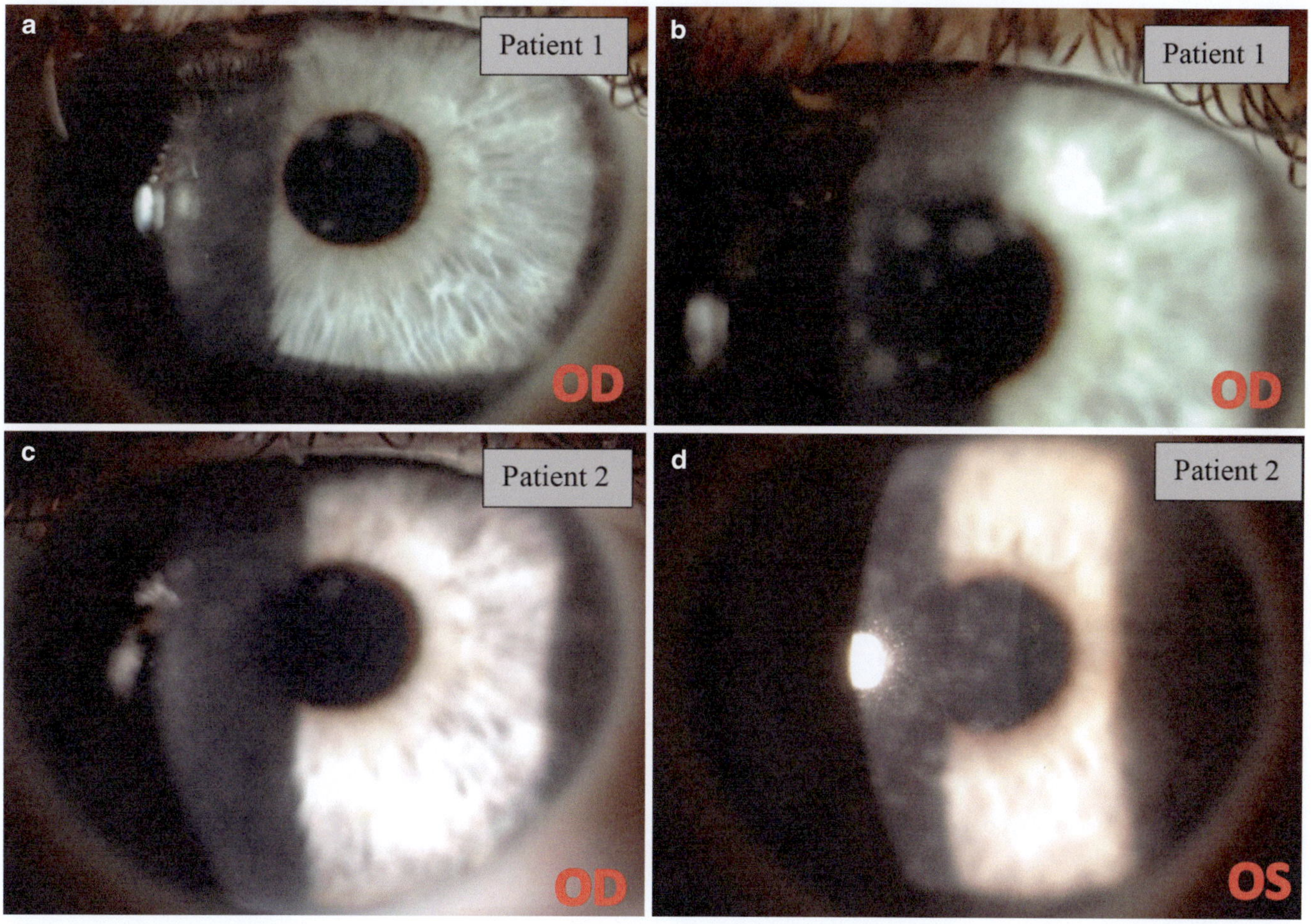

Fig. 8.6 Nummular lesions

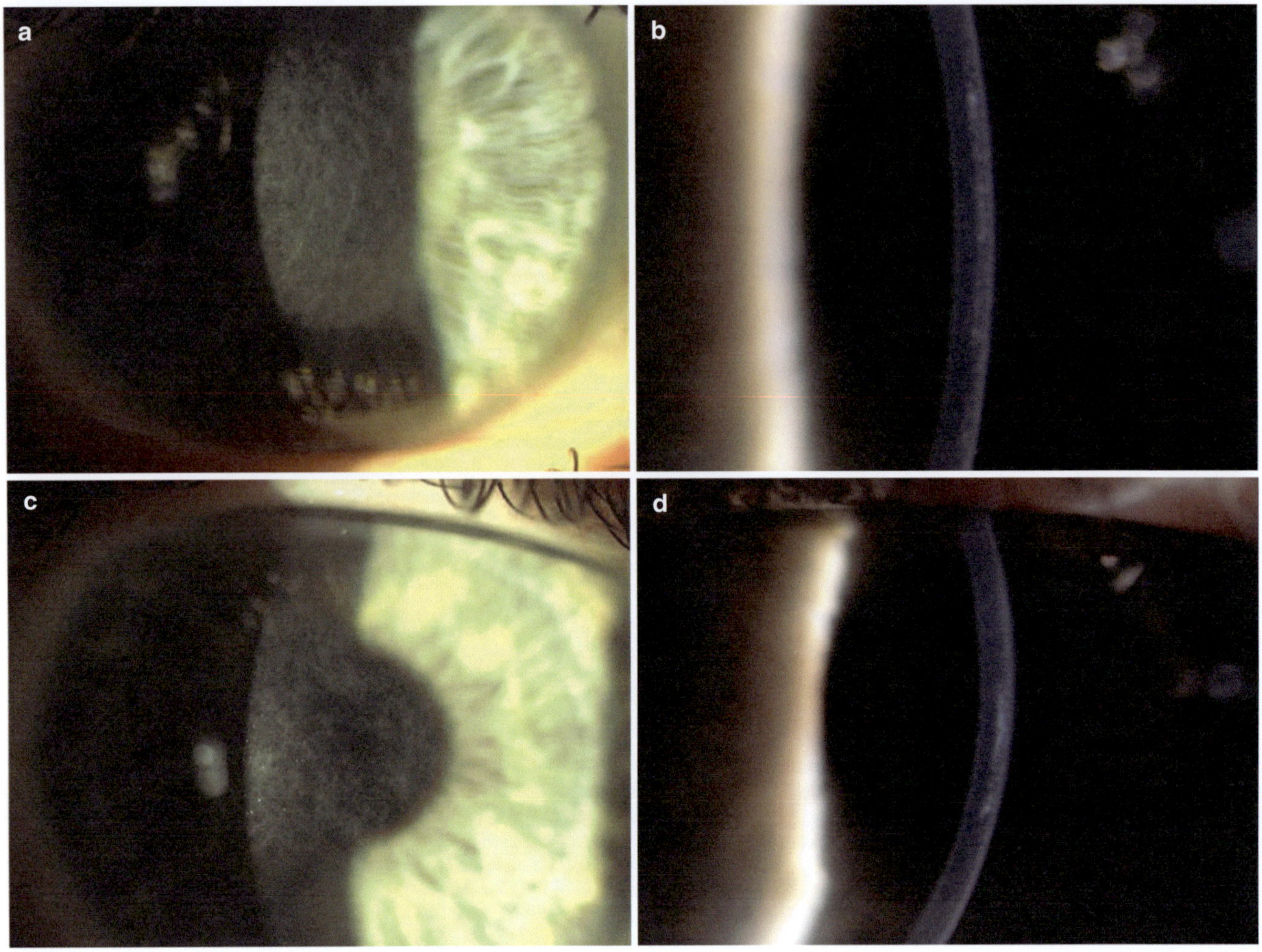

Fig. 8.7 Depth of the scars

Management: Steroid eye drops were restarted and haze resolved over 1 month.

Extra Illustrations

See Figs. 8.11, 8.12, 8.13 and 8.14.

Take-Home Message

- Early haze is usually benign and responds well to topical steroids.
- Pre- and postoperative vitamin C decreases the risk of haze.
- Intraoperative mitomycin-C should be used following PRK, especially with high treatments and redo surgeries.
- Delayed epithelial healing should be managed promptly to avoid long term corneal damage.
- Topical steroid should be tapered slowly over 1 month following PRK procedure.
- Topical steroid should be restarted for Grade 2 haze and above.

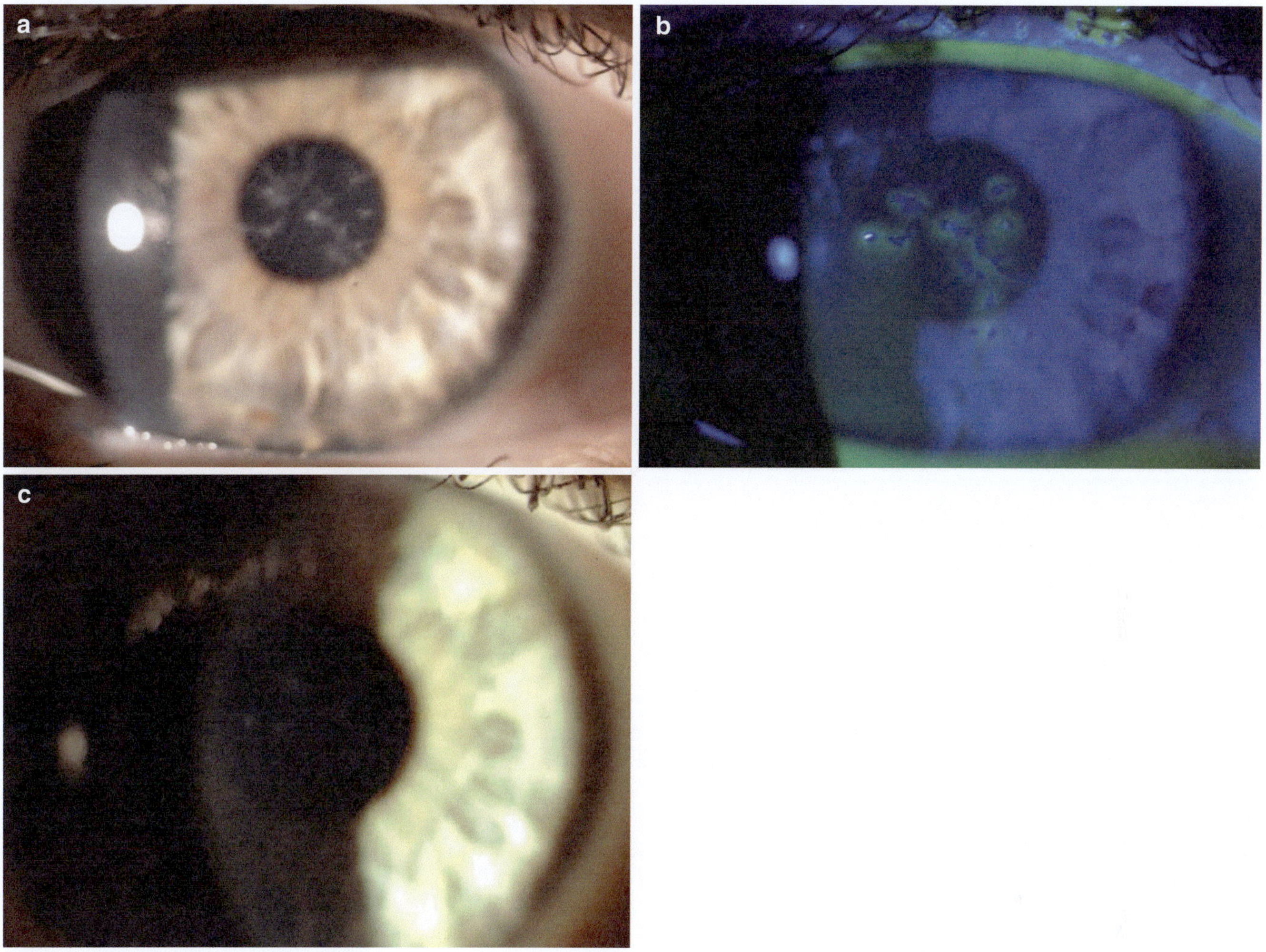

Fig. 8.8 Nodular scar

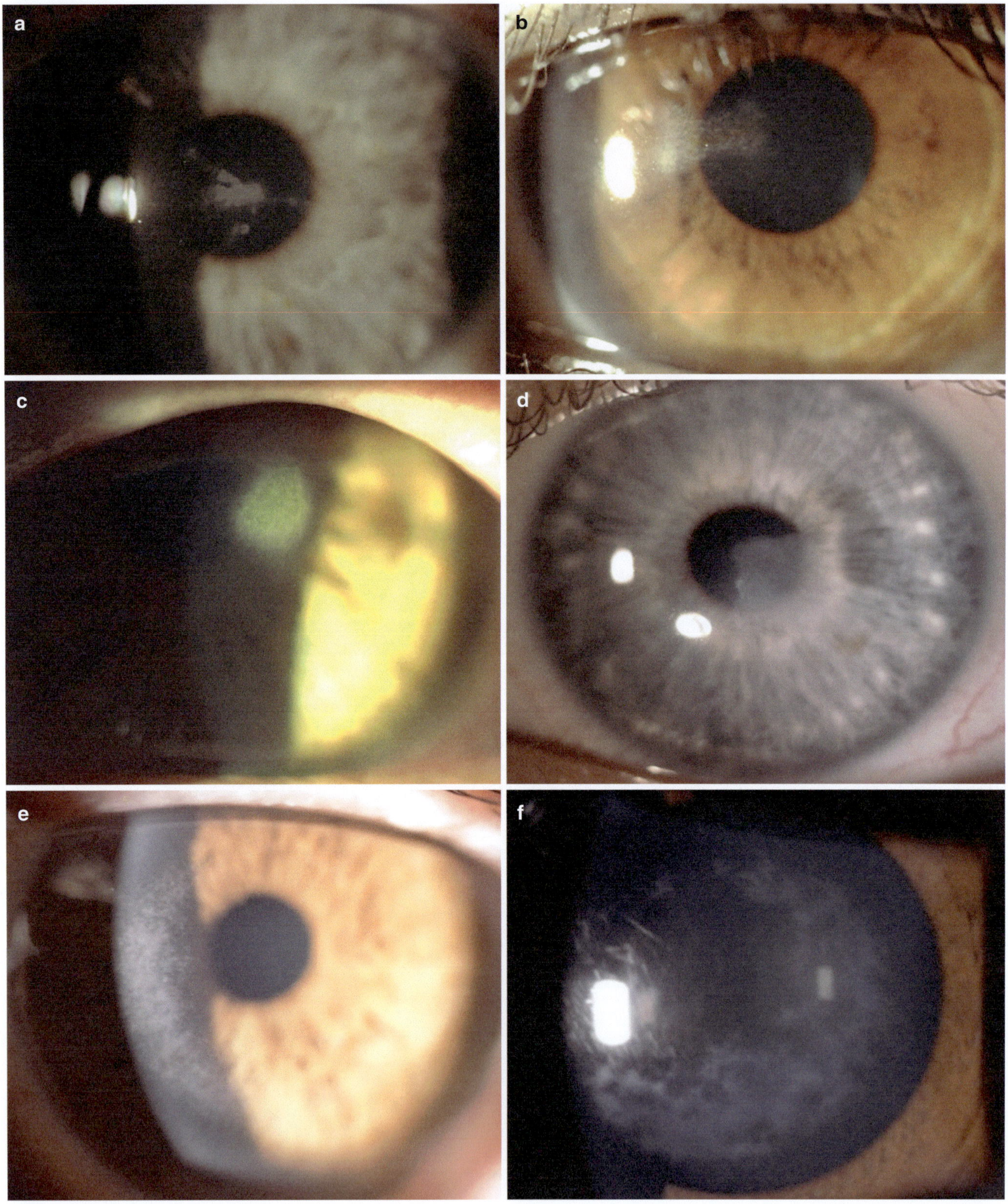

Fig. 8.9 Different shapes of corneal scarring

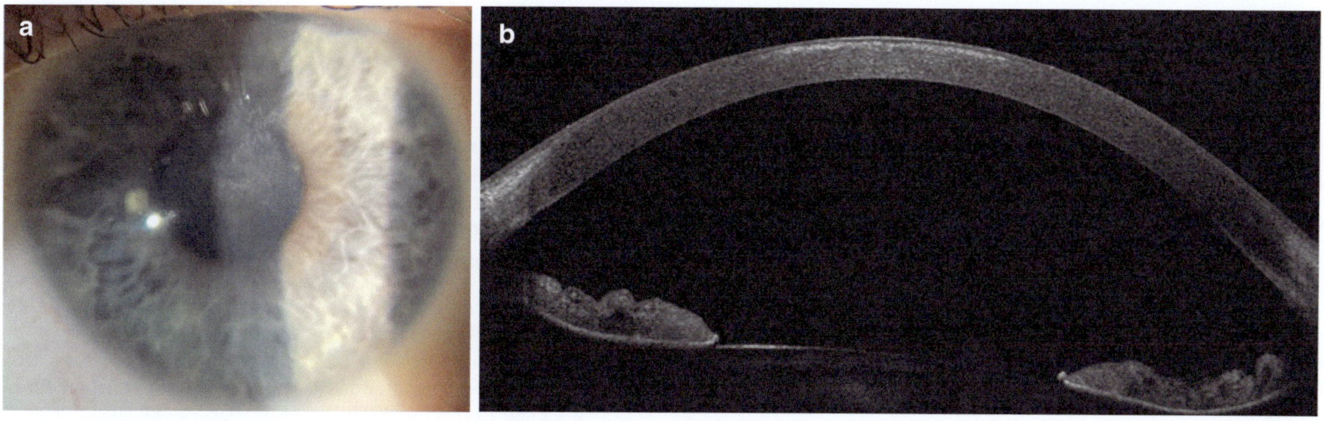

Fig. 8.10 Importance of steroid. (*Courtesy Willem-Martin Gerber, MD*)

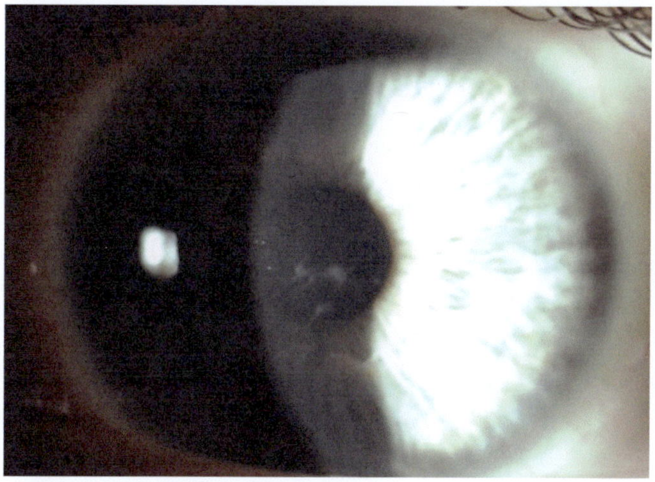

Fig. 8.11 Fine central corneal spicules

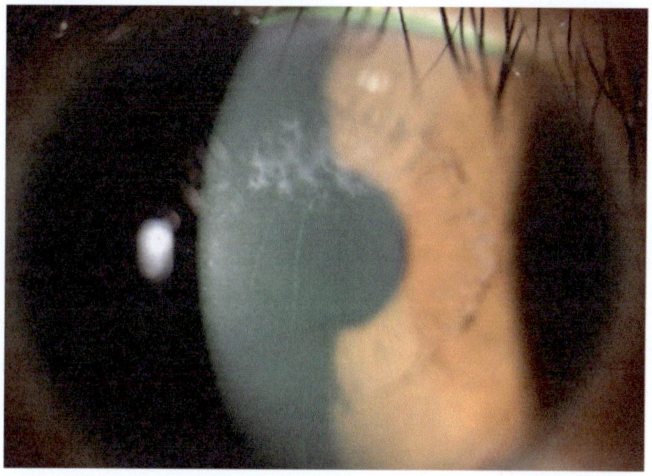

Fig. 8.13 Scarring superior to the visual axis

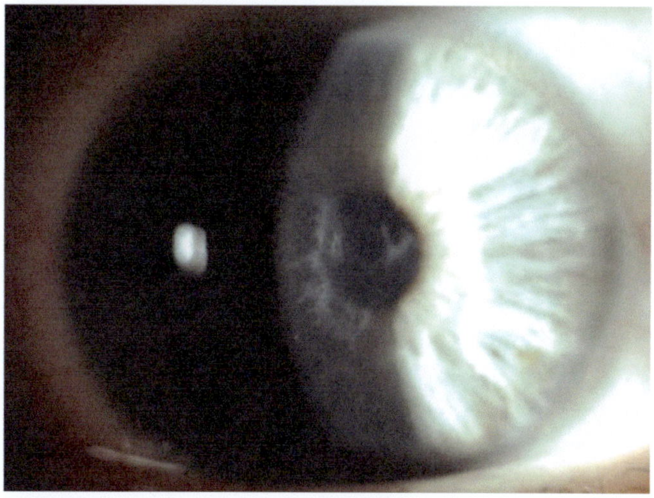

Fig. 8.12 Large specular scar at the pupillary border

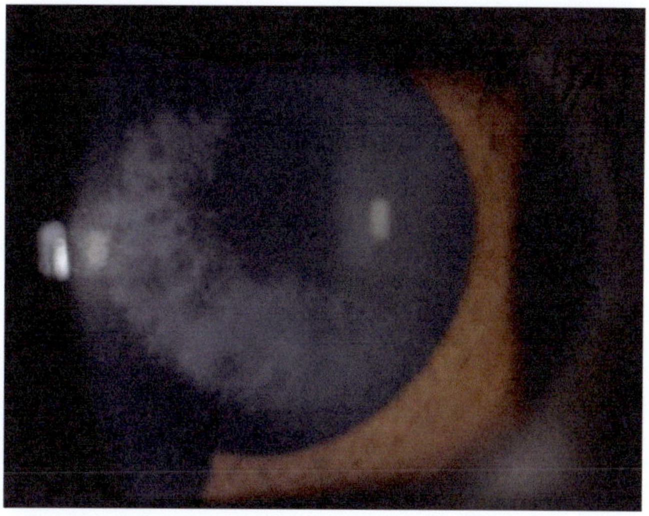

Fig. 8.14 Arcuate shape grade 3 corneal haze

Acknowledgments We would like to thank PhiYen Yasmin Nguyen M.P.P who provided extensive research assistance and helped to draft sections of the chapter.

References

1. Lipshitz I, Loewenstein A, Varssano D, Lazar M. Late onset corneal haze after photorefractive keratectomy for moderate and high myopia. Ophthalmology. 1997;104(3):369–74. https://doi.org/10.1016/s0161-6420(97)30306-6.
2. Murueta-Goyena A, Cañadas P. Visual outcomes and management after corneal refractive surgery: a review. J Optom. 2018;11(2):121–9.
3. Shojaei A, et al. Short-time mitomycin-C application during photorefractive keratectomy in patients with low myopia. J Cataract Refract Surg. 2013;39(2):197–203.
4. Bedei A, Marabotti A, Giannecchini I, Ferretti C, Montagnani M, Martinucci C, Barabesi L. Photorefractive keratectomy in high myopic defects with or without intraoperative mitomycin C: 1-year results. Eur J Ophthalmol. 2006;16(2):229–34.
5. Wilson S. Corneal myofibroblast biology and pathobiology: generation, persistence, and transparency. Exp Eye Res. 2012;99:78–88.
6. Vigo L, Scandola E, Carones F. Scraping and Mitomycin C to treat haze and regression after photorefractive keratectomy for myopia. J Refract Surg. 2003;19(4):449–54. https://doi.org/10.3928/1081-597x-20030701-12.
7. Gabler B, Winkler von Mohrenfels C, Dreiss AK, et al. Vitality of epithelial cells after alcohol exposure during laser-assisted subepithelial keratectomy flap preparation. J Cataract Refract Surg. 2002;28:1841–6.
8. Stojanovic A, Ringvold A, Nitter T. Ascorbate prophylaxis for corneal haze after photorefractive keratectomy. J Refract Surg. 2003;19(3):338–43.
9. Nien C, Flynn K, Chang M, Brown D, Jester J. Reducing peak corneal haze after photorefractive keratectomy in rabbits: prednisolone acetate 1.00% versus cyclosporine a 0.05%. J Cataract Refract Surg. 2011;37(5):937–44.
10. Tomás-Juan J, Murueta-Goyena Larrañaga A, Hanneken L. Corneal regeneration after photorefractive keratectomy: a review. J Optom. 2015;8(3):149–69.
11. Fantes F. Wound healing after excimer laser Keratomileusis (photorefractive keratectomy) in monkeys. Arch Ophthalmol. 1990;108(5):665.

Infectious Keratitis

9

Samir A. Melki, Jason Brenner, and Wassef Chanbour

See Tables 9.1 and 9.2.

Case: 30-year-old patient presenting one week following PRK surgery. He was reported to be non-compliant with the postoperative eye drop regiment (Fig. 9.1).

Exam: Large central corneal bacterial ulcer with a ring shape infiltrate (Fig. 9.1a).

Management: Culture was taken and results showed Group B strep; topical fortified antibiotics were given and followed with topical steroids. Ulcer healed within 2 months leaving a central corneal haze (Fig. 9.1b–d).

Core message: Postoperative topical antibiotics is a must after PRK until complete epithelial healing.

Case: 4 days following a PRK procedure, a patient presented with blurry vision, pain, and red eyes (Fig. 9.2).

Exam: Large ring shape infiltrates with central stromal infiltrate in addition to a hypopyon.

Management: Culture showed pseudomonas bacteria; topical fortified antibiotics were given followed by topical steroid a few days later.

Case: A patient presenting 4 weeks following a non-complicated PRK, reporting pain and blurry vision for a few days (Fig. 9.3).

Exam: Large central epithelial defect with underlying hazy cornea. The edge of the defect is smooth and corneal sensitivity is diminished (Fig. 9.3a, b).

Management: Herpes simplex keratitis is first on the differential, and oral or topical antivirals are recommended.

Case: Patient presented 4 months following a PRK procedure complicated with severe dryness and recurrent erosions in the morning when he wakes up (Fig. 9.4).

S. A. Melki (✉) · J. Brenner
Boston Vision, Department of Ophthalmology, Harvard Medical School, Boston, MA, USA
e-mail: melki@bostonvision.com; brenner@bostonvision.com

W. Chanbour
Department of Ophthalmology and Visual Neurosciences, University of Minnesota, Minneapolis, MN, USA
e-mail: chanb013@umn.edu

Exam: Para-central corneal infiltrate of 1mm with surrounding edematous cornea (Fig. 9.4a, b).

Management: Cultures were positive for staphylococci and fortified antibiotics were started.

Core message: Dryness and recurrent erosion should always be well managed, and antibiotics should be started early.

Case: One week following a non-complicated PRK, a patient presented with a non-healing epithelial defect following the removal of contact lens (Fig. 9.5).

Exam: Central dendritic lesion with terminal bulbs (Fig. 9.5a, b).

Management: Topical or oral antiviral should be started and topical steroids to be tapered.

Core message: Dendrites should be differentiated from pseudo-dendrites; the latter can occur with late epithelial healing following PRK and does not have terminal light bulb shape on fluorescein staining. Also, as recent PRK procedure impairs corneal sensitivity, this test is not specific for Herpetic keratitis.

Case: Patient presented 4 days following LASIK with blurry vision (Fig. 9.6).

Exam: Whitish large paracentral infiltrate with surrounding edema and no epithelial defect.

Management: Flap lift, irrigation, and cultures were performed. Cultures came back negative, and patient improved when topical steroids were added.

Core message: Grade 3 DLK may be mistaken for an infectious keratitis; flap lift and cultures are indicated when the diagnosis is not clear.

Case: 37-year-old female patient had an uneventful PRK. Postoperatively she had a delayed epithelial healing. The patient went daily to different hospitals for pain management. She presented to clinic 3 weeks later with bilateral corneal infiltrates consistent with bilateral Pseudomonas keratitis (Fig. 9.7).

Exam: Residual epithelial defect staining with fluorescein following PRK (Fig. 9.7a). Patient developed later

S. A. Melki et al. (eds.), *Refractive Surgery Atlas*, https://doi.org/10.1007/978-3-031-60661-8_9

Table 9.1 Characteristics risk factors and management of infection keratitis following refractive surgery

Onset	Early onset <1 week Late onset >1 week [1]
Rate	0.02%–0.8% after PRK [2] 0%–1.5% in LASIK [2]
Pathology	Early onset: Staphylococci, Streptococci, Herpes Late onset: Atypical mycobacteria, nocardia, acanthamoeba, and fungi
Risk factors	Dry eyes, blepharitis, Meibomian gland dysfunction (MGD), history of previous healed keratitis, and previous corneal surgeries
Clinical features	PRK: Bacterial infections present as single dense white infiltrates or multiple patchy infiltrates LASIK: Interface infiltrates, flap margin infiltrates, surface ulceration [2]
Sample collection	PRK: easily accessible for sampling; blade or spatula can be used to scrape the lesions LASIK: Flap lifting, scraping [3]
Stain and culture media	• Gram's stain, Ziegl Neelsen, KOH mount • Blood agar, Chocolate agar, Lowensteing-Jensen, Sabouraud • Viral PCR
Antibiotics	• Bacterial: Fortified preparation of drugs, such as vancomycin, cefazolin, tobramycin, and ceftazidime • Viral: topical acyclovir/ganciclovir or oral acyclovir/valacyclovir • Fungal: natamycin, voriconazole, amphotericin B
Flap management	• Depending on the severity of the flap melting, flap can be left in place, lifted and irrigated with antibiotics, or amputated as a last resort
Prevention	• Betadine 10% preparation and cleaning around eyelids, periocular region, and eye lashes • Clean blades and instruments should be used for each eye • Postoperative antibiotic eye drops
Outcomes	50%–75% resolution with a best corrected visual acuity >20/40 [2, 4]

Table 9.2 Measures to reduce infectious keratitis

Stage	Risk factor	Management/prevention
Before surgery	Dry eyes	Artificial tears +/− Cyclosporine
	Blepharitis	Warm compress +/− Antibiotic ointment +/− Doxycycline
During surgery	Surgical trauma	• Careful flap lift to avoid epithelial injury • Avoid high energy ablations
	Sterility	• 10% Povidone iodine scrub • Disposable gloves/surgical drape • Autoclave quality check every 3 months • Use different set of instruments for each eye
After surgery	Epithelial defects	• Bandage contact lens • Topical 4th generation fluoroquinolones • Decrease corticosteroids
	Poor follow up	• Regular follow up for the first 3 months • Thorough exam • Eye drops review

corneal ring infiltrate in the right eye (Fig. 9.7b) and a hypopyon with central infiltrate in the left eye (Fig. 9.7c).

Management: Fortified antibiotics were given as soon as the infiltrates were noticed, and patient healed completely in the right eye (Fig. 9.7d) but had residual scarring, limiting her vision to 20/200 in the left eye (Fig. 9.7e).

Core message: Patients who develop delayed epithelial healing following PRK should be followed closely and treated aggressively until complete healing.

Case: A 37-year-old woman developed severe suppurative keratitis immediately after having a PRK in her left eye. The patient reported exposure, swimming in freshwater that might have been contaminated (Fig. 9.8).

Exam: Stromal ring infiltrate noted on slit lamp exam (Fig. 9.8a); subsequent histopathologic examination showed double-walled cyst structure of Acanthamoeba (Fig. 9.8b).

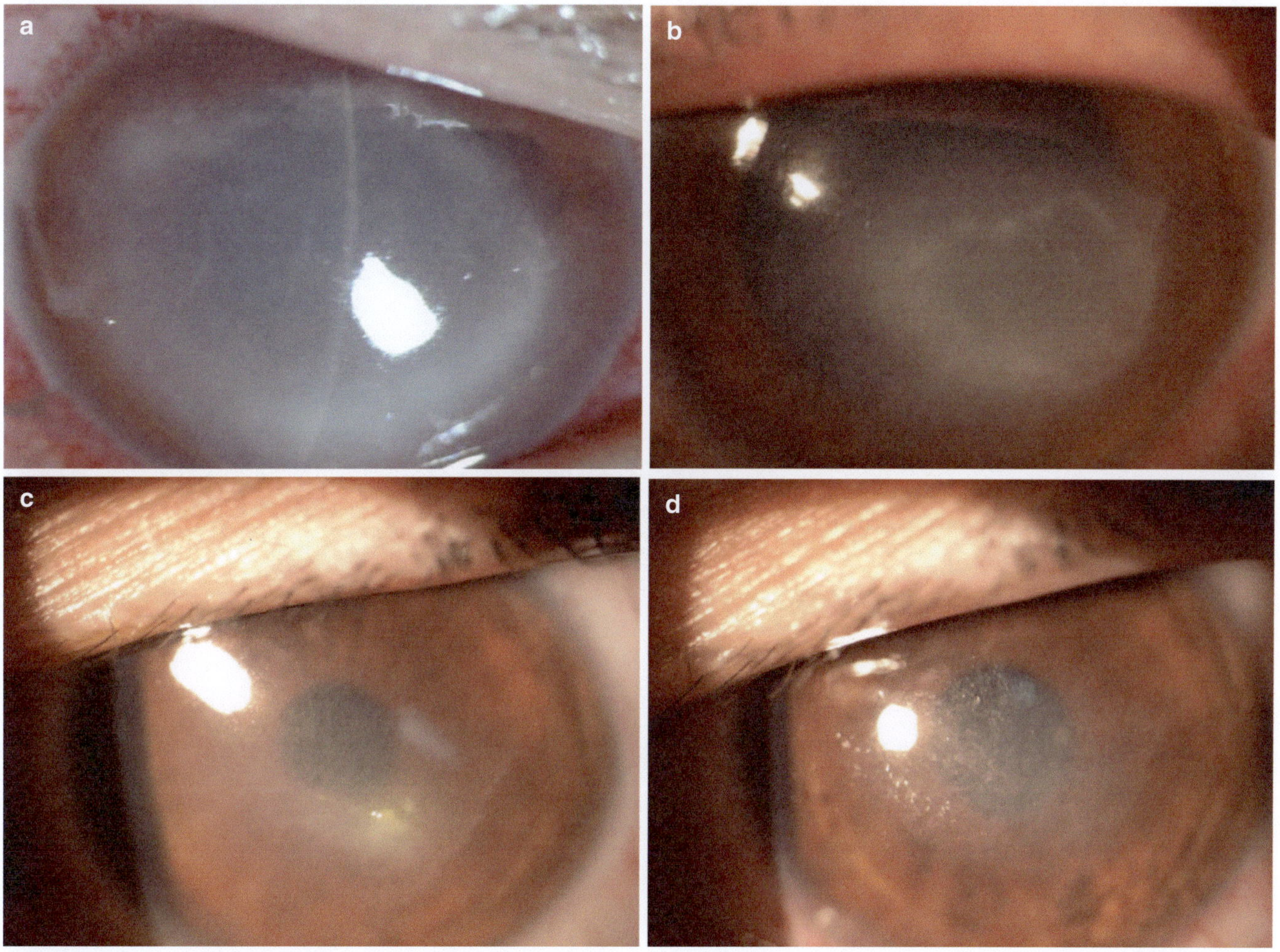

Fig. 9.1 Bacterial ulcer. (**a**) Large ring-shaped infiltrate, (**b–d**) progressively healing throughout 2 months with central haze

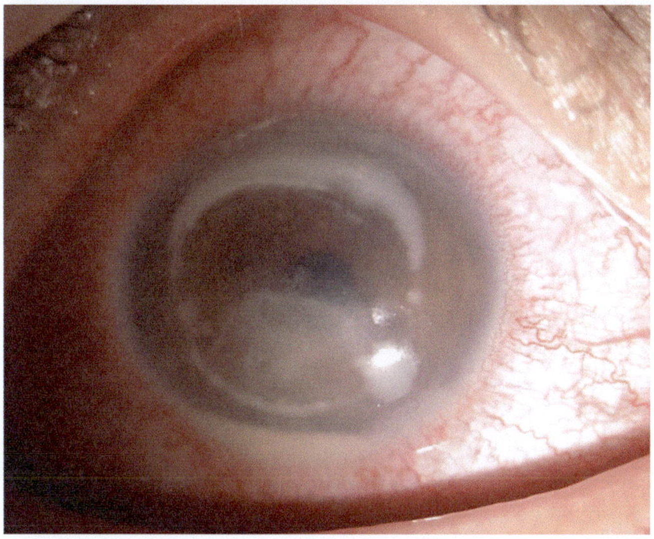

Fig. 9.2 Ring infiltrate

Management: Intensive chlorhexidine (0.02%) drop treatment was started and led to complete recovery from the infectious keratitis.

Core Message: All patients should avoid water exposure until complete healing from refractive surgery.

Case: 12 days following PRK, a patient presented to the ED with increasing pain and blurry vision. Bandage contact lens was removed at postoperative day 5 and patient continued using ofloxacin and loteprednol eye drops (Fig. 9.9).

Exam: Central corneal ulcer with clear infiltrates (Fig. 9.9a); epithelial defect noted on fluorescein staining (Fig. 9.9b). Cultures showed only a few staph and strep species, unclear if contaminant.

Management: Intensive fortified vancomycin and tobramycin eye drops were given and patient improved.

Core Message: Infectious keratitis can occur while using antibiotic eye drops, as new resistant species are arising.

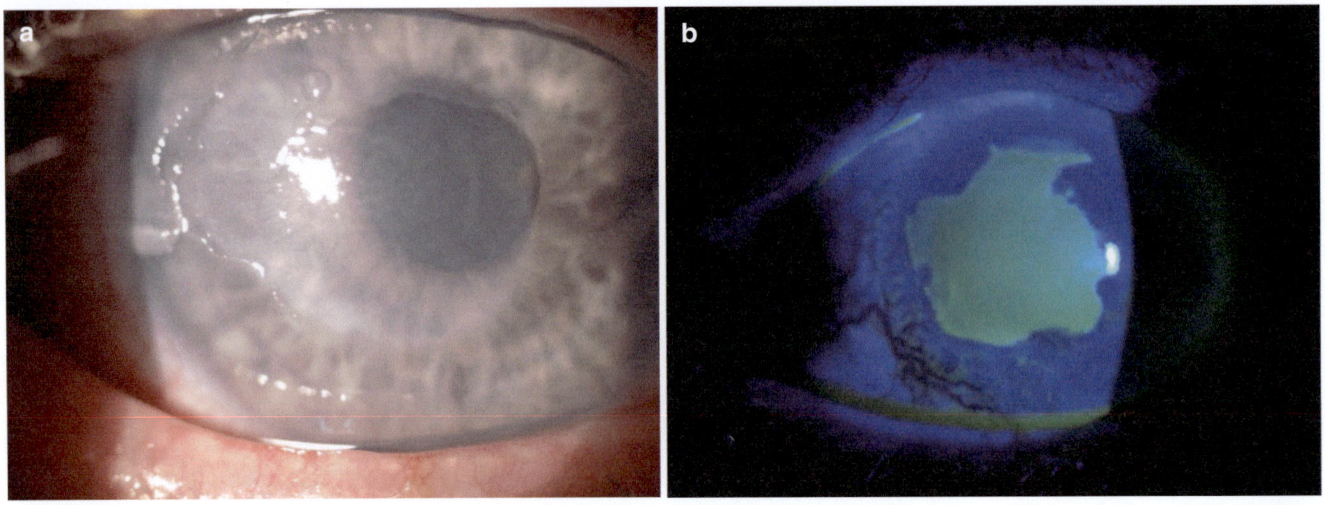

Fig. 9.3 Geographic ulcer without (**a**) and with (**b**) fluorescein stain

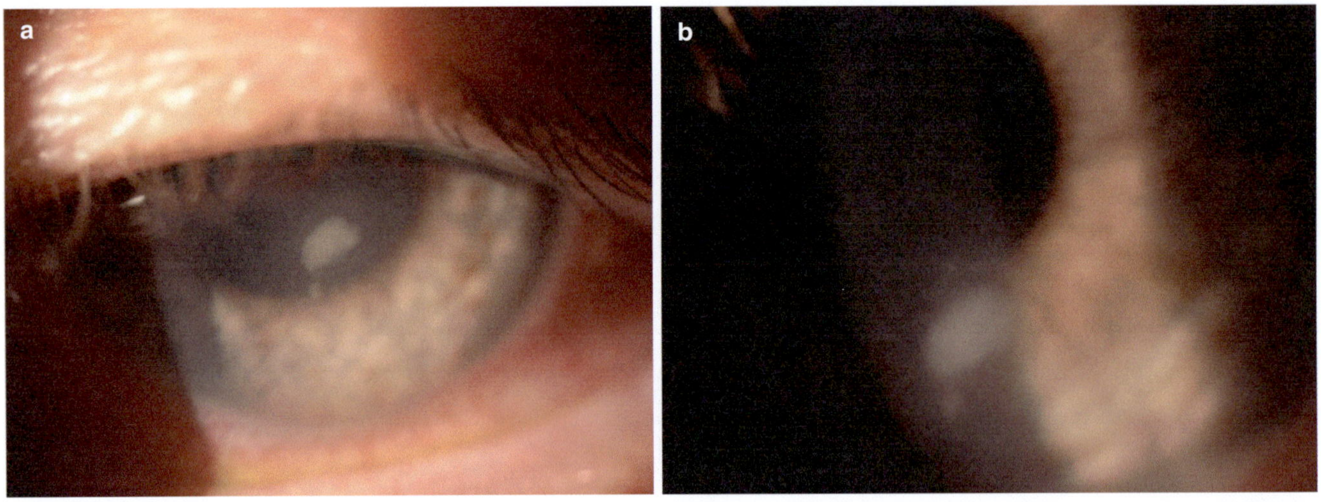

Fig. 9.4 Late infection. (**a**) Paracentral infiltrate, (**b**) enlarged

Case: Patient presented to clinic for recurrent ocular pain, redness, and blurry vision years following a LASIK surgery (Fig. 9.10).

Exam: Central corneal epithelial defect with whitish infiltration at the edge of a large vascular bundle extending from the limbus

Management: Patient started on HSV treatment and topical steroid drops were added later. Residual neovascularization persisted following treatment.

Case: A 50-year-old patient (S/p LASIK 20 years ago) had a trauma with vegetable materials causing flap dislocation. Flap was repositioned elsewhere and patient presented to clinic 10 days later with blurry vision and photophobia (Fig. 9.11).

Exam: Slit lamp exam shows a paracentral epithelial defect, a <1 mm vegetable material was noted under the flap *(red arrow),* with associated flap edema (Fig. 9.11a).

Management: Flap was lifted for culture, foreign body removal, and antibacterial and antifungal irrigation. Culture came back negative. Patient's condition worsened with hypopyon and worsening stromal infiltration despite using fortified antibacterial and antifungal eye drops (Fig. 9.11b).

Then, the flap was completely amputated; flap culture came back positive for Alternaria species. Patient's condition improved on topical voriconazole, leaving a central corneal haze 1 month later (Fig. 9.11c). Final uncorrected visual acuity was 20/50.

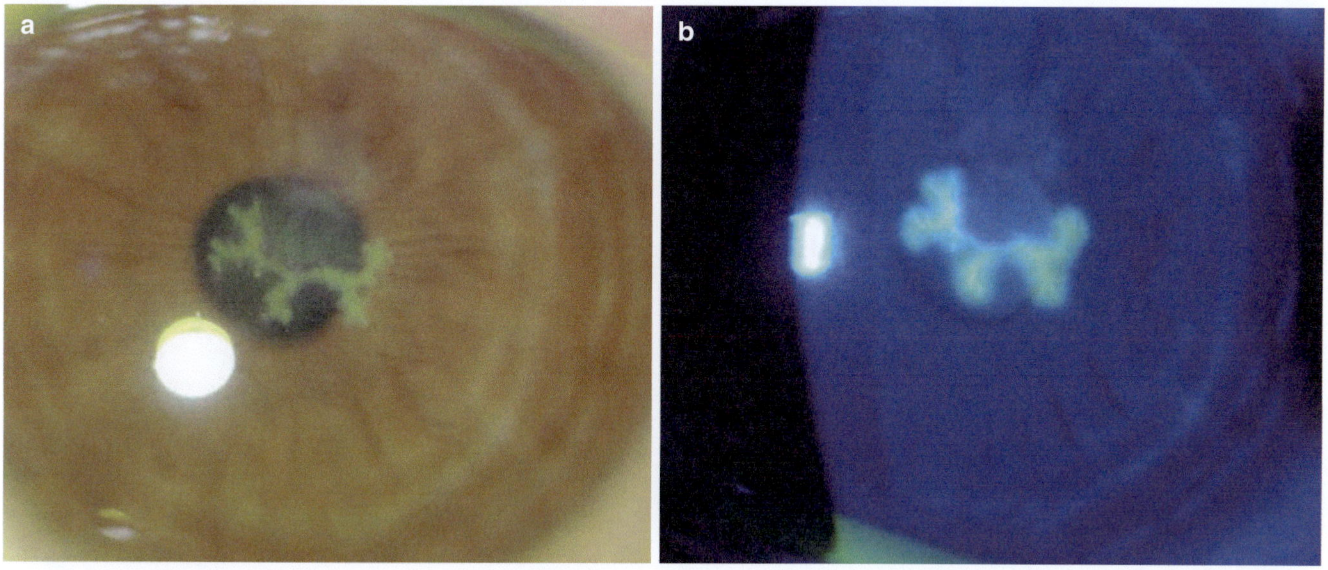

Fig. 9.5 Dendritic ulcer without (**a**) and with (**b**) fluorescein stain

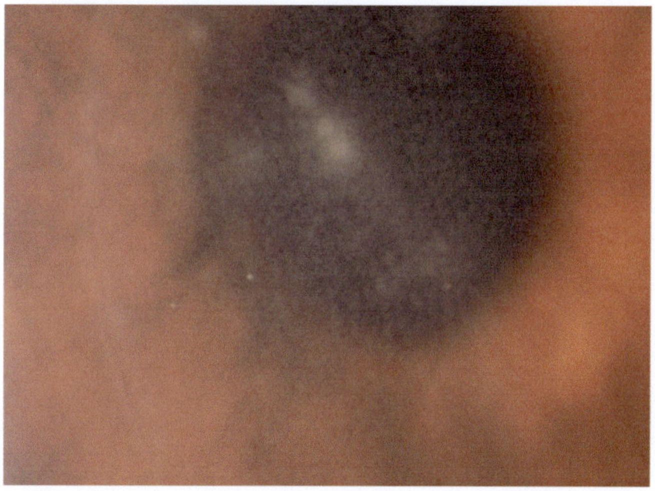

Fig. 9.6 Flap interface

Core Message:

- No foreign, unsterile material should be left under the flap.
- Care must be taken to remove all material by scraping the underside of the flap in case of trauma with foreign body.
- Consider antibiotic or betadine flushing of the interface after foreign body removal.
- Flap can still be dislodged years following LASIK

Case: Patient presented with pain, redness, and blurry vision for 2 days. There was no history of trauma but reported morning dryness and working in his garden for the prior week. Patient had uncomplicated LASIK 5 years prior. UCVA: 20/70 (Fig. 9.12).

Exam: A corneal ulcer was noted with diffuse flap inflammation and clumps of inflammatory cells (stage 3 DLK) (Fig. 9.12a). No epithelial defect was present at the first evaluation in the ED.

Management: Flap lift, scraping for culture and irrigation with antibiotics were performed (Fig. 9.12b, c). A full thickness hole was noted in a melted area due to the infection *(red arrow)* (Fig. 9.12b). Culture came back negative but the patient was kept on fortified anti-bacterial eye drops.

Postoperative follow up: Day 1, an epithelial defect was noted with minimal residual DLK (Fig. 9.12d, e). Week 2, complete healing and epithelization. UCVA was 20/25 (Fig. 9.12f, g).

Case: A 68-year-old female patient presented with pain, blurry vision, and photo sensitivity 4 months following a non-complicated cataract surgery. Her UCVA was 20/125. Her recent UCVA following surgery was 20/30. She had a LASIK few years ago complicated with dry eyes (Fig 9.13).

Exam: Para-central superficial corneal ulcer of 1mm was noted. It involves the flap with adjacent flap interface whitish material (Fig 9.13a). Scraping and culture showed Cutibacterium (Propionibacterium) acnes.

Management: Patient was started on fortified antibiotics and steroid eye drops. Her condition improved over the next weeks (Fig. 9.13b, c) and left a paracentral scar (Fig. 9.13d). The interface deposits did not show a connection with the

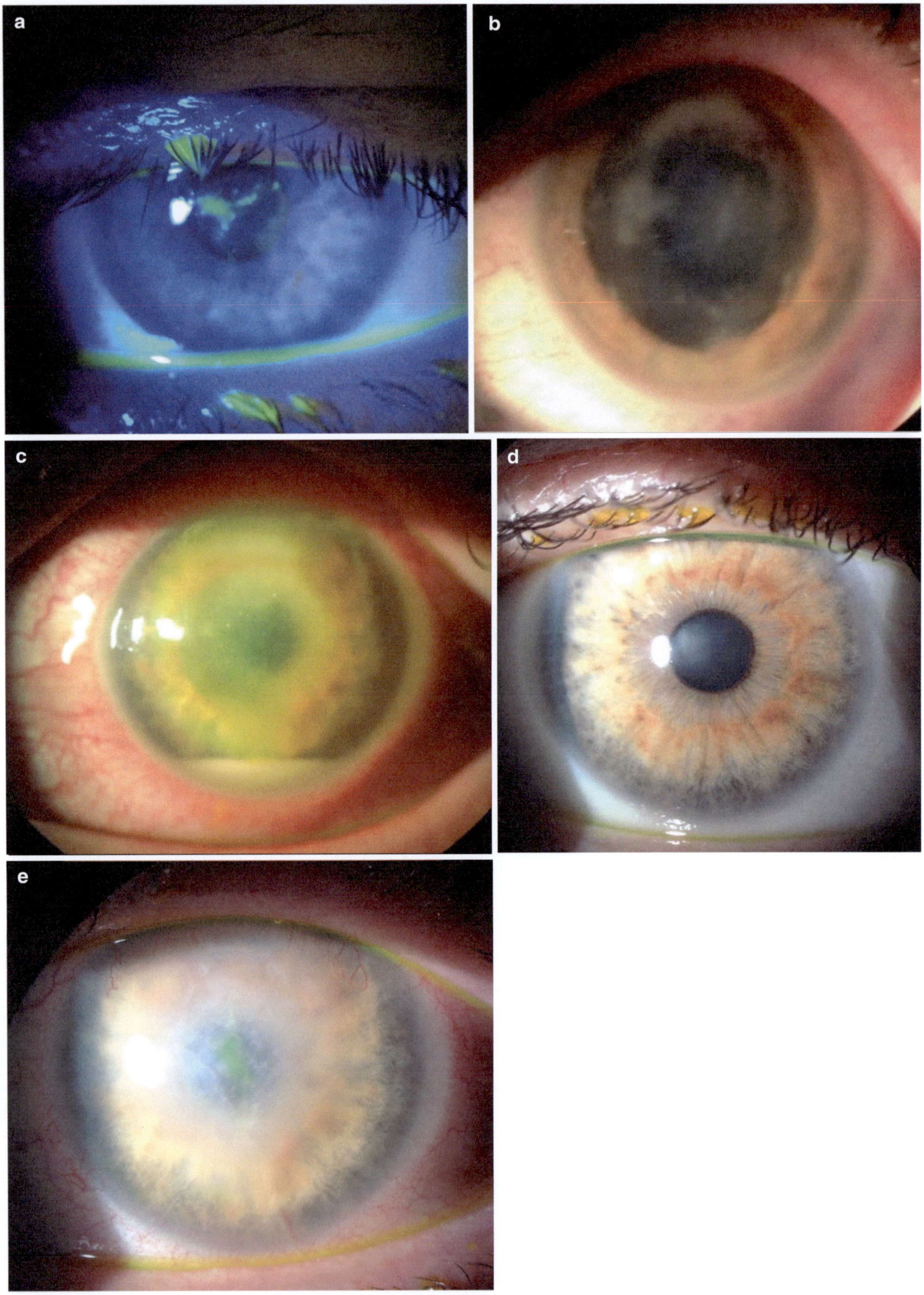

Fig. 9.7 Bilateral keratitis. (**a**) Persistent epithelial defect post PRK, (**b**) right eye corneal infiltrate, (**c**) left eye infiltrate with hypopyon, (**d**) healed right eye after fortified antibiotics, (**e**) residual scar in the left eye after antibiotics. (*Courtesy of Juliana Freitas, MD; Conselho Brasileiro de Oftalmologia, Brazil*)

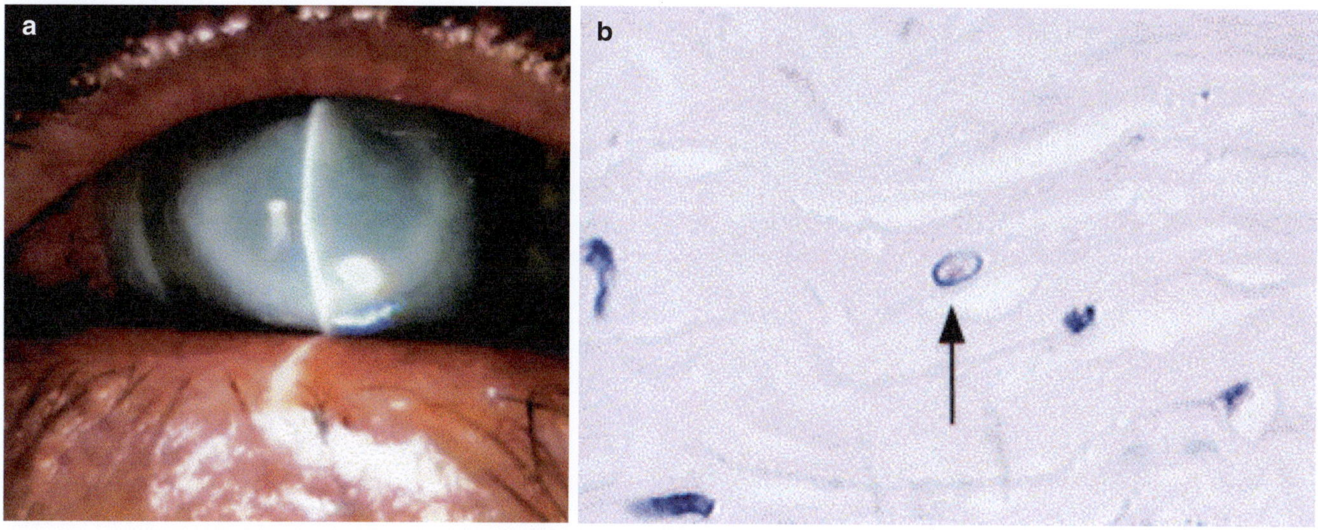

Fig. 9.8 Acanthamoeba keratitis. (**a**) Slit lamp photo showing ring infiltrate, (**b**) histopathologic exam show in double-walled cysts. (*Courtesy of Roger Kardawi, MD; Milford Franklin Eye Center, Massachusetts, USA*)

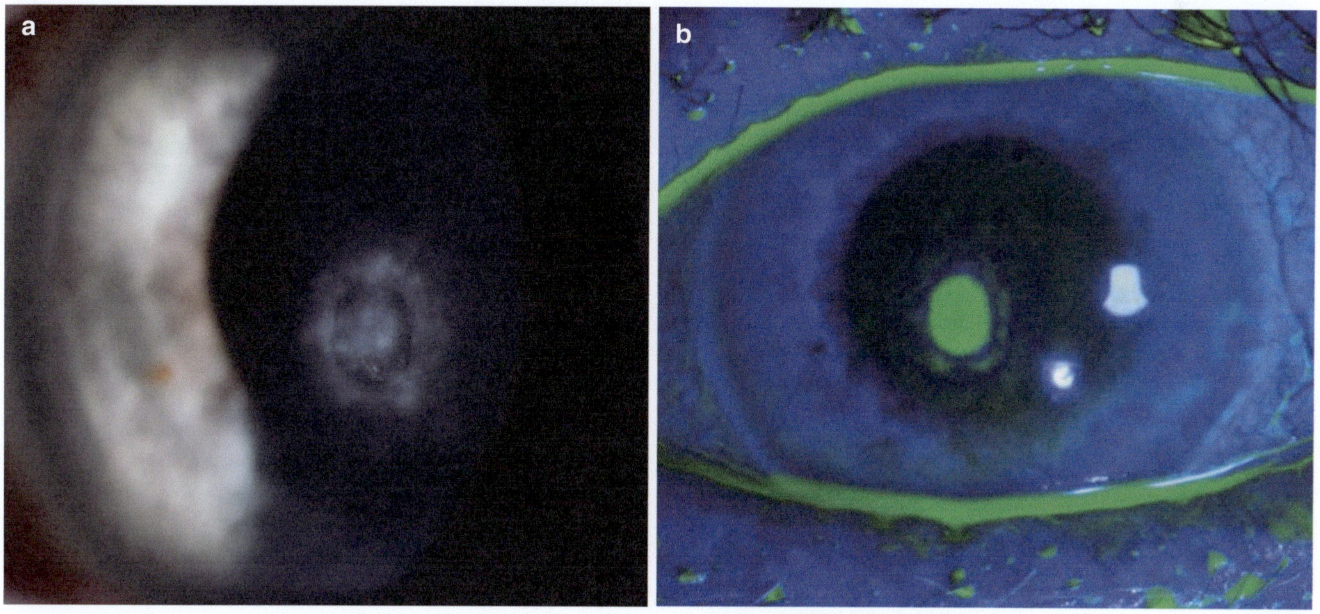

Fig. 9.9 Central corneal ulcer without (**a**) and with (b0 fluorescein stain. (*Courtesy of Catherine Liu, MD*)

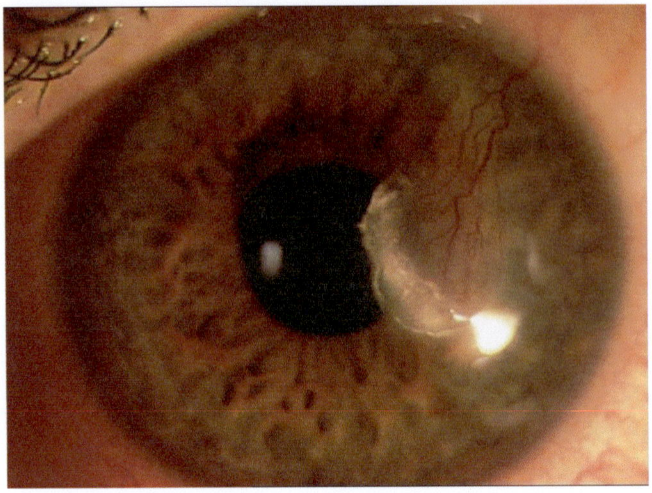

Fig. 9.10 Central corneal neovascularisation

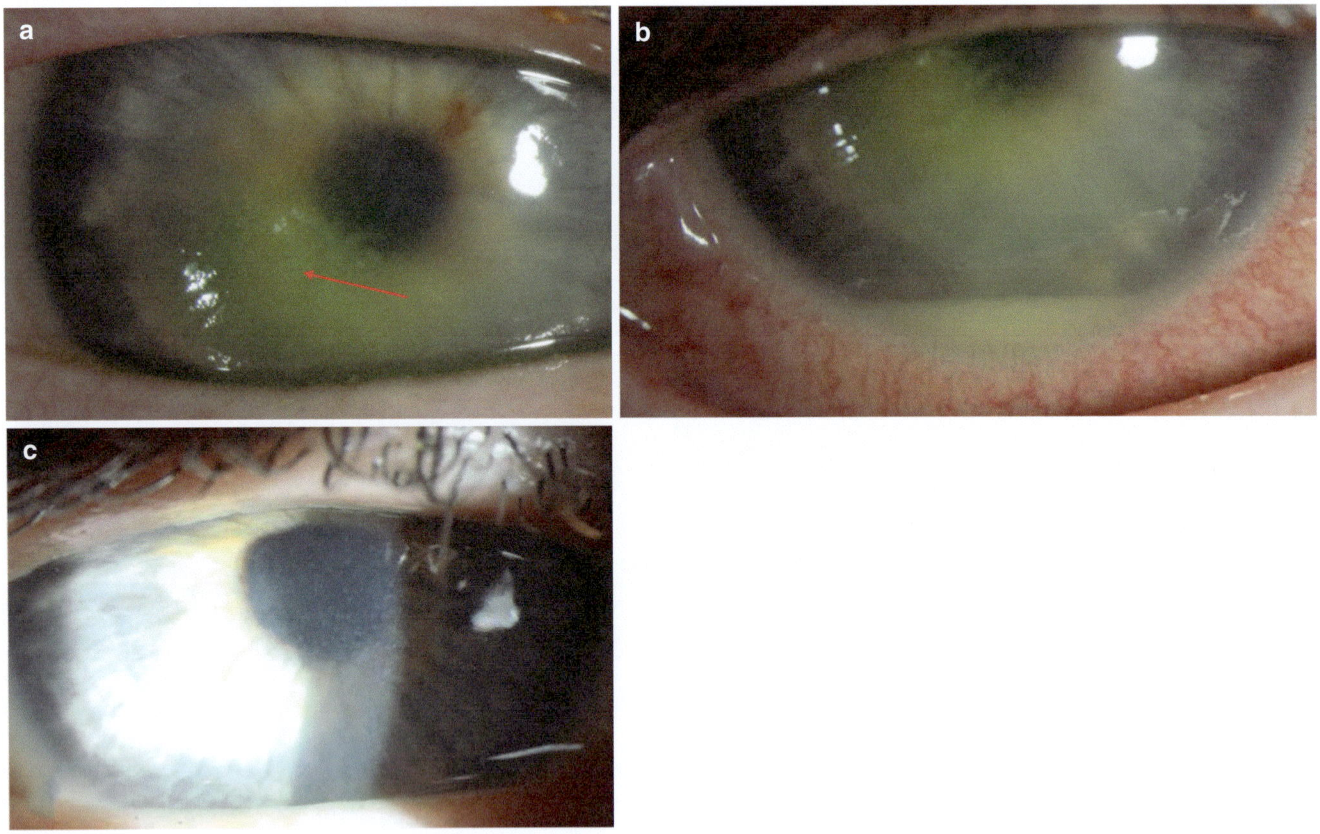

Fig. 9.11 Interface foreign body. (**a**) Initial presentation, (**b**) worsening with hypopyon, (**c**) healing after flap amputation and voriconazole use

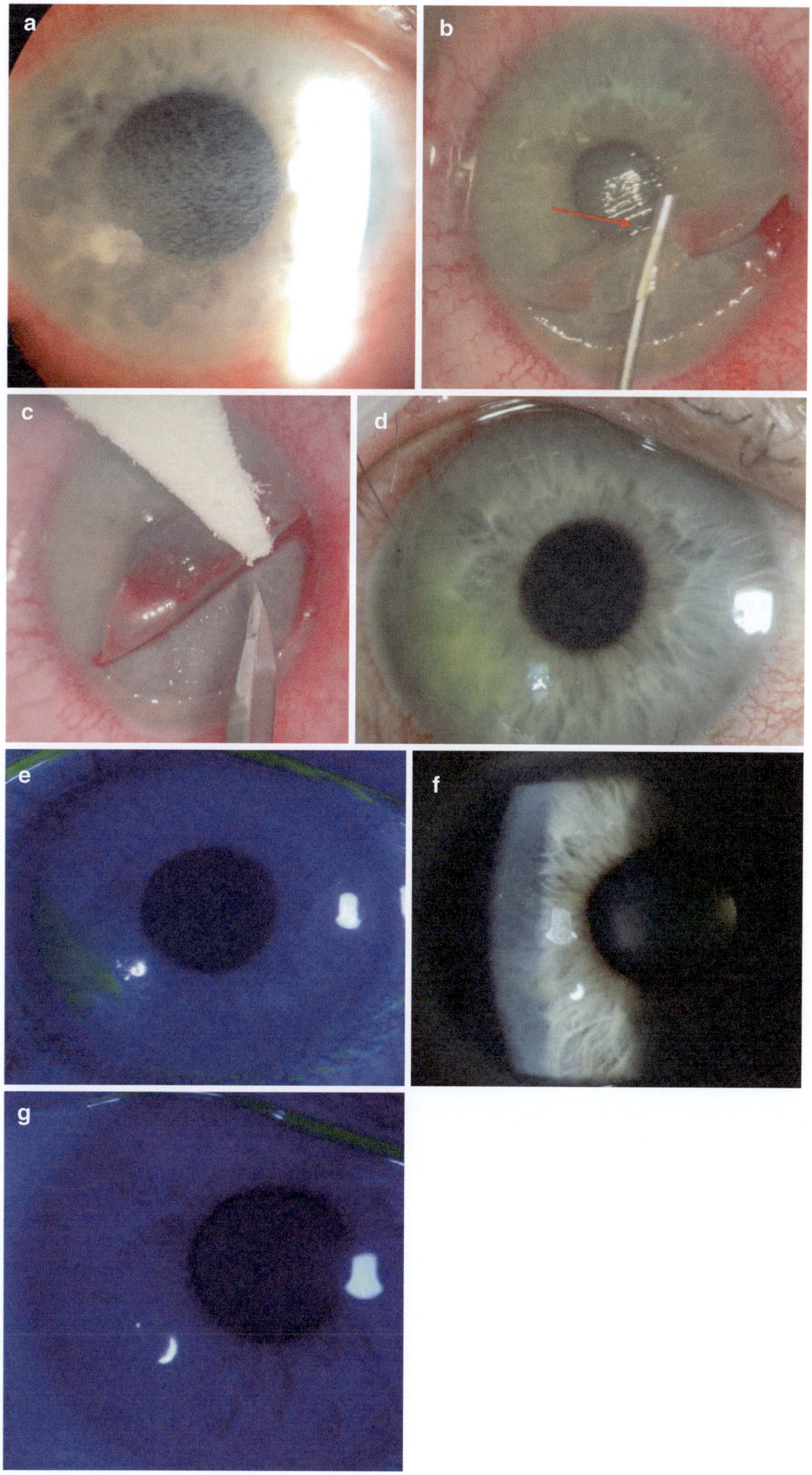

Fig. 9.12 Corneal ulcer with melting and DLK. (**a**) Stage 3 DLK, (**b**) flap lifted, full thickness hole (red arrow) noted, (**c**) cultures taken, (**d**, **e**) day 1 post flap lift, (**f**, **g**) week 2 after flap lift

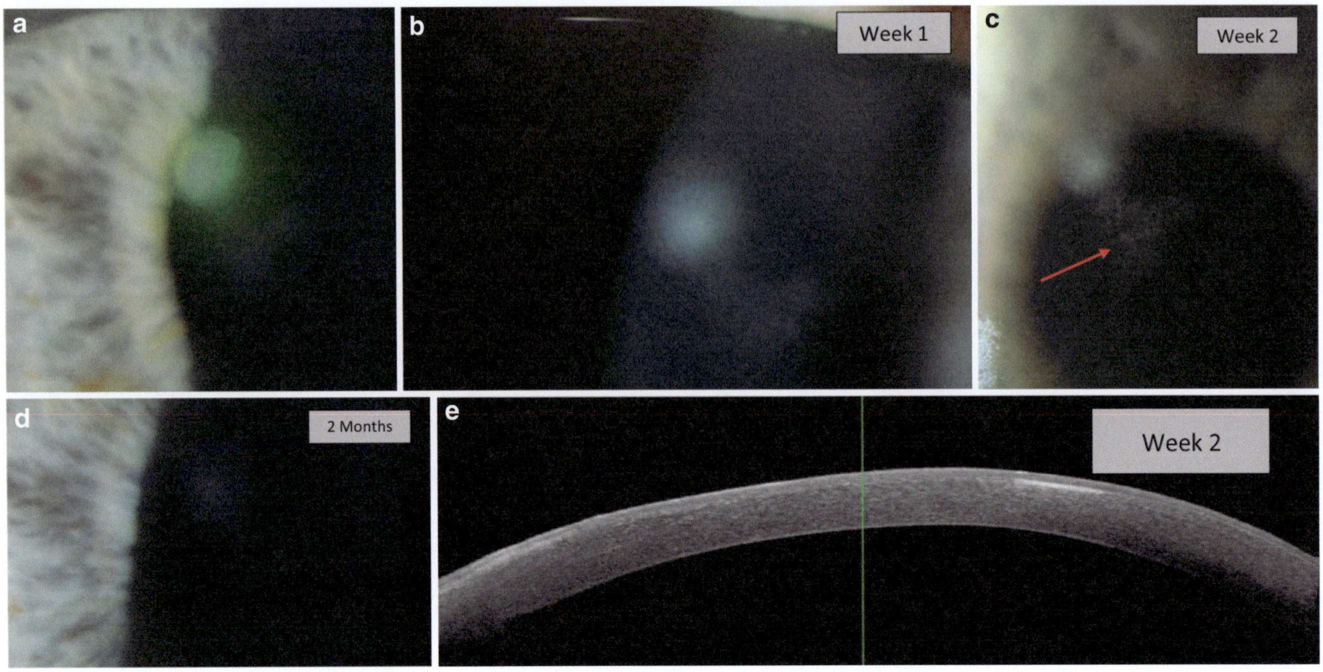

Fig. 9.13 Interface collection. Slit lamp photos showing paracentral ulcer (**a**) day 1, (**b**) week 1, (**c**) week 2, (**d**) month 2. (**e**) OCT at week 2

epithelium on corneal OCT (Fig. 9.13e). It formed aggregates at 2 weeks (*red arrow*) and it is most likely inflammatory material rather than epithelial ingrowth. UCVA improved to 20/30 after 2 months.

Take-Home Message

- Pre- and postoperative management of dry eye speeds up the recovery and may be preventive from bacterial keratitis following refractive procedures.
- Corneal sensitivity testing is not accurate following refractive surgeries.
- Patients known to have herpes simplex keratitis should have no recurrence for over a year before considering refractive surgery. Antivirals should be started before the procedure to prevent recurrence due to the epithelial injury and the use of topical steroids eye drops.
- Herpes simplex keratitis should be considered in non-healing postoperative epithelial defects.
- The LASIK flap never heals completely. Fluid can still accumulate in the interface in case of infections or endothelial failure, and there is a lifelong risk of dislocation with severe trauma.
- It is possible that the flap-stroma interface prevents antibiotic eye drop from penetrating deep into the cornea; therefore, the flap can be sacrificed to allow antibiotics to penetrate deeper in the cornea in case of deep stromal infections.
- When the flap is thinned/melted due to an infectious keratitis, there is a high risk of flap perforation if it is lifted for irrigation and culture. It is better to avoid flap lift in advanced central corneal ulcers.
- In resistant cases, with negative surface and interface cultures, the LASIK flap may be excised to get accurate cultures, decrease the infectious load, and to allow antibiotic penetration deeper in the cornea.

References

1. Llovet F, de Rojas V, Interlandi E, Martín C. Infectious keratitis in 204 586 LASIK procedures. Ophthalmology. 2010;117(2):232–8.e1-4.
2. Chang MA, Jain S, Review ADT. Infections following laser in situ keratomileusis: an integration of the published literature. Surv Ophthalmol. 2004;49(3):269–80.
3. Haq Z, Farooq AV, Huang AJ, Review. Infections after refractive surgery. Curr Opin Ophthalmol. 2016;27(4):367–72.
4. Moshirfar M, Welling JD, Feiz V, Holz H, Clinch T. Infectious and noninfectious keratitis after laser in situ keratomileusis. Occurrence, management, and visual outcomes. J Cataract Refract Surg. 2007;33(3):474–83.

Non-Infectious Keratitis

10

Jason Brenner, Wassef Chanbour, and Samir A. Melki

See Table 10.1.

Case: One day following PRK surgery (Fig. 10.1).

Exam: OD: Corneal swelling and Descemet folds were noticed in addition to the epithelial defect (Fig. 10.1a, b).

OS: Diffuse swelling and Descemet folds (Fig. 10.1c).

Management: No change in the management is recommended as the condition heals spontaneously within 2 weeks following PRK, rarely causing long term damage (Fig. 10.1d, e).

Core message: Corneal swelling is common following PRK, it is a self-limiting disease.

Case: 4 days following a non-complicated LASIK procedure, a patient presented with blurry vision and light sensitivity (Fig. 10.2).

Exam: Inferior flap and peripheral stromal opacification (Fig. 10.2a) in addition to an epithelial defect (Fig. 10.2b).

Management: Flap lift and irrigation was performed; cultures were taken and were negative. Steroids were increased and inflammation resolved over 2 weeks leaving some peripheral scarring and astigmatism (Fig. 10.2c, d).

Case: One day following LASIK, a patient presented for follow up. UDVA: 20/20 (Fig. 10.3).

Exam: 360-degree dense inflammatory peripheral white flap infiltrates (Fig. 10.3a, b)**,** lesions can be considered a stage 4 DLK.

Management: Intensive topical steroid application. Patient recovered completely in 2 weeks.

Core message: Infections are less likely to occur day one post LASIK.

J. Brenner (✉) · S. A. Melki
Boston Vision, Department of Ophthalmology, Harvard Medical School, Boston, MA, USA
e-mail: brenner@bostonvision.com; Melki@bostonvision.com

W. Chanbour
Department of Ophthalmology and Visual Neurosciences, University of Minnesota, Minneapolis, MN, USA

Cases: One week following a PRK procedure, patient presented with pain and foreign body sensation (Fig. 10.4).

Exam: Multiple peripheral stromal white infiltrates without overlying epithelial defect (Fig. 10.4a, b).

Management: Steroid drops were increased and patient healed within one month.

Case: A patient presented two weeks following a non-complicated PRK (Fig. 10.5).

Exam: 3 white peripheral infiltrates <1 mm each with an overlying epithelial defect.

Management: The patient's topical steroids were increased, and post operative antibiotics were continued. Healing occurred within one week.

Case: One month following a PRK procedure, a patient presented with red eye and burning for a few days. (Fig. 10.6).

Exam: Inferior peripheral dense stromal infiltrate was noticed over 90 degrees of arc (Fig. 10.6a) and inferior Blepharitis (Fig. 10.6b).

Management: Warm compress, topical steroids, and antibiotics should be started.

Core message:

– Early corneal infiltrates related to surgery should be differentiated from late infiltrates which can be an isolated local event, not related to the refractive procedure.
– Marginal keratitis should be suspected if the patient has blepharitis and symptoms are not as severe as typical infectious keratitis. Cultures are not necessary for every case.

Case: A 33-year-old male patient presented with recurrent pain and redness in the left eye. Patient had LASIK surgery 8 years prior to presentation (Fig. 10.7).

Exam: Paracentral inflammatory infiltrate involving the flap with peripheral corneal neovascularization (Fig. 10.7a, b) and overlying epithelial defect on fluorescein staining (Fig. 10.7c).

S. A. Melki et al. (eds.), *Refractive Surgery Atlas*, https://doi.org/10.1007/978-3-031-60661-8_10

Table 10.1 Diagnosis and management of common non-infectious causes of keratitis following refractive surgery

Onset	Early onset <1 week Late onset >1 week	
Rate	2.34% following refractive procedures [1]	
Pathology and clinical features	**Marginal keratitis**	localized corneal hypersensitivity reaction to toxins produced by bacteria colonizing the eyelid margins **Etiology:** localized corneal hypersensitivity reaction to toxins produced by bacteria colonizing the eyelid margin causing antigen-antibody complexes deposits in the stroma [2] **Clinical diagnosis:** Sluggish onset of redness and irritation. Localized peripheral circular stromal infiltrate. The epithelium is usually intact. There is typically an associated blepharitis **Treatment:** Steroid eye drops +/− antibiotics
	Rosacea/ phlyctenular keratitis	**Possible etiologies:** Overstimulation of the innate immune system by microbes, UV light, or autoimmunity, leading to keratinocyte activation [3] **Clinical Diagnosis:** Peripheral corneal neovascularization extending into a scar in the middle of the flap associated with blepharitis **Ocular Treatment:** Topical steroid eye drops, Topical azithromycin, topical tacrolimus, oral doxycycline, intense pulsed light treatment (IPL)
	Diffuse lamellar keratitis	**Etiologies:** Blepharitis, interface toxins and deposits **Clinical Diagnosis:** Starting 24 h after LASIK with flap interface inflammation **Ocular Treatment:** Topical steroid eye drops and flap lift with irrigation depending on the stage of the disease (Refer to Chap. 11 for more detailed information)
	Others	Thygeson's superficial punctate keratitis, sterile keratitis, and peripheral ulcerative keratitis have also been reported in case reports following refractive procedures
Prevention	• Same as infectious keratitis (Chap. 9, Table 9.1)	
Outcomes	• 89% achieve 20/40 vision and better.1 • Better outcome than infectious keratitis	

Management: After failing to improve with HSV treatment, symptoms resolved with topical steroids. But patient had multiple recurrences later and he was diagnosed with phlyctenular keratitis.

Core message: Corneal neovascularization following lasik can be infectious (viral, bacterial, fungal), inflammatory (atopic, phlyctenular, etc.), degenerative (pterygium), or traumatic.

Case: 4 months following a non-complicated LASIK, a 36-year-old patient presented with tearing and light sensitivity for 3 weeks duration (Fig. 10.8).

Exam: Diffuse small nummular shape subepithelial infiltrates (Fig. 10.7a, b).

Management: Inflammation was resistant to topical steroids. Cyclosporin was later effective in alleviating the patient symptoms and stabilizing the disease.

Core message: Subepithelial infiltrates may require longer suppressive treatment and they most likely follow a viral infection that is unrelated to the LASIK surgery.

Case: A 34-year-old patient presented 5 years following LASIK with new onset photophobia and blurry vision of 20/40 in both eyes worsening since few months (Fig. 10.9).

Exam: Corneal deposit like material in the superficial stroma (Fig. 10.9a) of both eyes OD (Fig. 10.9b), and OS (Fig. 10.9c).

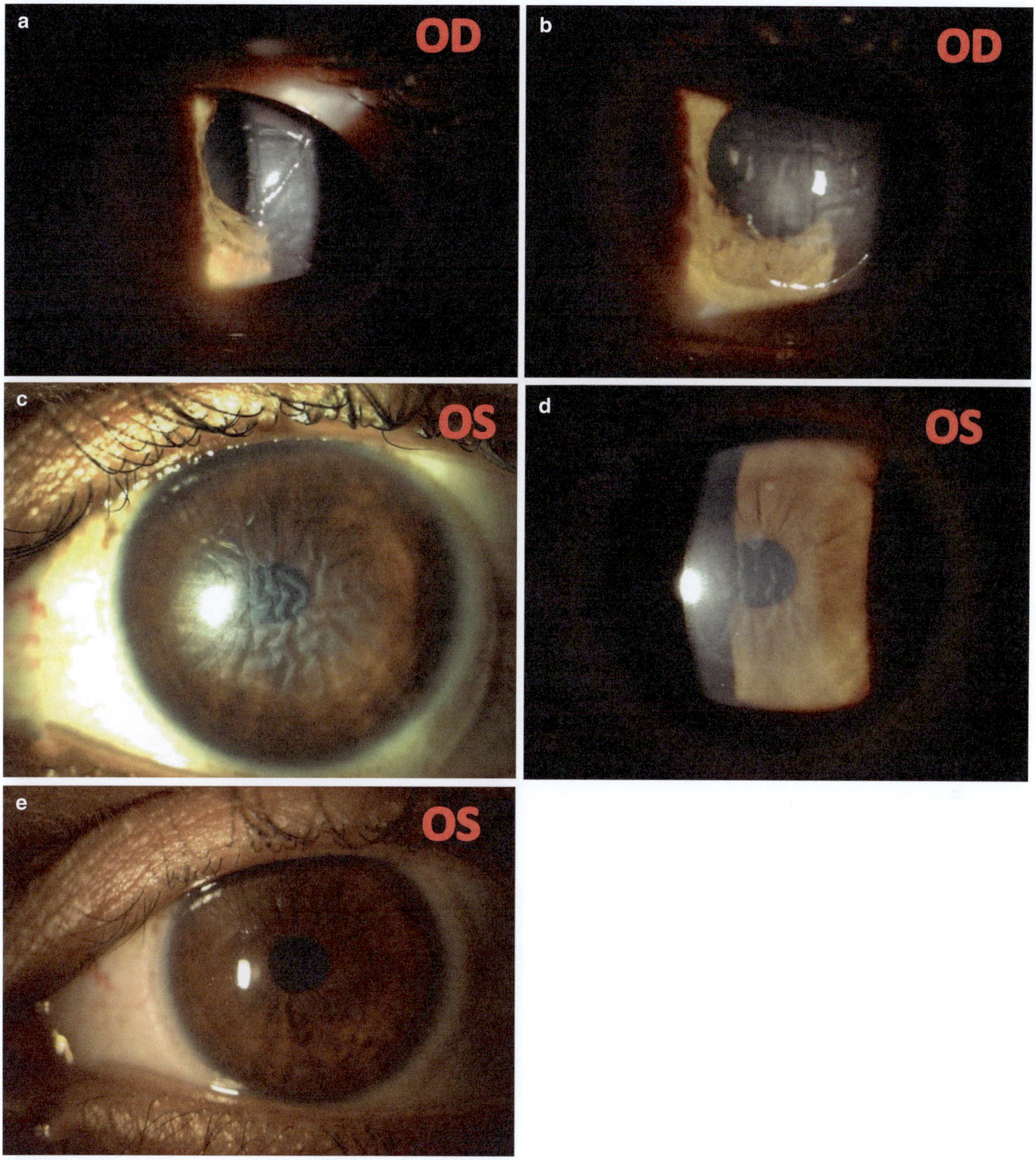

Fig. 10.1 Excessive corneal swelling after uncomplicated PRK

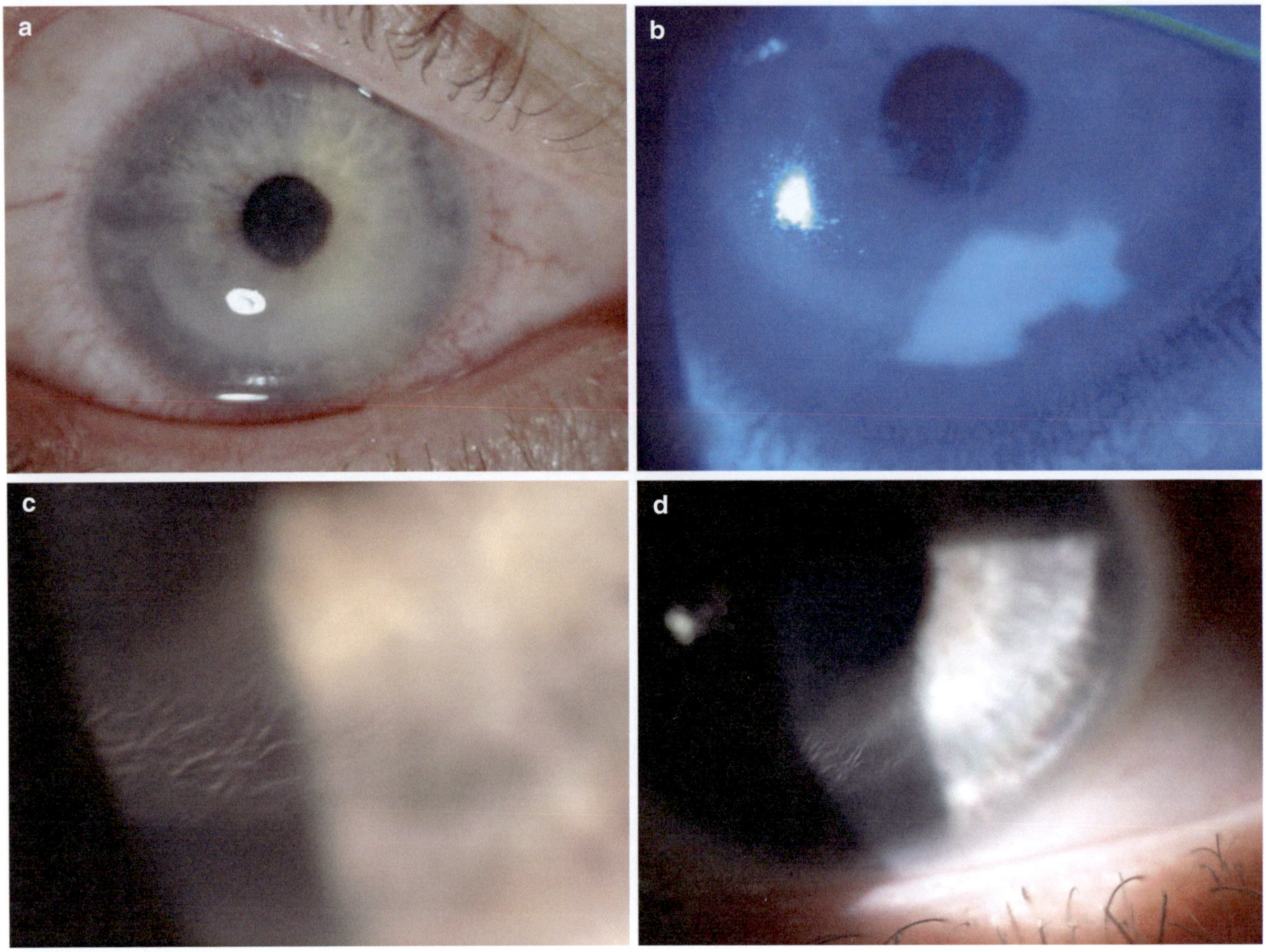

Fig. 10.2 Localized keratitis

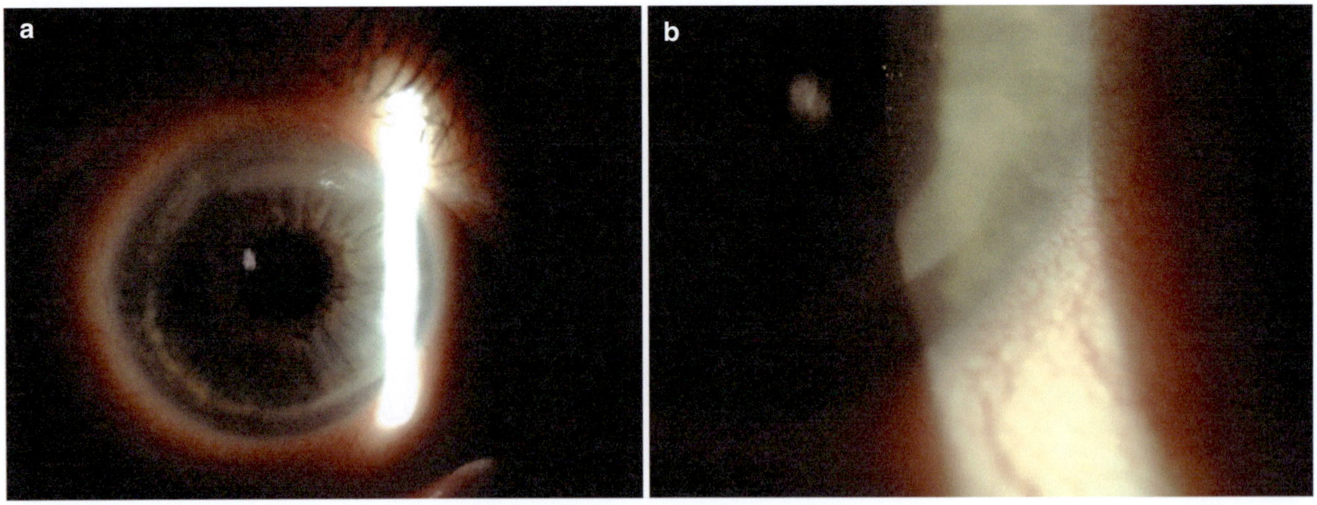

Fig. 10.3 Dense white infiltrates

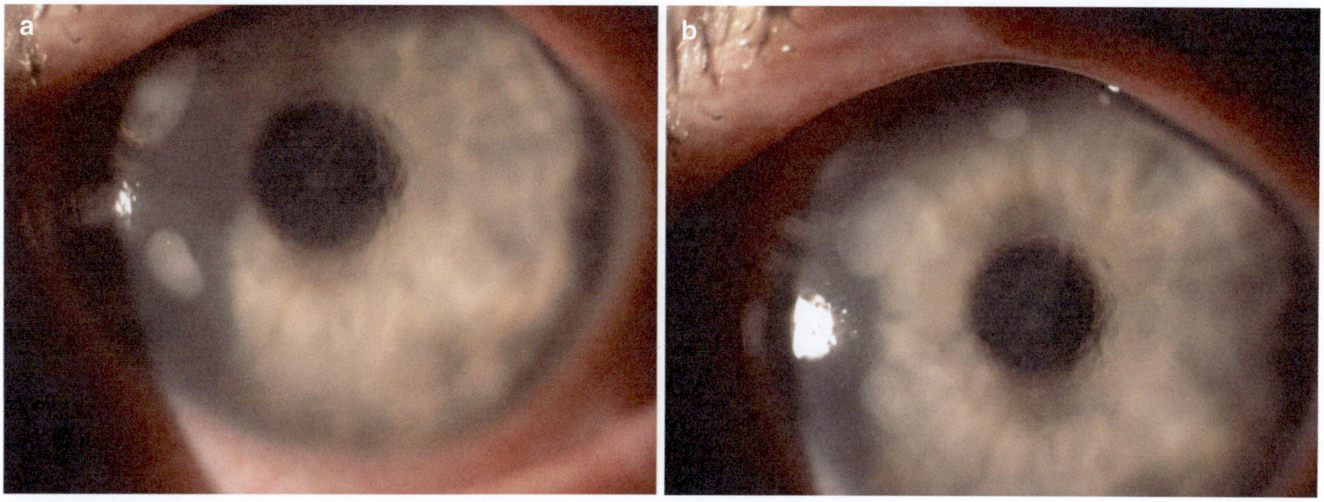

Fig. 10.4 Early sterile infiltrates

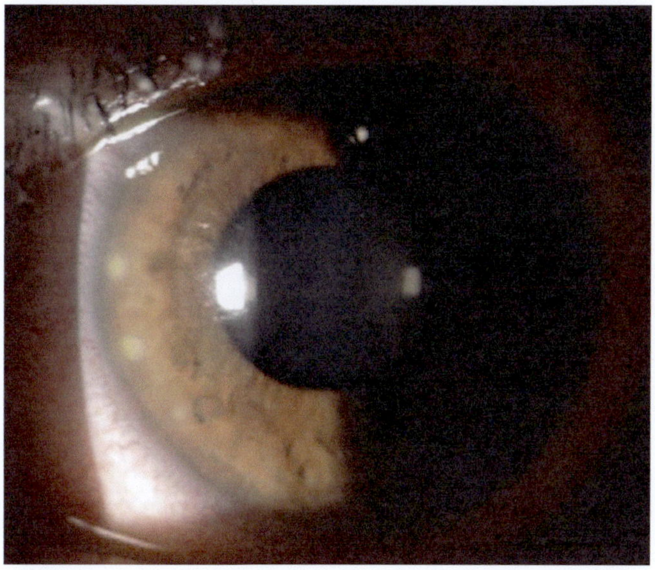

Fig. 10.5 Multiple sterile keratitis

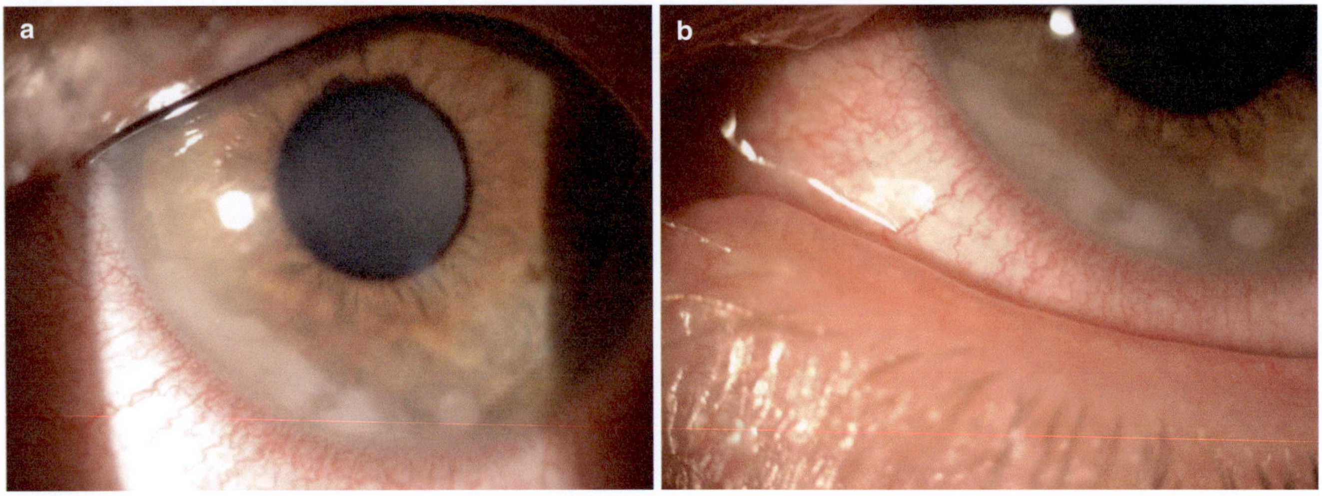

Fig. 10.6 Marginal keratitis

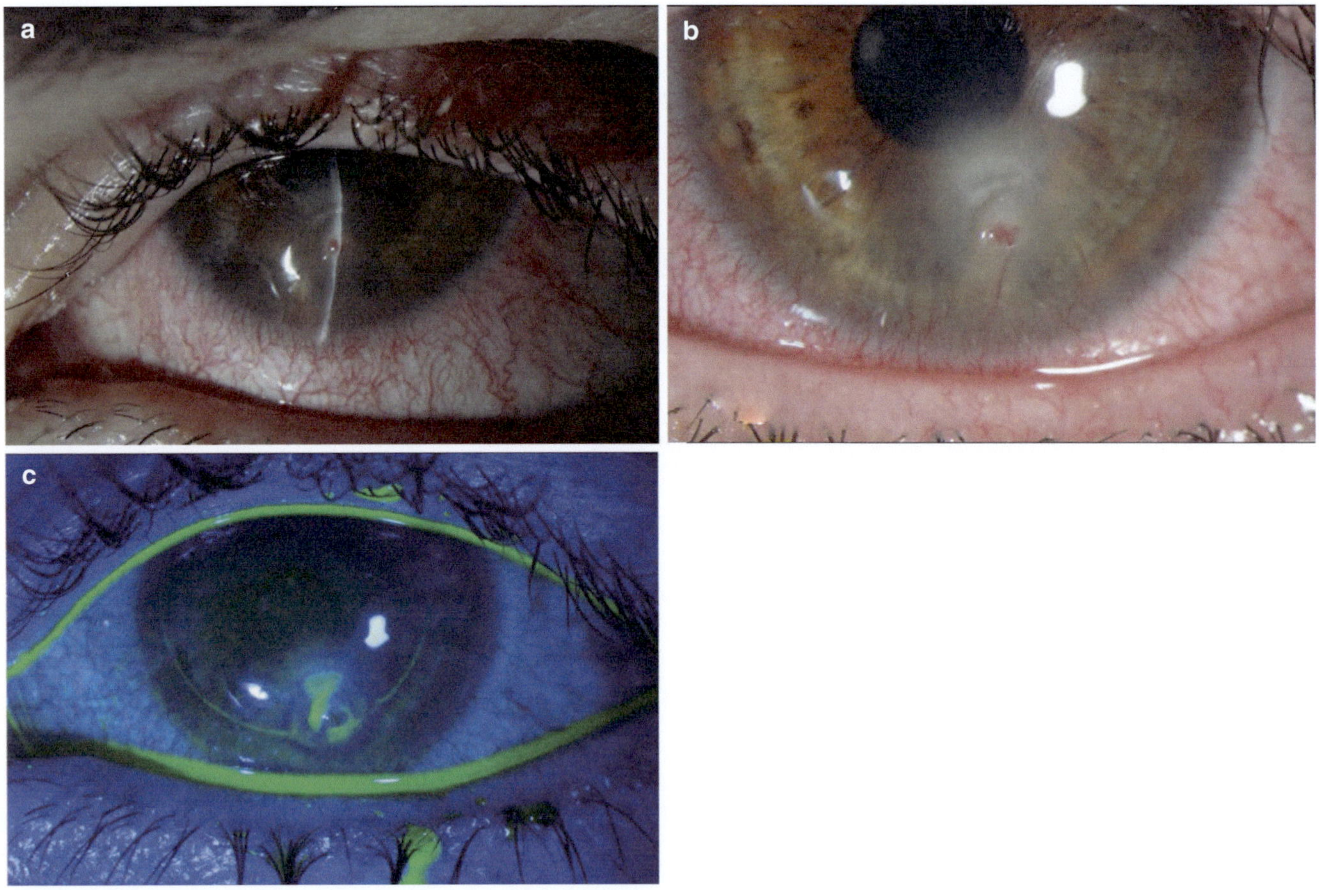

Fig. 10.7 Phlyctenular keratitis. (*Courtesy of Deborah S. Jacobs, MD. Mass Eye and Ear, Massachussets, USA*)

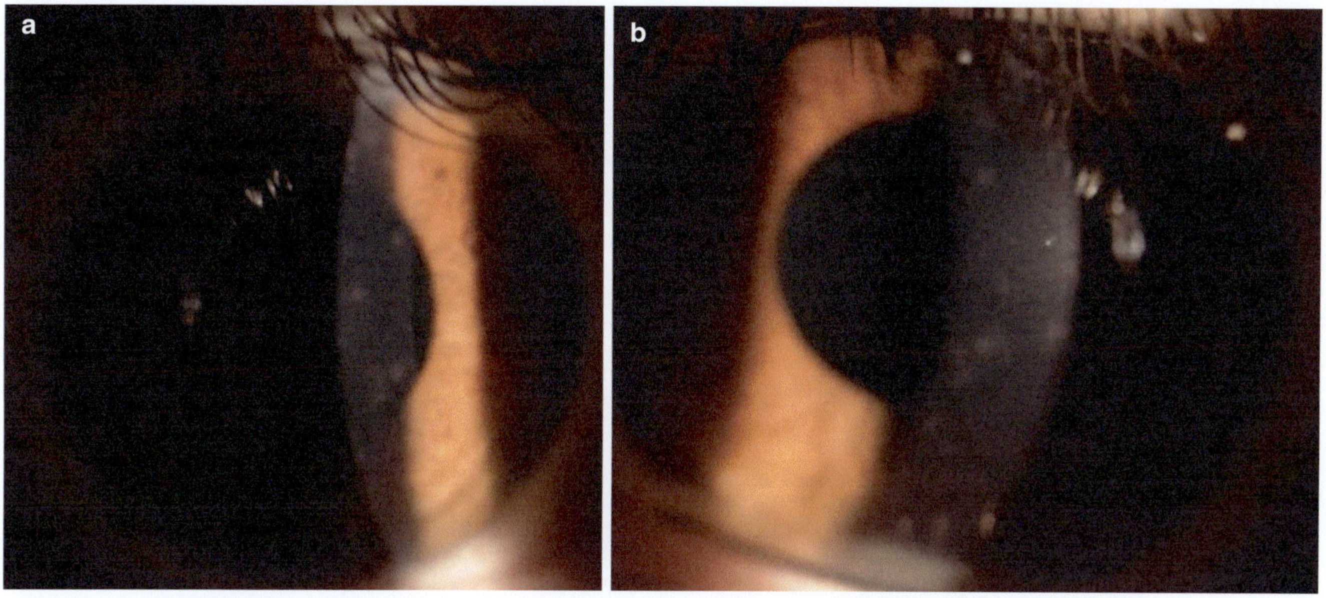

Fig. 10.8 Subepithelial infiltrates

Fluorescein staining showed diffuse superficial punctate keratitis, some were noted on top of the stromal deposits.

Genetic test for corneal dystrophies came back negative for mutations in TGFBI gene.

Management: Patient was given a trial of steroids. Photophobia decreased, visual acuity improved to 20/20, and deposits decreased in densities 3 weeks after treatment in the right and left eye, respectively (Fig. 10.9d, e). The patient was diagnosed with Thygeson's superficial punctate keratitis and was given topical cyclosporine as a long-term treatment without recurrence.

Core message: Thygeson superficial punctate keratitis may have different presentation following LASIK; subepithelial scars and deposits may be noted.

Take-Home Message

- Blepharitis is better addressed before refractive surgery to avoid dry eyes and marginal keratitis.
- Stromal sterile infiltrates are common following PRK, visual acuity is rarely affected when they are peripheral.
- When the diagnosis is clear, cultures are not always necessary in case of inflammatory stromal infiltrates.
- Inflammatory keratitis may have a different clinical picture following LASIK.
- Flap lift and irrigation can be performed in severe DLK, but it should be avoided when there is clear evidence of corneal melt.

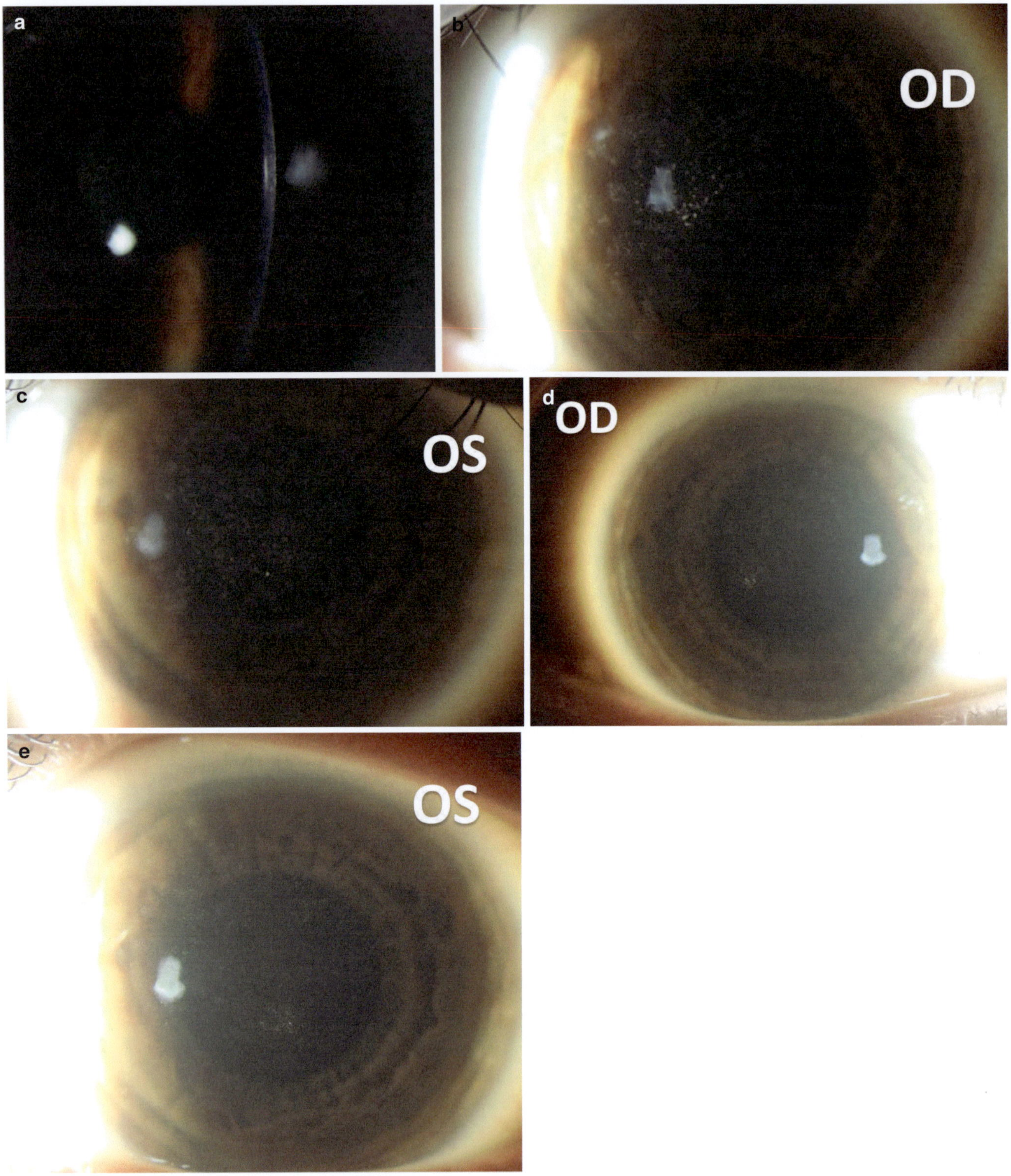

Fig. 10.9 Uncommon keratitis

References

1. Moshirfar M, Welling JD, Feiz V, Holz H, Clinch TE. Infectious and noninfectious keratitis after laser *in situ* keratomileusis. Occurrence, management, and visual outcomes. J Cataract Refract Surg. 2007;33:474–83.
2. Robin JB, Dugel R, Robin SB. Immunologic disorders of the cornea and conjunctiva. In: Kaufman HE, Barron BA, McDonal MB, editors. The Cornea. 2nd ed. Boston: Butterworth-Heinemann; 1998. p. 551–95.
3. Emer J, Weinkle A, Doktor V. Update on the management of rosacea. Clin Cosmet Investig Dermatol. 2015;8:159.

11 Diffuse Lamellar Keratitis

Karen Matar, Jason Brenner, Wassef Chanbour, and Samir A. Melki

See Tables 11.1 and 11.2.

Case: An asymptomatic 31-year-old male presented for routine follow-up 1 day after LASIK surgery (Fig. 11.1).

Exam: Stage 1 DLK; white faint granular cells in the periphery; not reaching the central visual axis (Fig. 11.1a, b).

Management: Topical steroids every 2 h and follow-up after 48 h.

Core message: In stage 1, DLK occurs at the periphery and does not affect visual acuity.

Case: A patient examined 1 day after a non-complicated LASIK procedure. UDVA: 20/20 (Fig. 11.2).

Exam: Stage 1 DLK; fine powdery cellular infiltrates originating near the flap border and migrating towards the center of the cornea; not reaching the visual axis.

Management: Topical steroids used every 2 h. Complete resolution of inflammation occurred 1 week later and steroids were tapered.

Core message: Early stages of DLK do not require any surgical intervention and can resolve with intensive topical corticosteroids.

Case: A 56-year-old male presented for follow-up 1 day after LASIK surgery (Fig. 11.3).

Exam: Arc-shaped dense white area on the flap, extending to the periphery (Fig. 11.3a), and the presence of white granular deposits outside the flap (Fig. 11.3b), consistent with arcus senilis.

Management: No treatment is recommended.

Core message: Pre-operative documentation of corneal findings is important. In arcus senilis the stromal deposits are well defined and extend beyond the flap.

Case: Patient diagnosed with stage 1 DLK presenting for worsening vision in the right eye 3 days after LASIK procedure. UDVA: 20/20 (Fig. 11.4).

Exam: Slit-lamp examination shows grade 1 DLK at postoperative day 1 (Fig. 11.4a). At day 3, DLK progressed to grade 2 DLK; white granular cells migrated from the periphery to the center in the right eye; involving the central visual axis (Fig. 11.4b).

Management: Increase steroids from every 2 h to every 1 h.

Core message: Frequent follow-up is necessary in all patients with DLK as worsening can still occur with steroid drops.

Case: Patient examined 2 days following a non-complicated LASIK surgery (Fig. 11.5). UDVA: 20/25

Exam: Diffuse white granular cells (Fig. 11.5a) with microfolds ***(red arrows)*** (Fig. 11.5b) in the central visual axis, consistent with stage 2 DLK.

Management: Hourly topical steroids with close observation as visual acuity is still preserved.

Case: Day 1 following a non-complicated LASIK procedure, patient presented with blurriness and UDVA of 20/30 (Fig. 11.6).

Exam: Diffuse lamellar keratitis stage 2 with inflammatory infiltrates across the visual axis (Fig. 11.6a, b).

Management: Hourly topical steroids with close observation. DLK improved at day 4 (Fig. 11.6c), and it resolved completely at day 8 (Fig. 11.6d).

Core message: Stage 2 DLK does not require flap lift.

Case: Patient presented with decreased vision following a blunt trauma to his eye. UDVA: 20/40 (Fig. 11.7).

Exam: Diffuse lamellar keratitis stage 2 with granular infiltration across the central visual axis (Fig. 11.7a–c).

Management: Topical corticosteroids were started and the patient healed completely within a week.

K. Matar
Cole Eye Institute, Cleveland Clinic Foundation, Cleveland, OH, USA

J. Brenner (✉) · S. A. Melki
Boston Vision, Department of Ophthalmology, Harvard Medical School, Boston, MA, USA
e-mail: brenner@bostonvision.com; Melki@bostonvision.com

W. Chanbour
Department of Ophthalmology and Visual Neurosciences, University of Minnesota, Minneapolis, MN, USA

S. A. Melki et al. (eds.), *Refractive Surgery Atlas*, https://doi.org/10.1007/978-3-031-60661-8_11

Table 11.1 Diagnosis and management of diffuse lamellar keratitis following LASIK

Onset	24–72 h after LASIK; however some findings are usually present on the first postoperative day [1]
Rate	0.1–7.7% after primary treatment with microkeratome [2] 0.2–19.4% after primary treatment with femtosecond laser [2]
Mechanism	• Noninfectious inflammatory process of unknown exact etiology at the lamellar interface [3] • Infiltration of cells is due to the accumulation of mononuclear cells and granulocytes in the lamellar interface [4] • Polymorphonuclear leukocytes can release destructive collagenases and may lead to stromal melting and scarring [3]
Symptoms	Asymptomatic; becomes symptomatic with decreased visual acuity [3] if: • It involves central visual axis • Stromal melting • Irregular astigmatism
Monitoring	Slit-lamp examination on the first postoperative day, fluorescein staining (no stain) [1]
Risk factors	• Preoperative: Preexisting dry eyes, blepharitis, Meibomian gland dysfunction (MGD), history of previously healed keratitis, previous corneal surgery [5] • Perioperative: Epithelial defects, oil, wax, metallic and other foreign particles in the lamellar interface, chemical toxin and bacterial endotoxin on instruments, trauma [5–7], glove talc, marking pen, old microkeratome blade, small suction ring, high energy FSL, large-diameter flap, povidone-iodine [1, 2, 8, 9]
Prevention	• Careful cleaning techniques and avoidance of contaminants [7] • Prevent tear film debris from reaching interface [8] • Using lower energy femtosecond lasers [10] • Preoperative screening and management of ocular surface diseases [11] • Use of powder-free gloves and drapes to cover lid margin [11] • Irrigating the interface after flap repositioning [11]
Indications for medical treatment	Stages 1 and 2
Medical treatment	Frequent topical corticosteroid application [1, 6–8]
Indications for surgical treatment	• Stage 3: Lifting the flap can blunt the inflammatory response and prevent scarring [1] • Stage 4: Lifting the flap at this stage could still be possible, however in some cases it would be of little benefit due to the stromal volume loss that can be worsened with any tissue manipulation. Early identification of stage 3 is the best prevention for this stage [1, 8]
Surgical technique	• Flap lift, scraping, and irrigation with BSS [3] • Stage 4: If scarring has occurred, treatment depends on individual cases and may include: Phototherapeutic keratotomy, lamellar keratoplasty, or flap amputation [6]
Outcome	• The majority of the identified DLK are stage 1 and 2. With treatment, patients have excellent visual and refractive outcomes • Stage 3 and 4 are rare and may lead to scarring and irregular astigmatism

Table 11.2 Stages and treatment of diffuse lamellar keratitis

Stages	Linebarger et al. Staging [1]	Treatment
Stage 1	Fine, white, granular cells in the periphery, outside visual axis, self-limiting. Occurs on the first day	Intensive topical steroids. Follow-up 24–48 h
Stage 2	Fine, white, granular cells migrate from periphery to center, involves central visual axis, some cells still in periphery, shifting sands appearance, no decrease in BCVA. Occurs on the second or third day; occasionally on the first day	Intensive topical steroids Short course of oral steroid can be considered. Follow-up 24–48 h
Stage 3	Dense, white, clumped cells in the central visual axis with relative clearing in the periphery, 1–2 lines decrease in BCVA, subjective haze described by the patient. Threshold DLK. Occurs on the second or third day	Intensive topical steroids. Lift flap, irrigate bed and flap with BSS. Wipe gently with a moistened sponge. Follow-up in 24–48 h
Stage 4	Aggregation of inflammatory cells and increased collagenase activity resulting in fluid collection, bullae formation, stromal melting, and corneal scarring. Appearance of corrugated "mud cracks". Irregular astigmatism, hyperopic shift, and decreased BCVA	Intensive topical steroids Lifting the flap could still be considered if recognized in the acute stage. If scarring occurs, then treatment is individualized. Better to avoid this stage by early identification of stage 3

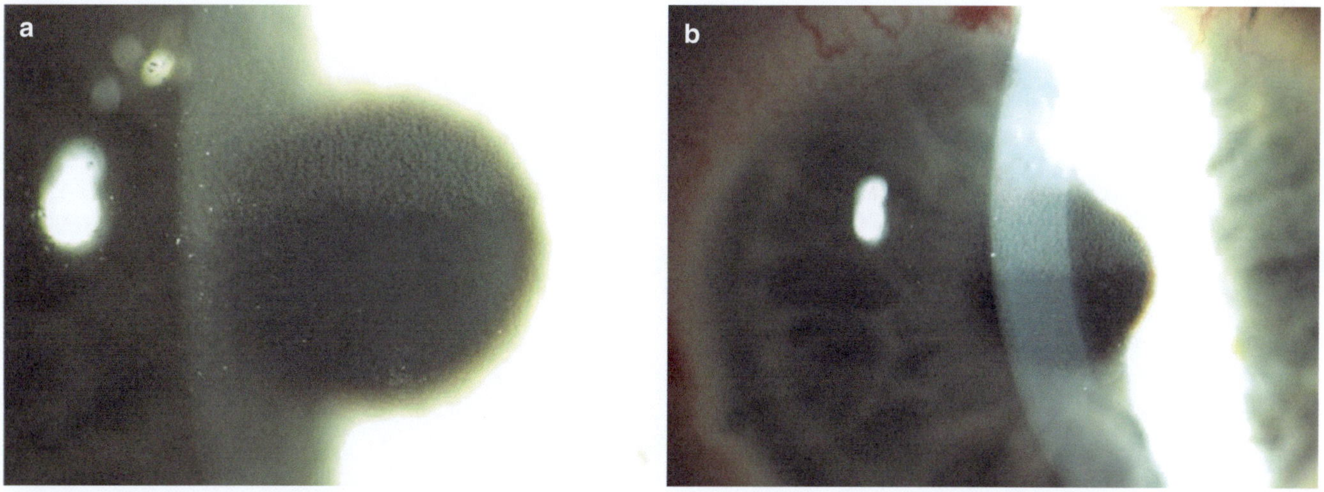

Fig. 11.1 Stage 1 DLK

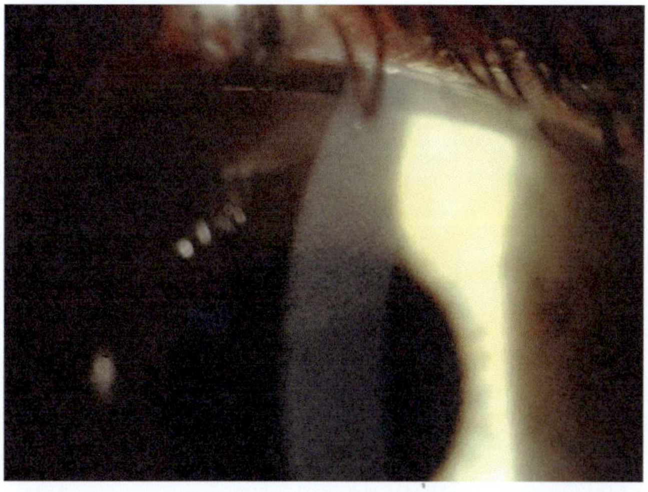

Fig. 11.2 Powdery infiltrates

Core message: Presence of cellular clumping warrants urgent surgical intervention to avoid progression to stromal melting and scarring.

Case: Patient seen next day following uncomplicated LASIK procedure (Fig. 11.8).

Exam: Stage 2 DLK; diffuse white granular cells with waves of increasing density across the central visual axis in the form of "sands of Sahara" (Fig. 11.7a, b).

Management: Intensive topical corticosteroid therapy with close follow-up.

Core message: DLK is also known as the "sands of Sahara" syndrome due to the appearance of waves of increasing cell density.

Case: Asymptomatic patients presenting for follow-up day 1 after LASIK surgery (Fig. 11.9).

Exam: Patient 1: Oily deposits on the interface corresponding to meibomian gland secretions (Fig. 11.9a).

Patient 2: Stage 1 DLK with whitish looking flap border (Fig. 11.9b).

Management: Patient 1: Observation

Patient 2: Increase topical steroid application

Core message: Meibomian gland secretions look like oil droplets that are well defined; it does not progress nor it affects the vision. It will never extend beyond the flap and tend to resolve within a few months.

Cases: Patient presented with light sensitivity and blurry vision day 1 following LASIK procedure (Fig. 11.10).

Exam: Stage 3 DLK with a horizontal line of inflammatory cells; the inflammation extends inferiorly to the flap edge (Fig. 11.10a).

Management: Flap lift and irrigation was performed on day 1 and patient given topical corticosteroids every 1 h with close observation. Inflammation decreased on day 2 postop (Fig. 11.10b), day 5 (Fig. 11.10c) and day 10 (Fig. 11.10d).

Core message: Presence of a large and dense clump of infiltrates warrants urgent surgical intervention to avoid progression to stromal melting and scarring.

Cases: Patient 1 presenting for a burning sensation and blurry vision 1 day after LASIK surgery.

Patient 2 presenting with mild discomfort after LASIK (Fig. 11.11).

Exam: Patient 1: A comma-shaped epithelial defect across the nasal border of the flap (Fig. 11.11a) with associated diffuse whitish cellular infiltration in the flap interface underlying the defect. Positive fluorescein staining of the epithelial defect with no staining over the diffuse lamellar keratitis area (Fig. 11.11b).

Patient 2: A healing peripheral epithelial defect surrounded by a stage 1 DLK (Fig. 11.11c, d).

Management: Treat epithelial defects with generous lubrication and DLK with topical steroid drops every hour. BCLs may be applied for larger epithelial defect.

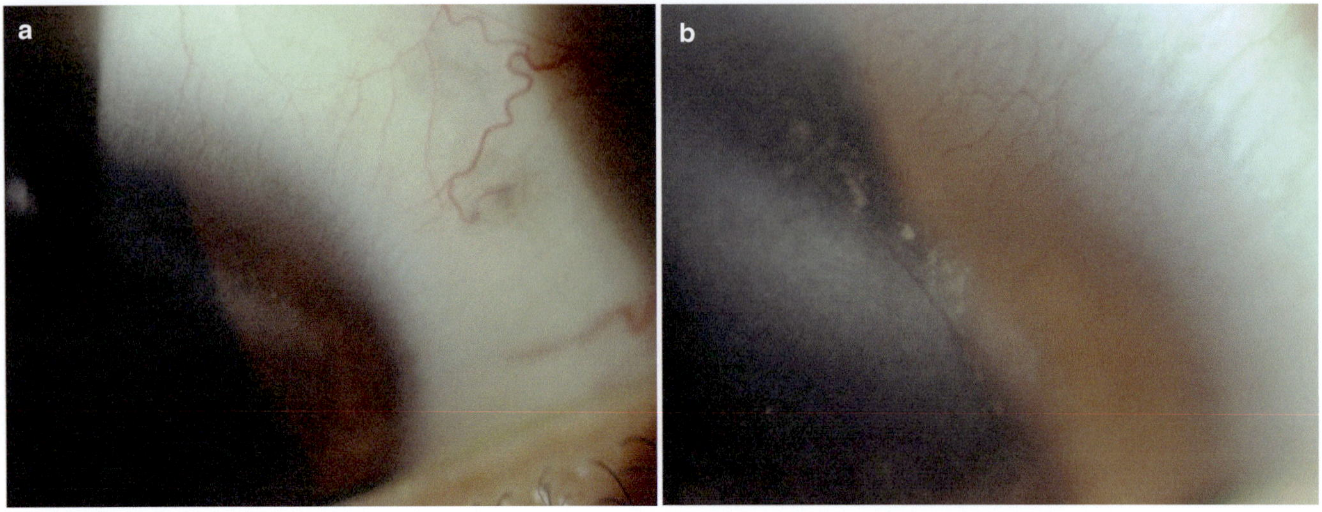

Fig. 11.3 DLK, or not?

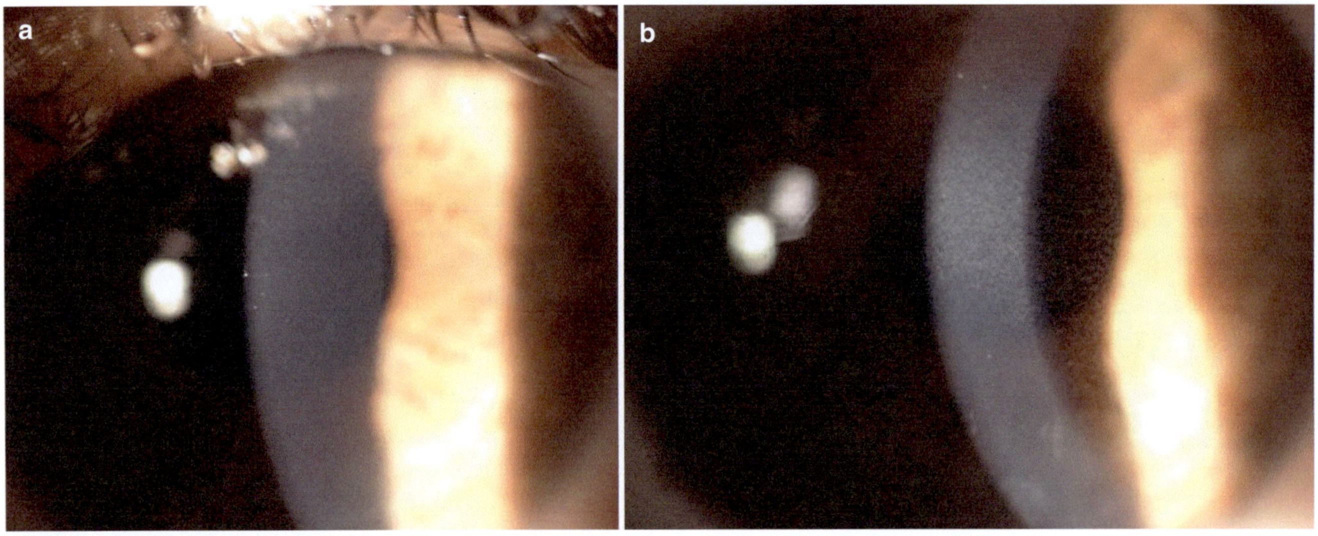

Fig 11.4 Progression to stage 2 DLK

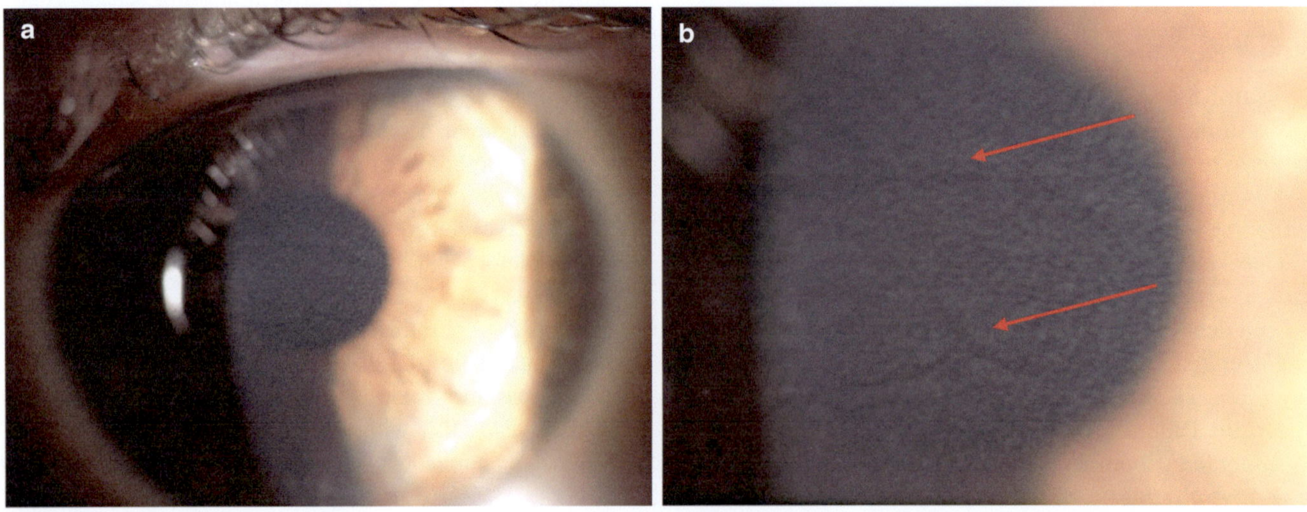

Fig. 11.5 Stage 2 DLK with microfolds

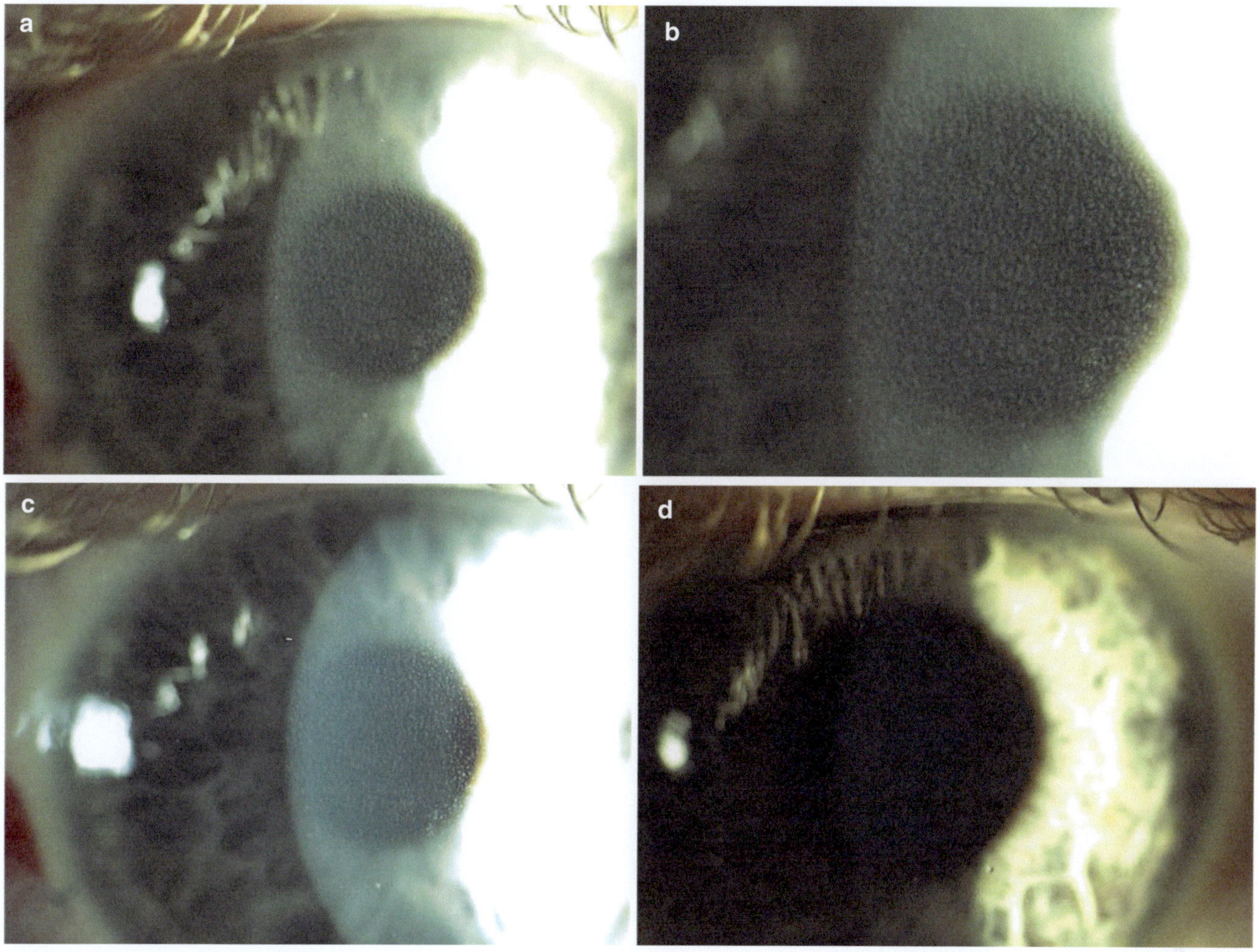

Fig. 11.6 Healing of stage 2 DLK

Core message: Presence of epithelial defects increases the risk of developing diffuse lamellar keratitis and epithelial ingrowth.

Case: A 30-year-old patient presented with blurry vision 1 day following a LASIK procedure (Fig. 11.12).

Exam: Dense white central stromal and flap opacification noted with cracked glass appearance (Fig. 11.12a).

Management: The patient was given topical and PO steroids. The cornea cleared progressively in 3 months leaving a central scar (Fig. 11.12b–e).

Case: 8 days following LASIK procedure, patient who underwent procedure elsewhere presented with blurry vision and light sensitivity (Fig. 11.13).

Exam: Central corneal stromal flap opacification with an overlying epithelial defect. Central stage 4 diffuse lamellar keratitis was suspected.

Management: Topical moxifloxacin and prednisolone were started and cornea healed with residual central scarring.

Extra Illustrations

See Figs. 11.14, 11.15, 11.16, 11.17 and 11.18.

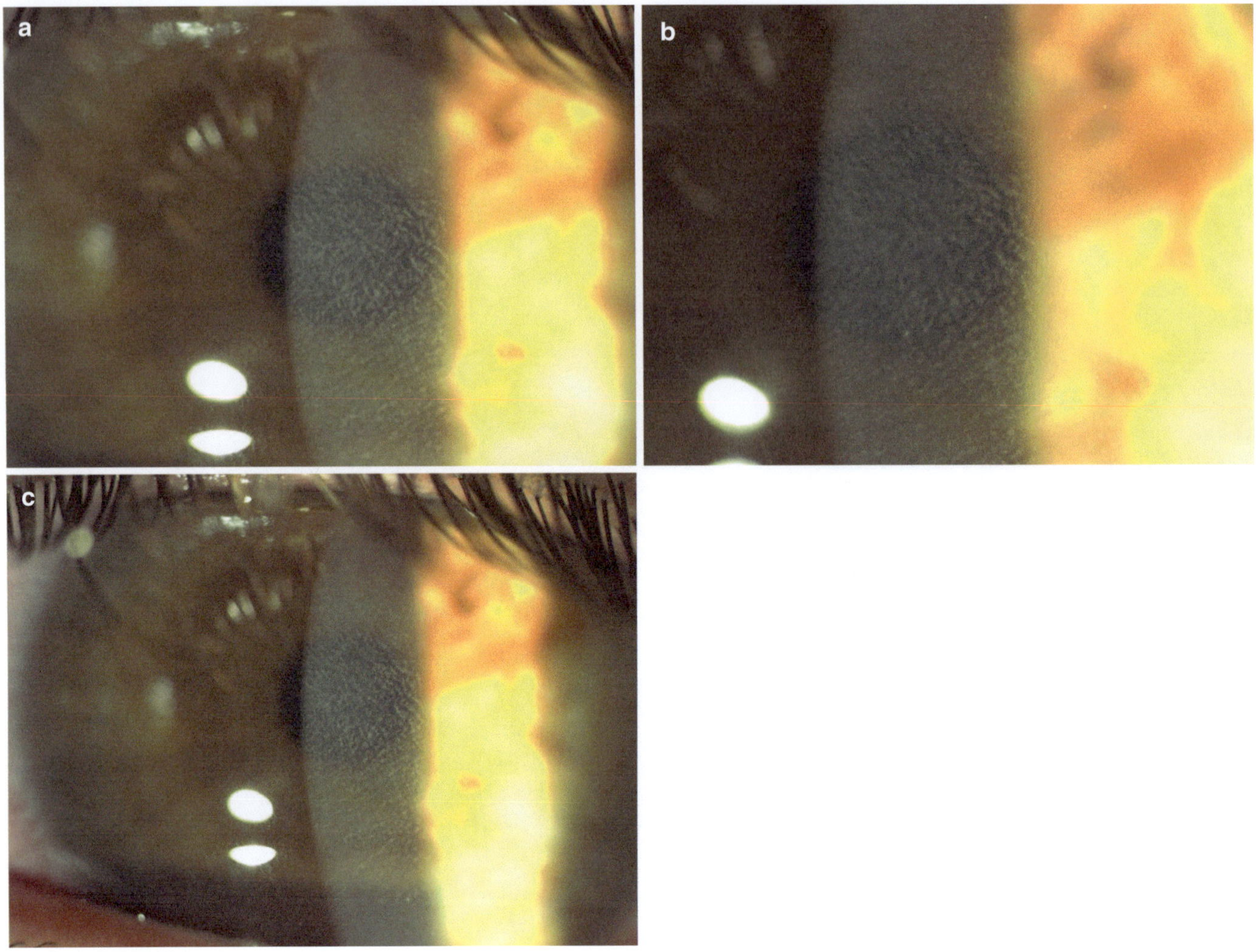

Fig. 11.7 Traumatic DLK

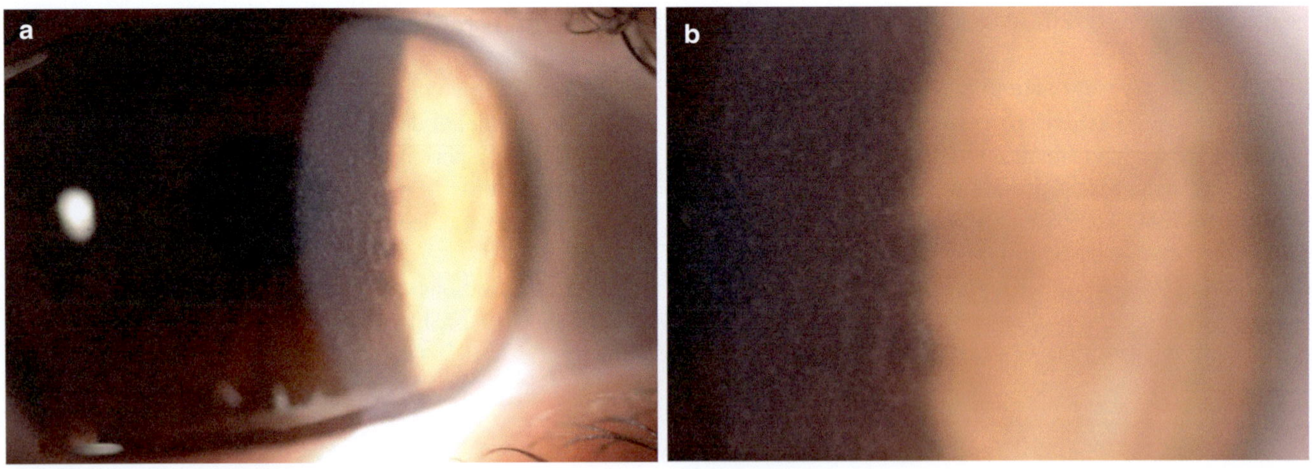

Fig. 11.8 Sands of Sahara

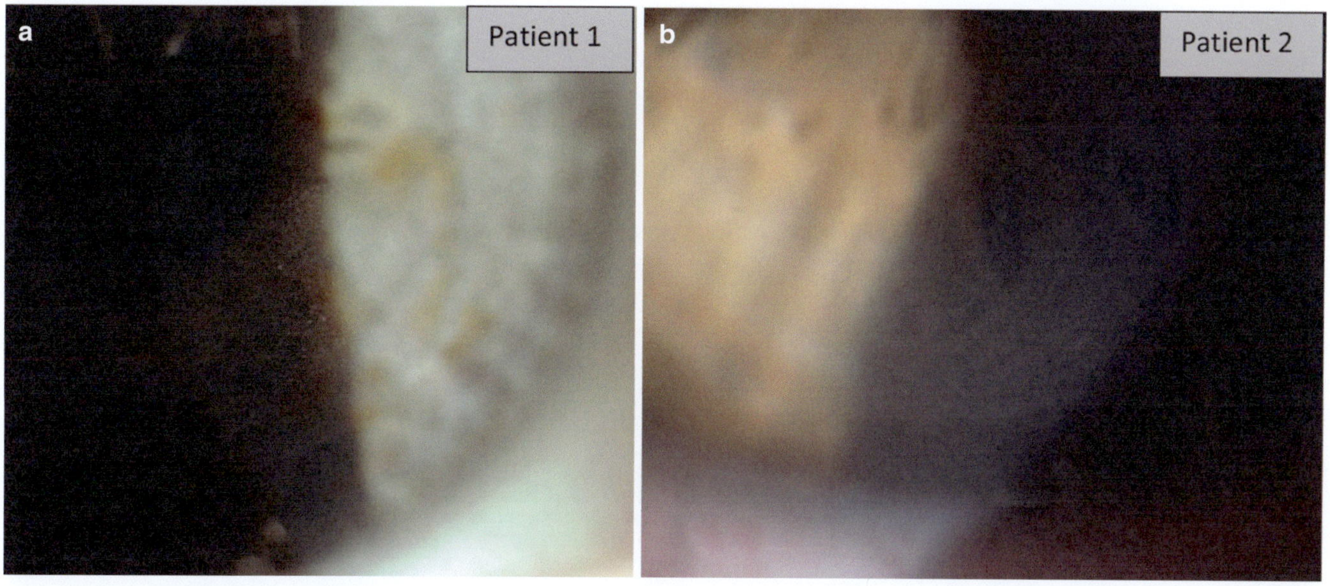

Fig. 11.9 Interface deposits vs. DLK

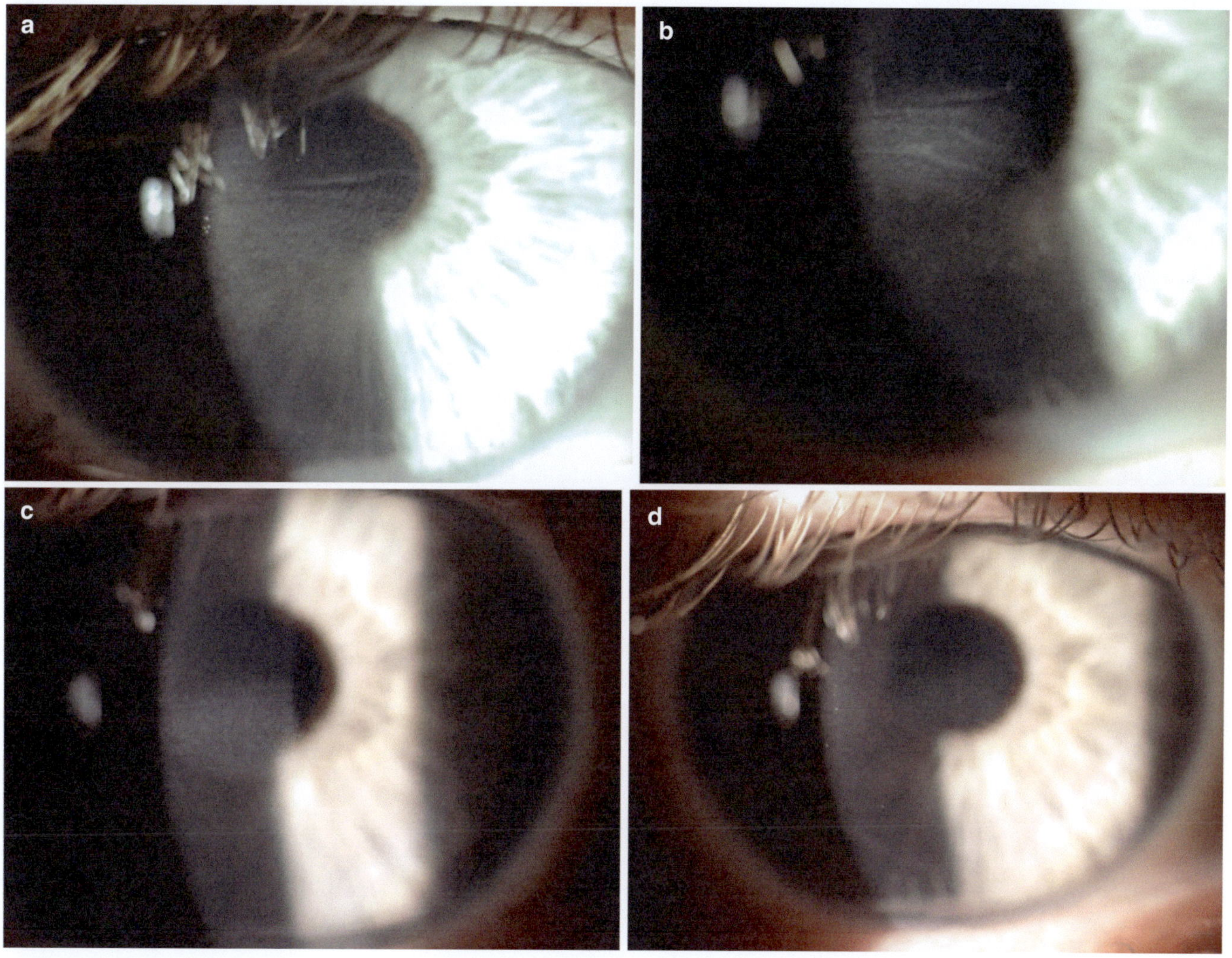

Fig. 11.10 Horizontal clumps

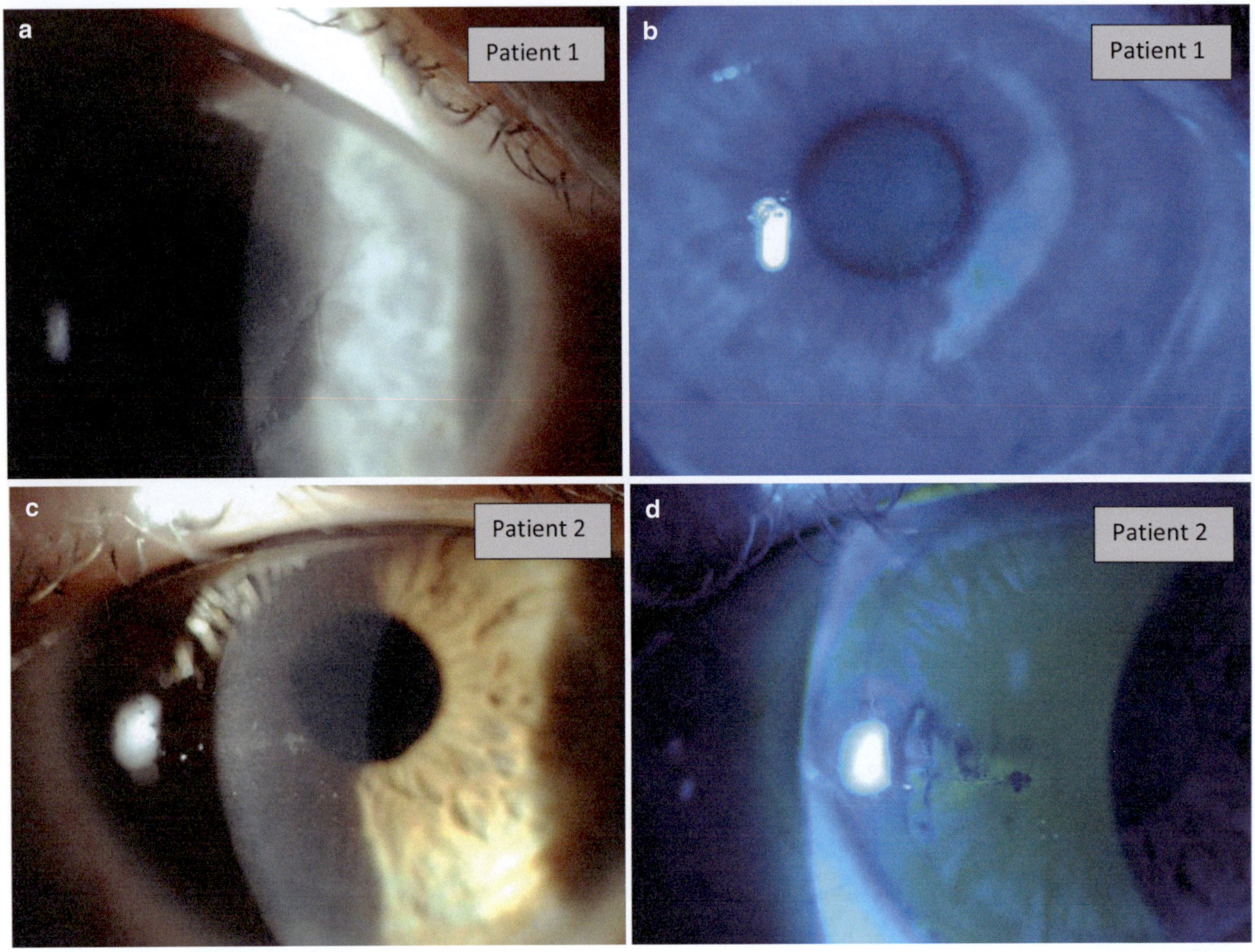

Fig. 11.11 Epithelial defects

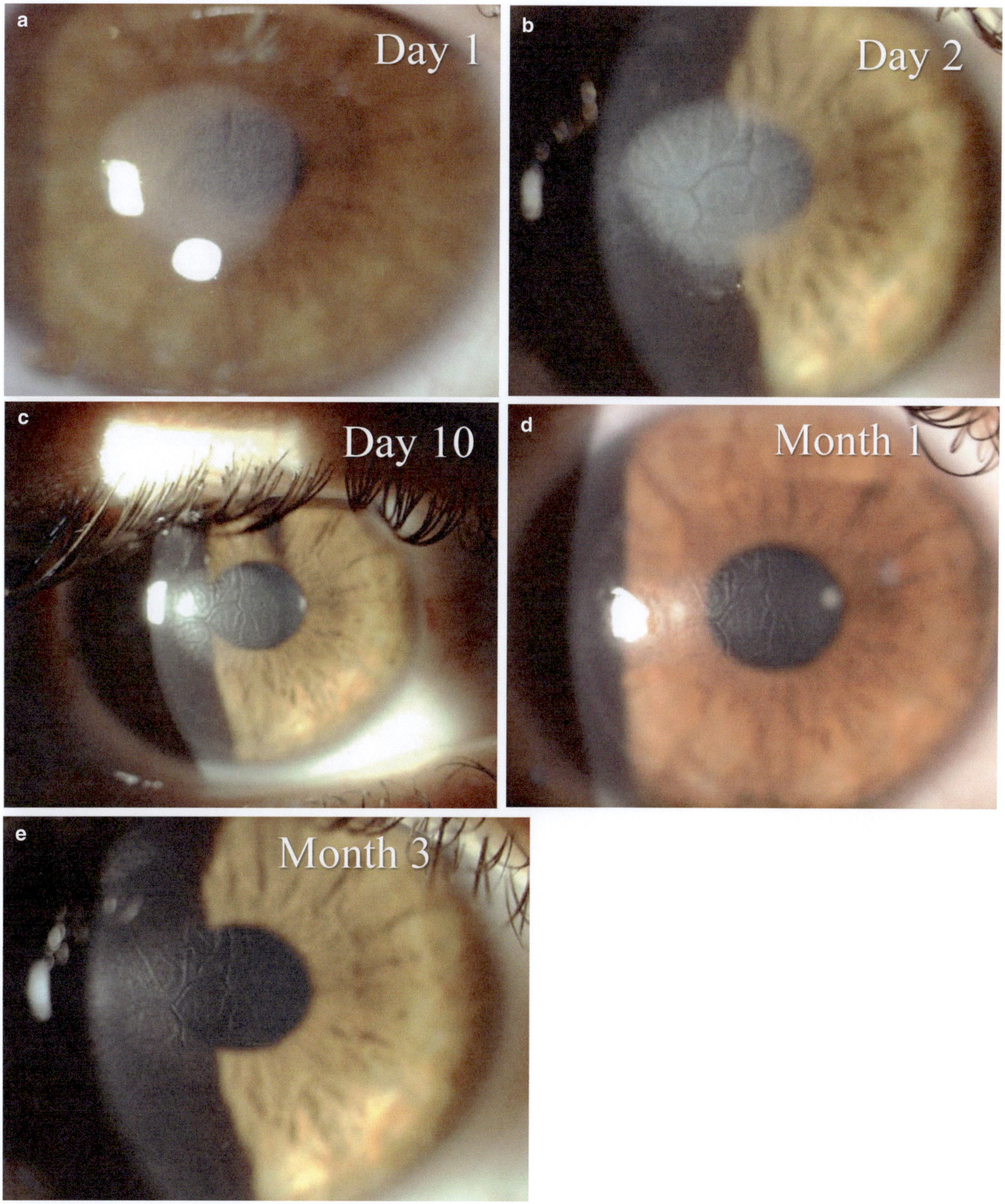

Fig. 11.12 Stage 4 DLK

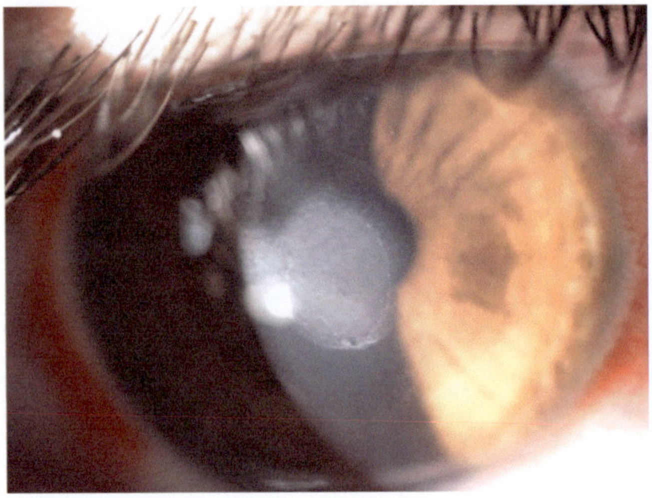

Fig. 11.13 Central corneal infiltrate (*Courtesy of Suphi Taneri, MD. Augenzentrum am St. Franziskus-hospital Münster, Münster, Germany*)

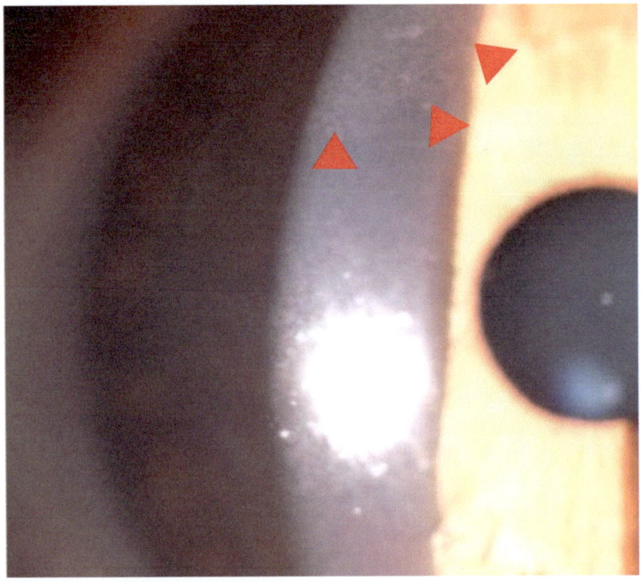

Fig. 11.14 Stage 1 DLK, white faint inflammatory cells in the periphery, not reaching the central visual axis ***(red arrowheads)***

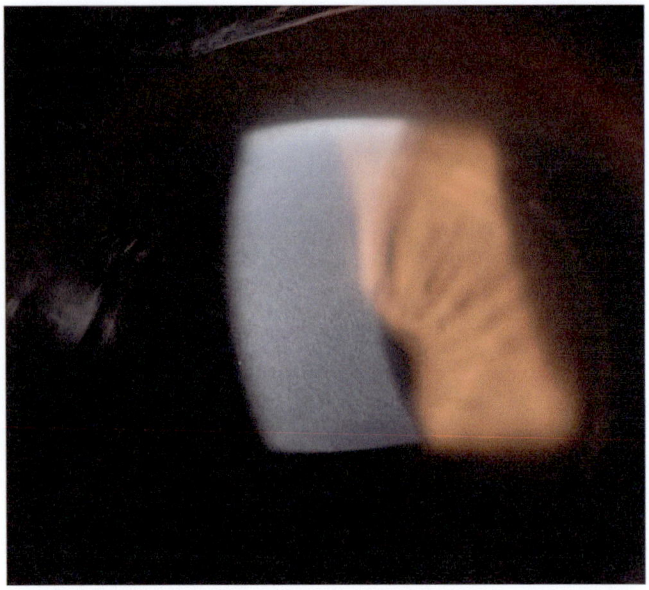

Fig. 11.15 Stage 2 DLK, granular cells involving the visual axis

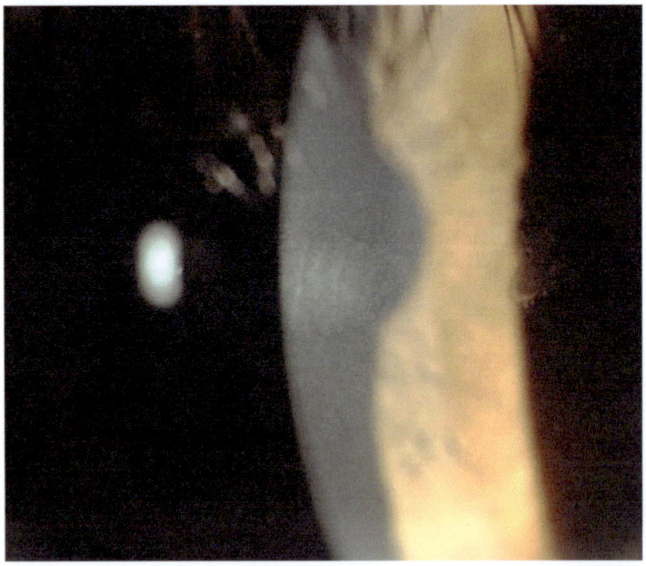

Fig. 11.16 Stage 3 DLK with dense white infiltrate involving the visual axis

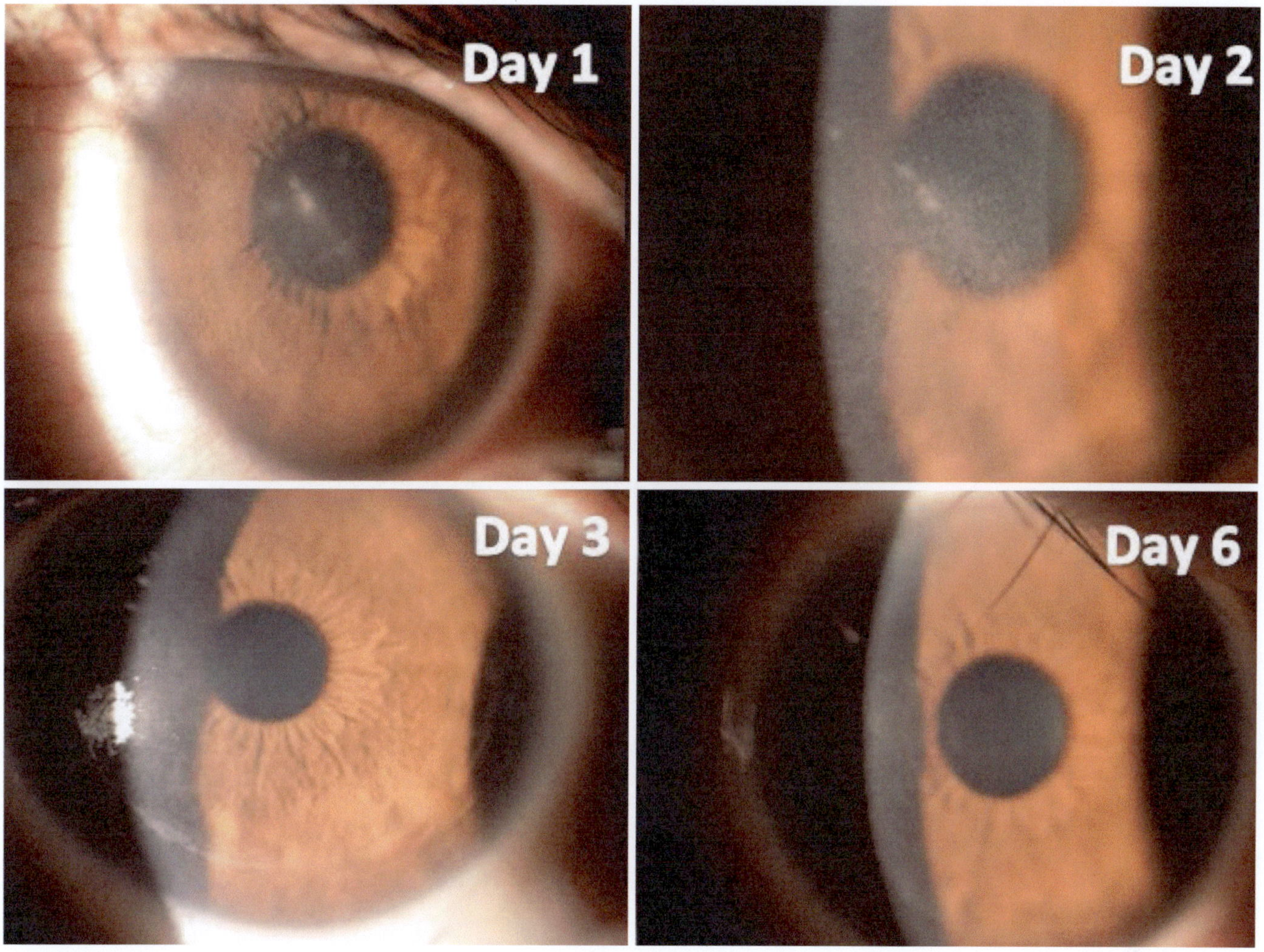

Fig. 11.17 Timeline showing Stage 3 DLK healing following flap lift and irrigation

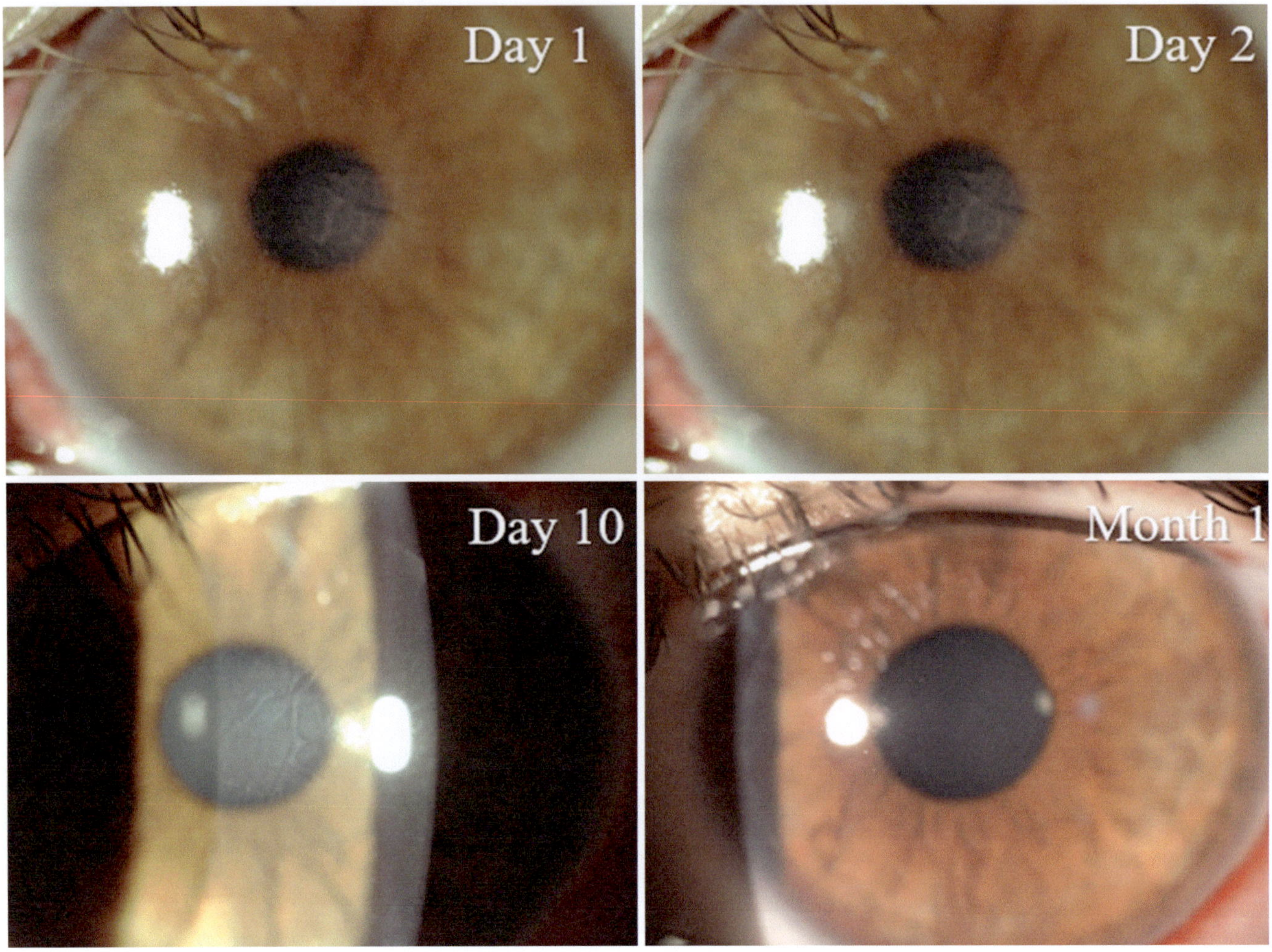

Fig. 11.18 Timeline showing stage 4 DLK healing following topical and oral steroid treatment

Take-Home Message

- Early postoperative follow-up and close observation are necessary to identify and treat diffuse lamellar keratitis.
- Diffuse lamellar keratitis progresses from stage 1 to stage 2 through the central migration of the cellular infiltrates.
- Most of the stage 1–2 diffuse lamellar keratitis will resolve with intensive topical corticosteroid treatment.
- Presence of large cellular clumping should be urgently managed with a flap lift and irrigation to prevent stromal melting and scarring. Cultures can be taken in these cases if there is a high suspicion for infectious keratitis.
- Epithelial defects increased risk of diffuse lamellar keratitis. Surgeons should be careful not to induce intraoperative epithelial defect and to avoid epithelial debridement in the early postoperative period.
- In the femtosecond era, stage 4 is an uncommon occurrence, and treatment is dependent upon individual cases and disease severity. In cases where severe melting is identified, lifting the flap can be complicated with flap perforation and epithelial ingrowth. Therefore, it is advisable to avoid lifting the flap in central stage 4 DLK with significant melting.

References

1. Linebarger EJ, Hardten DR, Lindstrom RL. Diffuse lamellar keratitis: diagnosis and management. J Cataract Refract Surg. 2000;26(7):1072–7.
2. de Paula FH, Khairallah CG, Niziol LM, Musch DC, Shtein RM. Diffuse lamellar keratitis after laser in situ keratomileusis with femtosecond laser flap creation. J Cataract Refract Surg. 2012;38(6):1014–9.
3. Sharma N, Vajpayee RB, Sullivan L, Melki S. Step by step LASIK surgery. 1st ed. New York: CRC Press; 2005. p. 190–2.
4. Bühren J, Baumeister M, Kohnen T. Diffuse lamellar keratitis after laser in situ keratomileusis imaged by confocal microscopy. Ophthalmology. 2001;108(6):1075–81.
5. Das S, Garg P, Mullick R, Annavajjhala S. Keratitis following laser refractive surgery: clinical spectrum, prevention and management. Indian J Ophthalmol. 2020;68(12):2813–8.
6. Melki S, Fava M. Cornea and refractive atlas of clinical wisdom. Thorofare: SLACK Incorporated; 2011. p. 207–10.
7. Alio JL, Azar DT. Management of complications in refractive surgery. Cham: Springer; 2018. p. 61–7.
8. Sridhar MS, Rao SK, Vajpayee RB, Aasuri MK, Hannush S, Sinha R. Complications of laser-in-situ-keratomileusis. Indian J Ophthalmol. 2002;50(4):265–82.
9. Segev F, Mimouni M, Sela T, Munzer G, Kaiserman I. Risk factors for sporadic diffuse lamellar keratitis after microkeratome laser-assisted in situ keratomileusis: a retrospective large database analysis. Cornea. 2018;37(9):1124–9.
10. Moshirfar M, Durnford KM, Lewis AL, et al. Five-year incidence, management, and visual outcomes of diffuse lamellar keratitis after femtosecond-assisted LASIK. J Clin Med. 2021;10(14):3067.
11. Sahay P, Bafna RK, Reddy JC, Vajpayee RB, Sharma N. Complications of laser-assisted in situ keratomileusis. Indian J Ophthalmol. 2021;69(7):1658–69.

12 Miscellaneous Refractive Surgery Complications

Francesca Kahale, Wassef Chanbour, Samir A. Melki, and Jason Brenner

Case: Patient presented 1 day following LASIK surgery with decrease in her superior visual field (Fig. 12.1).

Exam: Slit lamp exam showed superior hemorrhage under the flap forming a paracentral clot (Fig. 12.1a).

Management: After observation for a week, the patient reported worsening of her symptoms. The exam showed inferior migration of the blood covering half of the visual axis (Fig. 12.1b). Decision was made to irrigate the underside of the flap and the cornea cleared completely on day 1 following the irrigation (Fig. 12.1c).

Core message: Large superior blood clots resolve slowly and tend to move inferiorly under the flap.

Case: Scattered fine layer of red blood cells noted at the interface 1 day following LASIK procedure in two patients (Fig. 12.2a, b).

Management: Observation is acceptable and the corneas cleared in a few days.

Core message: Contrary to popular beliefs, red blood cells do not cause diffuse lamellar keratitis.

Case: Patient noted to have a white foreign body <1 mm ***(red arrow)*** at the flap interface; object is believed to be a sterile material from weck-cel (Fig. 12.3).

Management: Observation.

Core message: Inert and sterile foreign body material can be left under the flap.

Case: Two patients presented for yearly checkup following uncomplicated LASIK procedures (Fig. 12.4).

Exam: Inferior corneal neovascularization extending into the flap (**red arrow**) (Fig. 12.4a, b).

Management: Management of surface diseases (allergy, dry eye, etc.).

Core message: The cause for this neovascularization is unknown, but it is usually non progressive.

Case: An asymptomatic patient examined day 1 post LASIK (Fig. 12.5).

Exam: A Cilia was located in a small gap between the flap edge and the cornea (Fig. 12.5a).

Management: Cilia was removed with a forceps (Fig. 12.5b).

Case: Patient seen 1 day following a non-complicated LASIK procedure with an UCVA of 20/20 (Fig. 12.6).

Exam: Interface scattered oil deposits at the flap interface.

Management: Observation.

Core message: Interface Meibomian gland oil is typically not visually significant and will resolve spontaneously within weeks to months.

Case: Fiber material was noted at the mid peripheral flap interface in two patients following non-complicated LASIK procedures ***(red arrows)*** (Fig. 12.7a, b).

Management: Observation.

Case: Fiber material was noted at the flap interface and extruding to the surface (Fig. 12.8a).

Management: Fiber was removed as it can provide an entry point for germs (Fig. 12.8b, c).

Core message: Peripheral fibers are inert and can be left in place if it is small and completely covered by the flap. Larger fibers and fibers extruding through the flap edge should be removed.

Case: Patient with known ectasia post-LASIK presented with sudden onset of blurriness, pain, and photophobia (Fig. 12.9).

Exam: A localized circular area of corneal stromal and microcystic edema is noted without overlying epithelial defect (Fig. 12.9a, b).

Management: Topical sodium chloride, aqueous suppression, and steroid leads to resolution. Penetrating keratoplasty may be needed for visual rehabilitation.

F. Kahale
Mass Eye and Ear infirmary, Boston, MA, USA

W. Chanbour (✉)
Department of Ophthalmology and Visual Neurosciences, University of Minnesota, Minneapolis, MN, USA

S. A. Melki · J. Brenner
Boston Vision, Department of Ophthalmology, Harvard Medical School, Boston, MA, USA
e-mail: Melki@bostonvision.com; brenner@bostonvision.com

S. A. Melki et al. (eds.), *Refractive Surgery Atlas*, https://doi.org/10.1007/978-3-031-60661-8_12

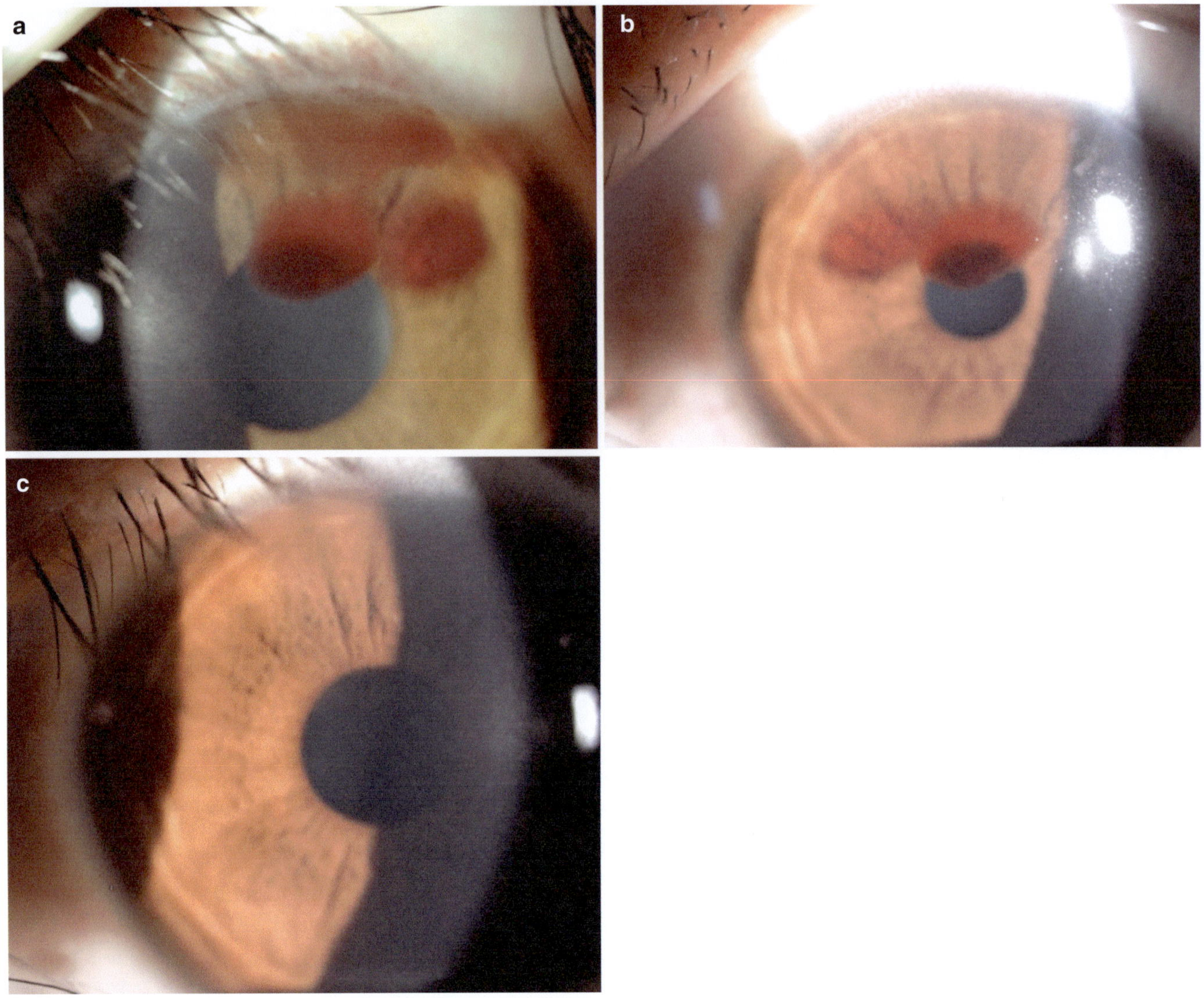

Fig. 12.1 Blood clot

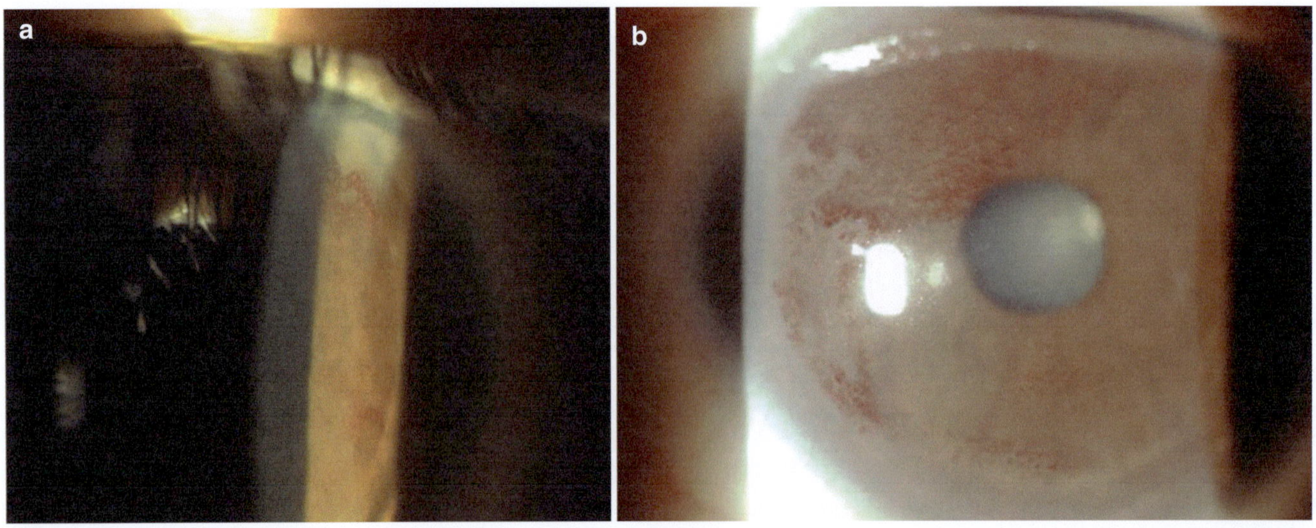

Fig. 12.2 Interface red blood cells

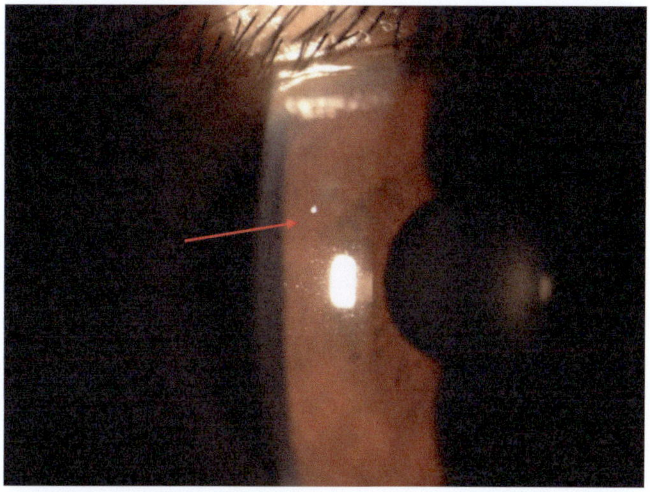

Fig. 12.3 Interface foreign body

Core message: Clinical exam should be correlated with patient clinical history as corneal hydrops can be mistaken for infectious keratitis.

Case: Patient with known post-LASIK ectasia presented with corneal edema leading to fluid accumulation in the interface and leakage of aqueous around the flap edge (Fig. 12.10).

Management: Topical sodium chloride, aqueous suppression, steroids, and corneal suturing failed to improve the swelling. Patient was operated with a penetrating keratoplasty eventually.

Core message: Hydrops in patients with post LASIK ectasia may present with interface fluid rather than the typical picture of white edematous cornea following hydrops in keratoconus.

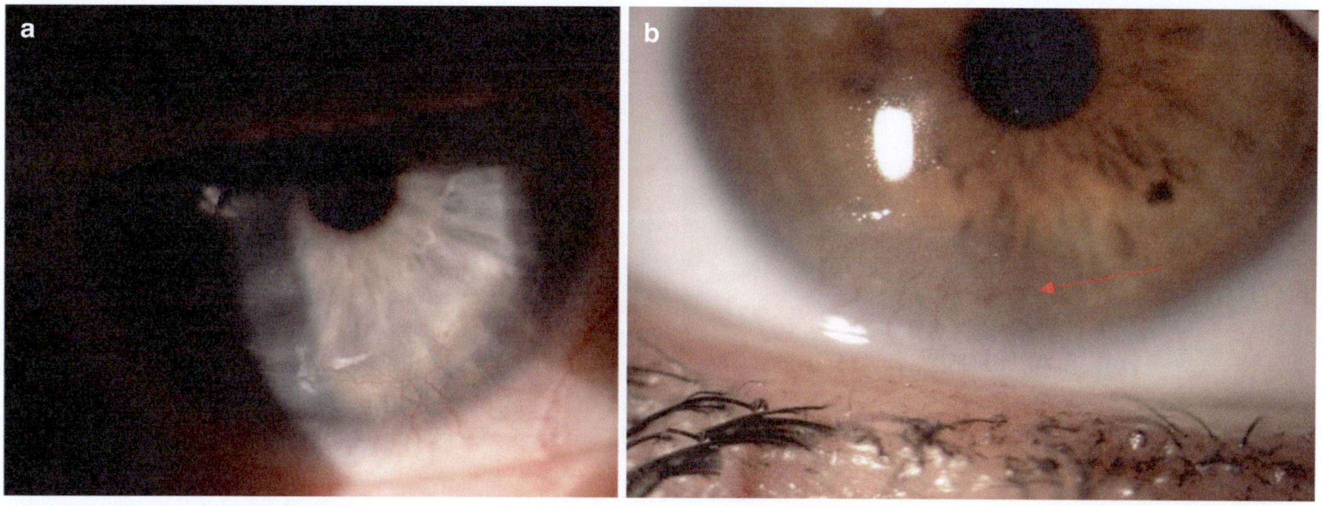

Fig. 12.4 Peripheral neovascularisation

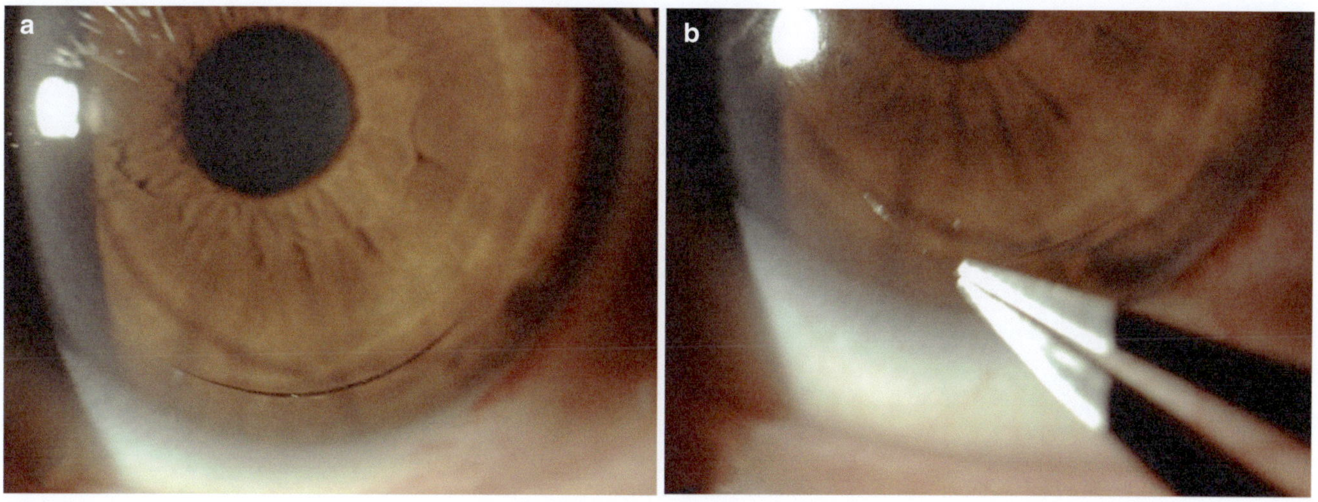

Fig. 12.5 Cilia

Case: Patient presented to clinic with progressive blurry vision after his intracore/LASIK procedure 8 years ago (Fig. 12.11).

Exam: Concentric ring corneal scarring related to the intracore treatment (Fig 12.11a), inferior corneal thinning due to post-LASIK ectasia (Fig 12.11b).

Management: Contact lens fitting to improve vision and CXL if patient has progression on topography.

Case: A 50-year-old patient was previously treated for recurrent erosion syndrome, due to a cat scratch, with 2 PTK and 1 PRK (last surgery 2 years prior). He presented to the clinic with persistent sharp pain in his right eye that was out of proportion to the physical exam (Fig. 12.12).

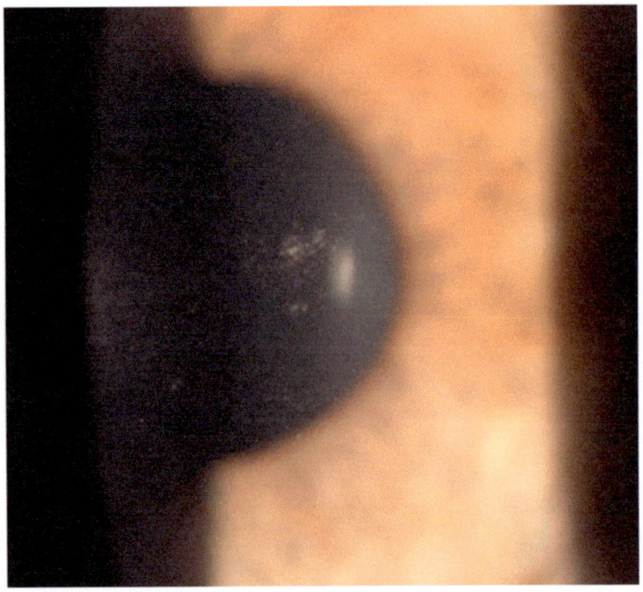

Fig. 12.6 Meibomian gland secretions

Exam: Confocal microscopy showing irregular branching pattern of the superficial sub basal nerve plexus in the right eye (Fig. 12.12a) compared to the normal left eye (Fig. 12.12b).

Management: The patient was given a trial of all the following treatments in addition to lubrication with mild improvement of his symptoms:

- Serum tears.
- Cyclosporine and lifitegrast eye drops.
- Punctal cautery.
- Cenegermin eye drops.
- Periorbital injections for pain control.
- Oral gabapentin, pregabalin, trazodone, and benzonatate.
- Scleral lenses.

Patient eventually felt better only with the intermittent use of bandage contact lens.

Core Message: Corneal neuralgia is one of the rare but drastic complications post refractive surgery. Patients have debilitating symptoms and increased risk of suicide. The response to therapy is variable between patients but all the previously mentioned treatments can be tried to improve their symptoms.

Case:

A 39-year-old lady with non-visually significant mild granular dystrophy and myopia underwent myopic LASIK 3 years ago to correct −4.5 D sphere in both eyes. She presented with gradual decreased vision more in the left eye for the past few months. Her BCVA was 20/20 in the right eye and 20/40 in the left eye. Her mother and younger sister also had mild non-visually significant granular dystrophy with 20/20 corrected vision in both eyes (Fig. 12.13).

Exam: At presentation, numerous confluent dense granular opacities are seen centrally in the interface between the flap and residual stromal bed of the right (Fig. 12.13a, c) and

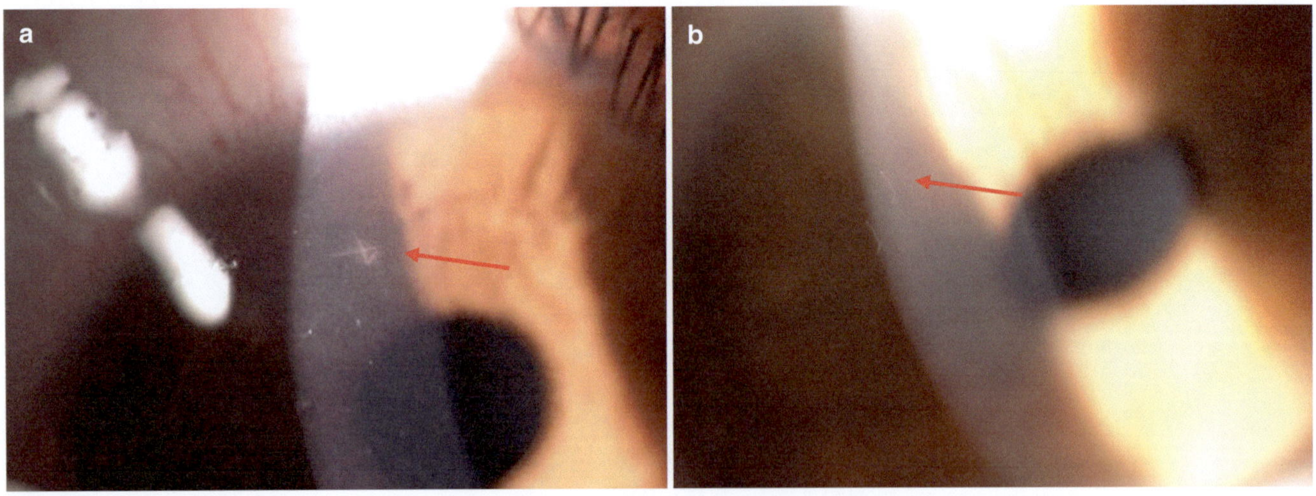

Fig. 12.7 Interface fiber

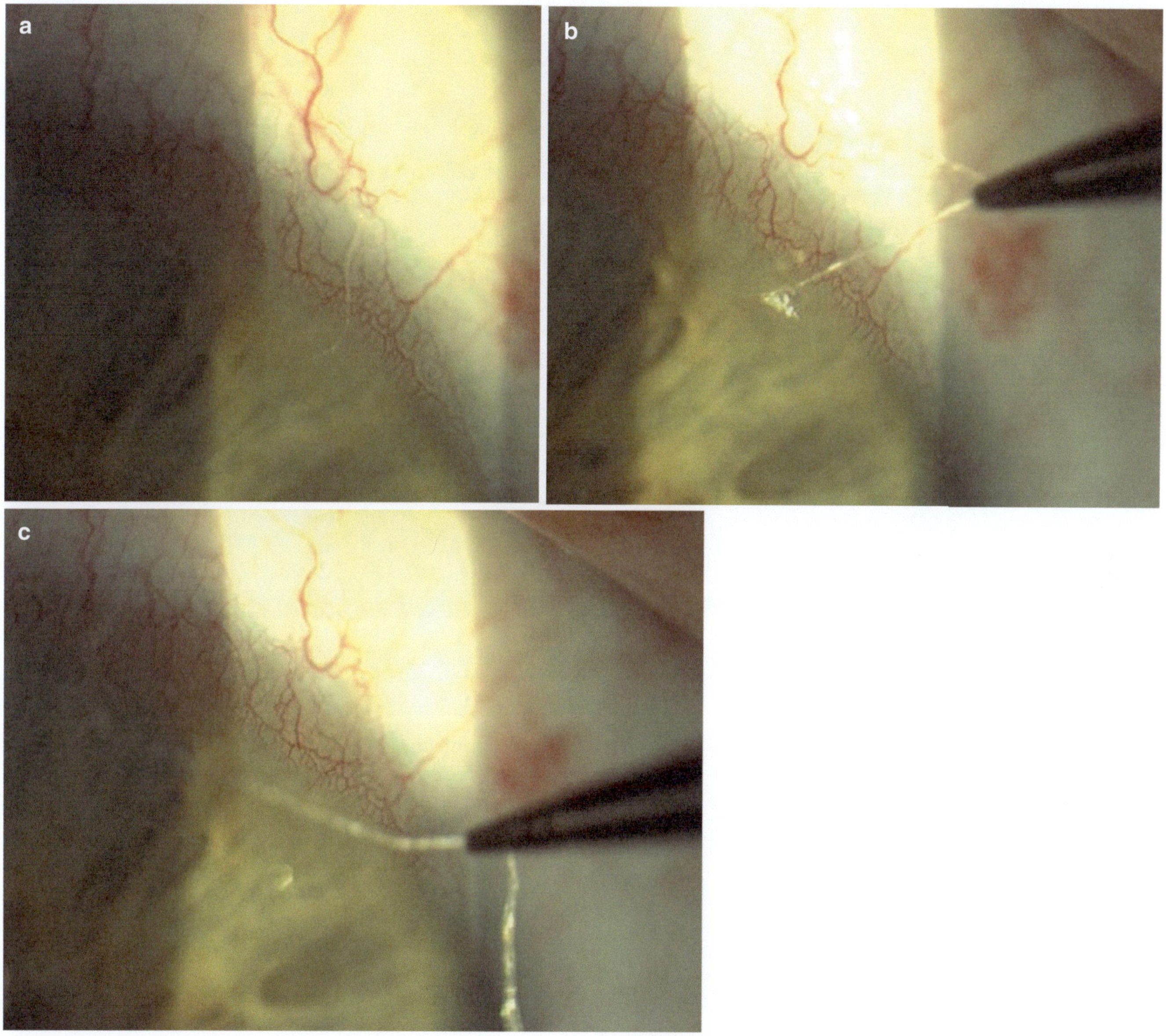

Fig. 12.8 Interface fiber

left eye (Fig. 12.13b, d). Unoperated right and left eye of the patient's mother had very few discrete granular lesions (Fig. 12.13e, f). Confocal microscopy showed interface deposits in the right and left eye of the operated patient respectively (Fig. 12.13g, h).

Management: Given the relatively good vision, observation is recommended for now. Otherwise, PTK may be considered to remove denser deposits.

Core message: Corneal dystrophies may worsen following LASIK procedures.

Case: Patient presented with blurry vision 2 months following a LASIK enhancement procedure, UDVA 20/80 (manifest refraction +1.25–0.75 × 135°, correctable to 20/30) (Fig. 12.14).

Exam: Topography showed inferior flattening (Fig. 12.14a). Multiple chronic chalazion were noted on the inferior palpebral conjunctiva (Fig. 12.14b).

Management: Lesions were excised and the topography improved 1 month later (Fig. 12.14c, d). UDVA improved to 20/25.

Case: Patient presenting for consult 20 years following a LASIK surgery. He is currently complaining of surface irritation. The patient had multiple unsuccessful retinal detachment surgeries. The latest was posterior pole vitrectomy, a

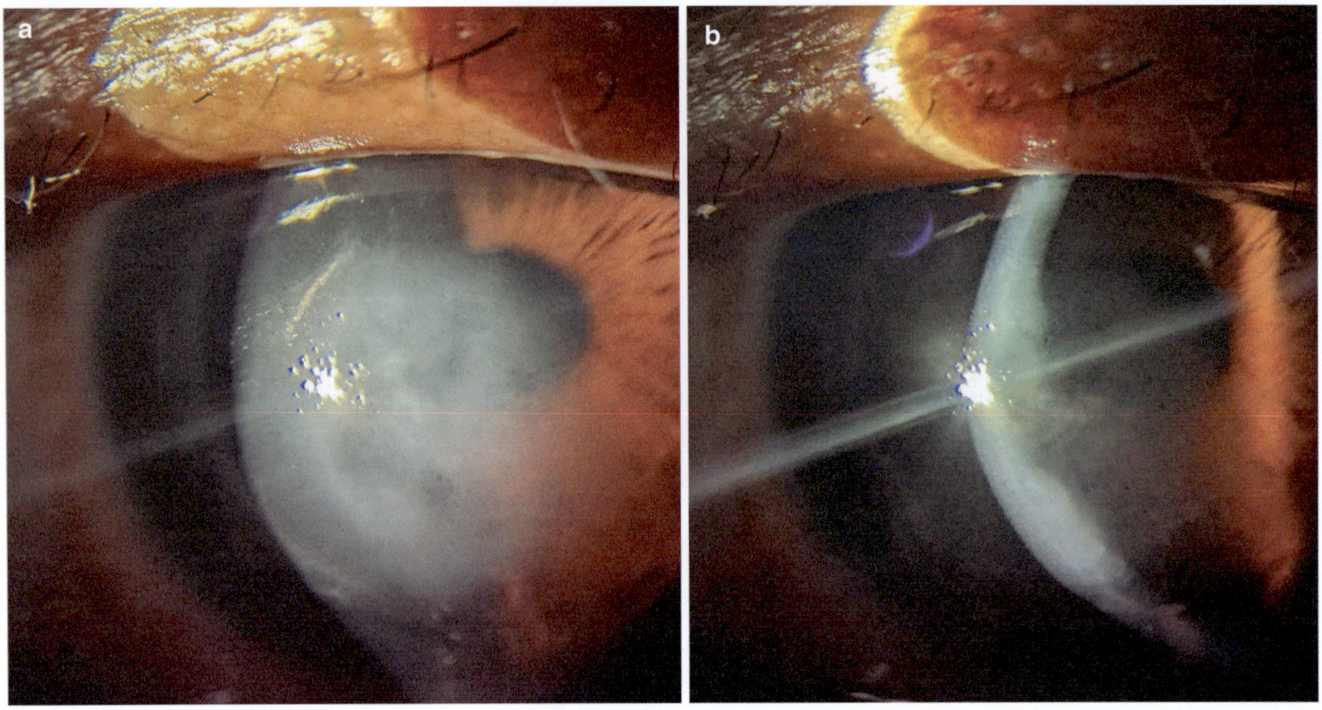

Fig. 12.9 Corneal hydrops in post-LASIK ectasia. (*Courtesy Jimmy Hu, MD. New York Eye and Ear Infirmary at Mt. Sinai, New York, USA*)

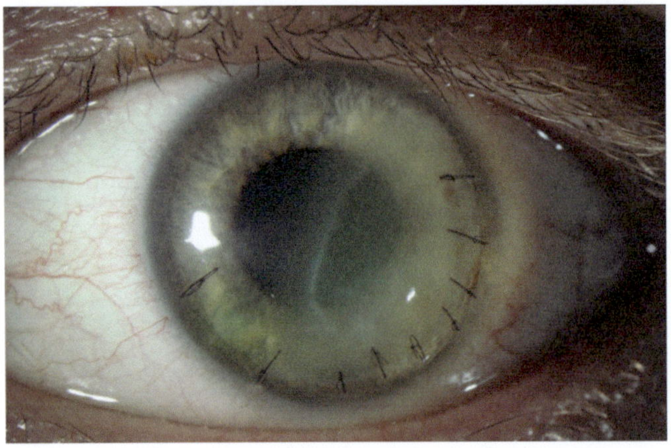

Fig. 12.10 Interface fluid in corneal hydrops. (*Courtesy of Joshua H. Hou, MD. University of Minnesota, Minnesota, USA*)

silicon oil injection. He had chronic retinal detachment and proliferative vitreoretinopathy (Fig. 12.15).

Exam: Diffusely calcified flap and peripheral cornea with inferior superficial keratitis.

Management: Topical lubricating drops and ointments. In case of worsening, EDTA can be used to remove the calcification or alternatively the flap can be amputated.

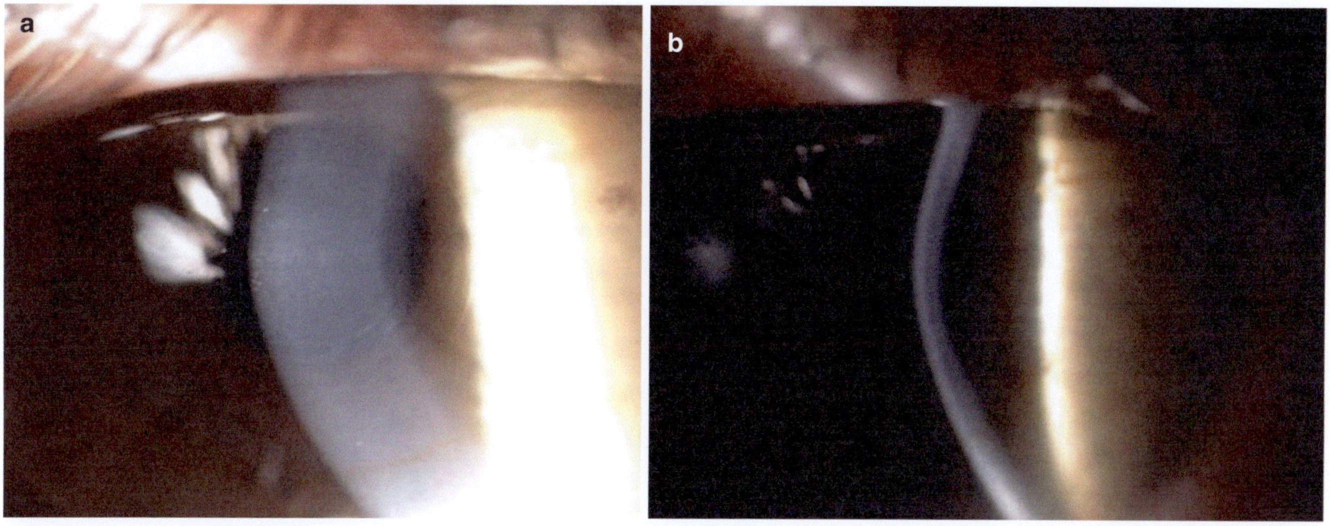

Fig. 12.11 Intracore. (*Courtesy of Suphi Taneri M.D. Augenzentrum am St. Franziskus Hospital Münster, Münster, Germany*)

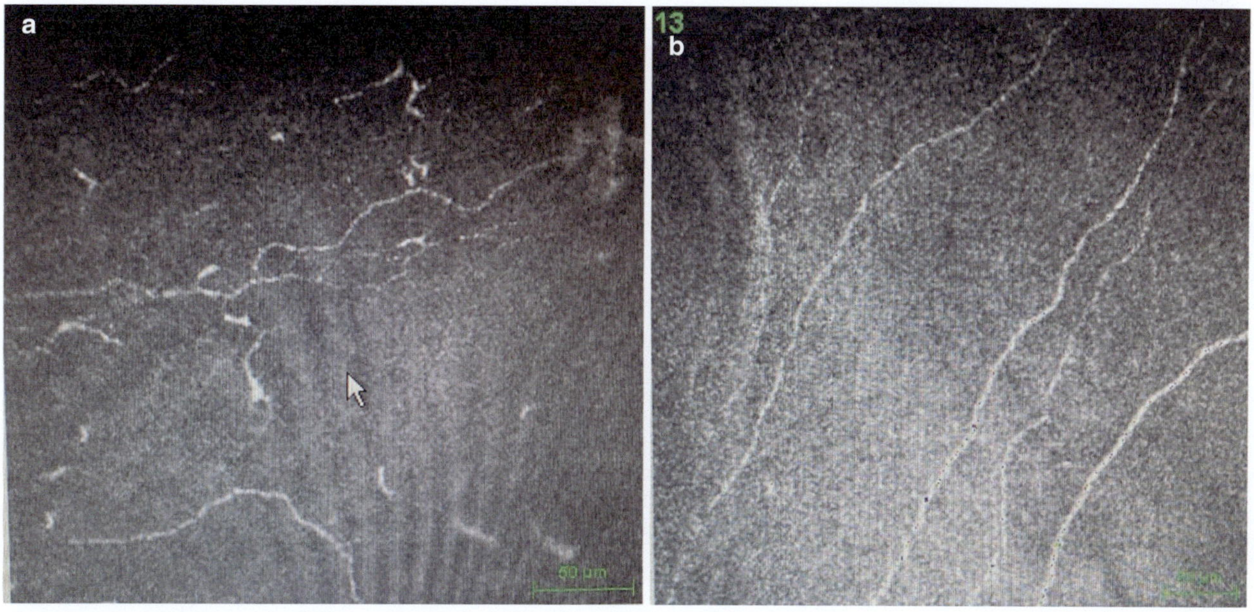

Fig. 12.12 Corneal neuralgia

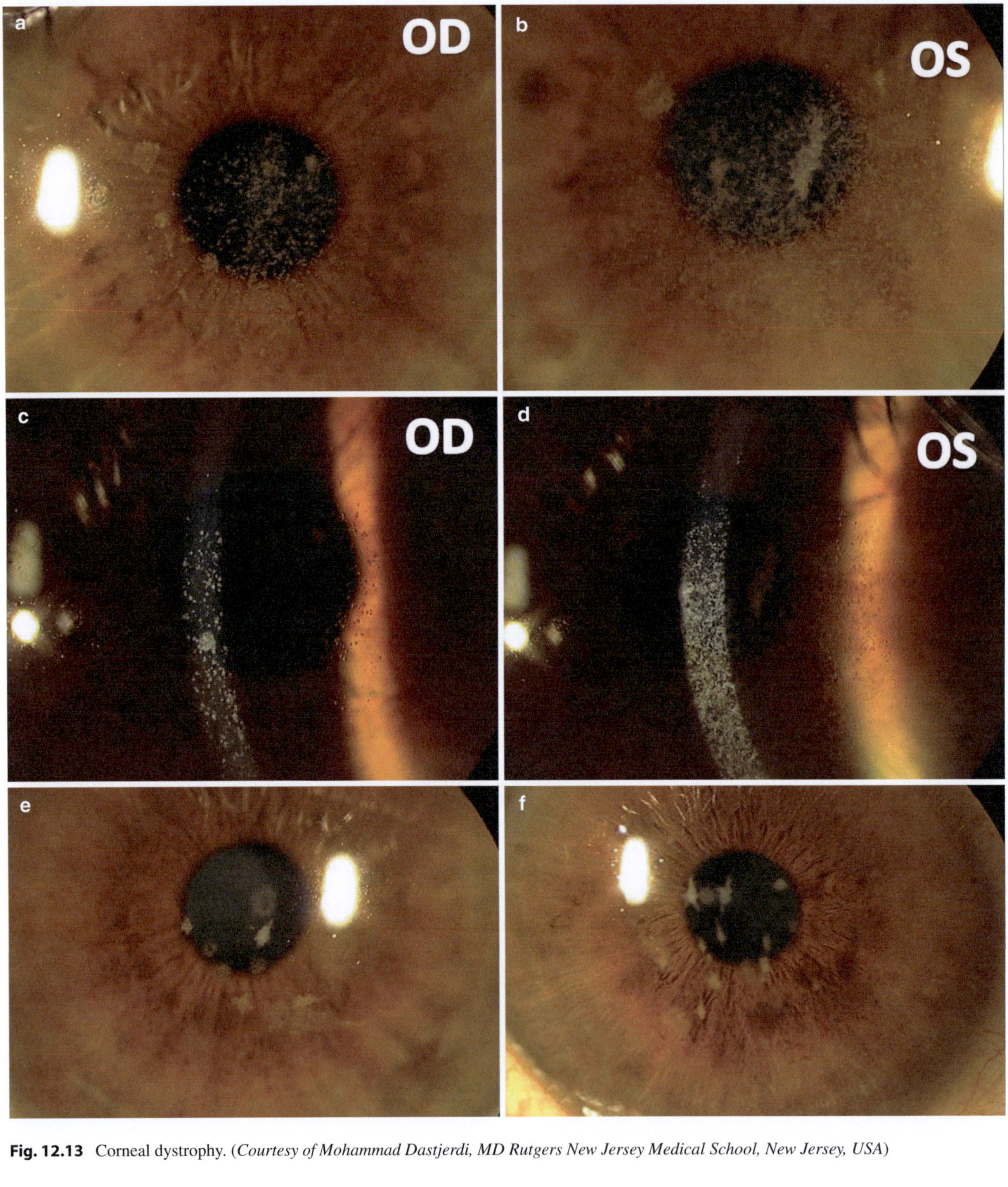

Fig. 12.13 Corneal dystrophy. (*Courtesy of Mohammad Dastjerdi, MD Rutgers New Jersey Medical School, New Jersey, USA*)

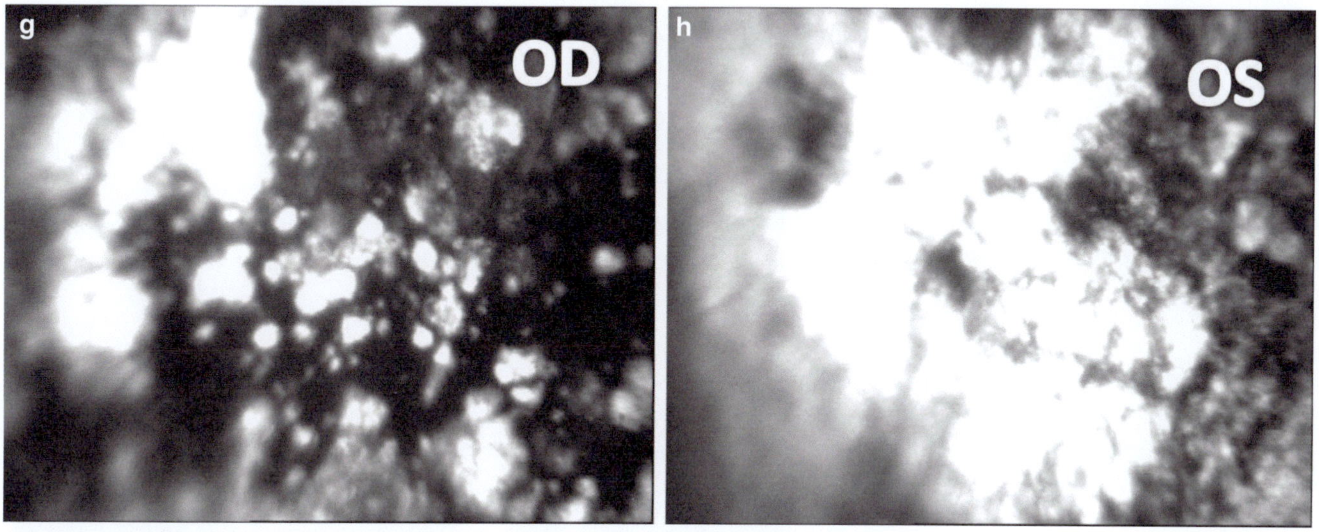

Fig. 12.13 (continued)

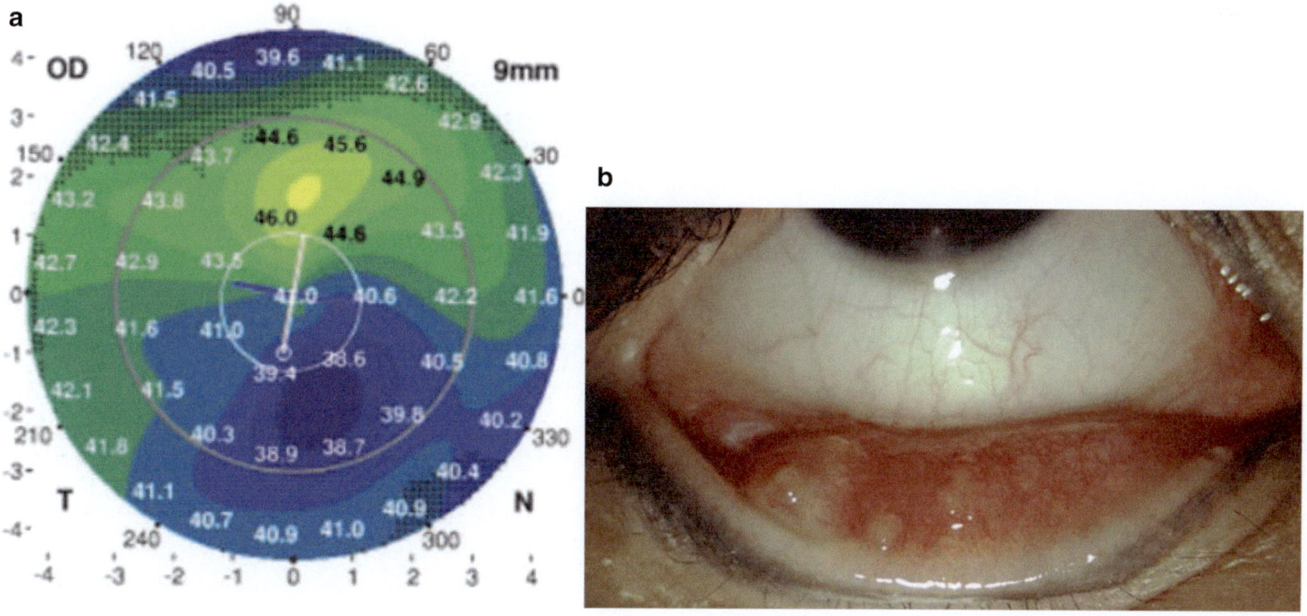

Fig. 12.14 Lid lesions induced irregular astigmatism. (*Chanbour, W., Brenner, J. and Melki, S. "Corneal irregularity after LASIK induced by eyelid disease," Journal of Refractive Surgery Case Reports, 2022; 2(1)*. Open Access article distributed under the terms of the Creative Commons Attribution - Non-Commercial 4.0 International)

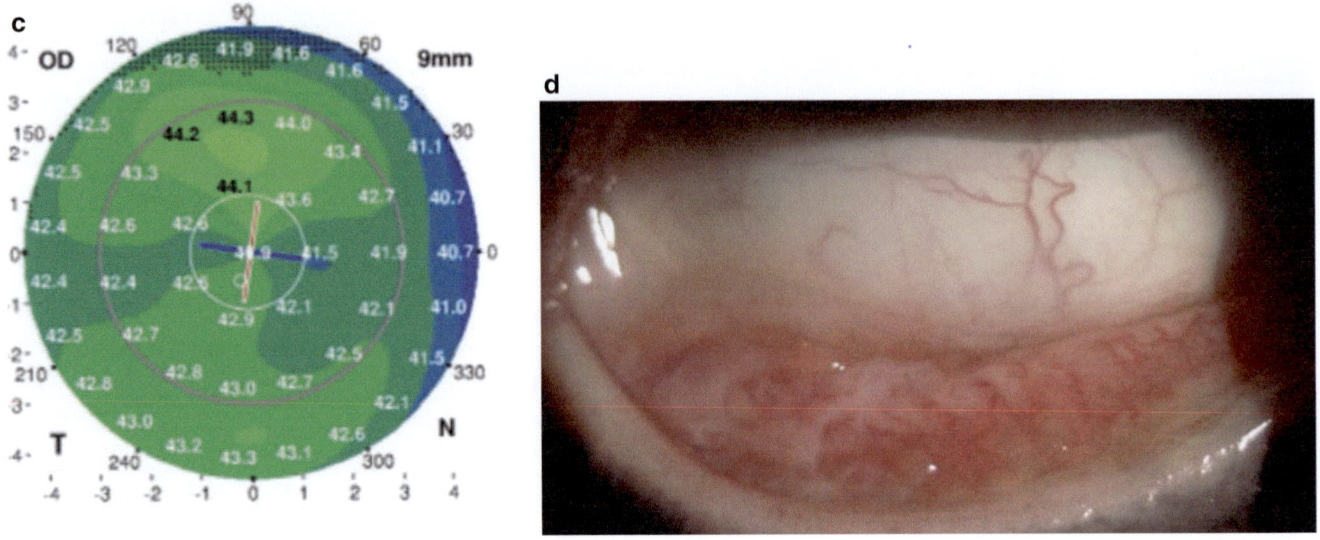

Fig. 12.14 (continued)

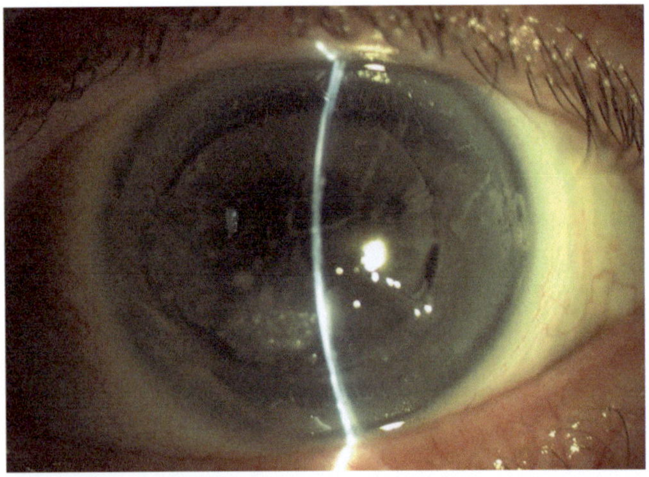

Fig. 12.15 Calcified flap

Take-Home Message

- Most of the non-metallic interface foreign body material (gauze, blood, fiber, etc.) are sterile and should be left in place to avoid additional surgical interventions and risks of LASIK complications (infections, epithelial ingrowth, flap dislocation, etc.).
- Sterile foreign body material should be removed if it is threatening the visual axis or extending outside the flap at the peripheral edge.
- Care should be taken to separate the surgical gauze and weck-cel from the flap lift instruments inside the surgical tray.
- Frequent intraoperative saline wash and flap interface irrigation are necessary in every LASIK procedure to avoid meibomian gland oil entrapment in the interface.
- Blood products do not cause diffuse lamellar keratitis.
- Managing surface diseases before and after LASIK procedures in addition to minimizing intraoperative trauma to the flap edge is advised to improve the epithelial healing and potentially prevent the occurrence of peripheral corneal neovascularization.
- Diseases affecting the endothelial cell function (high IOP, endothelial damage from glaucoma surgeries, corneal hydrops, etc.) can cause fluid collection in the interface. The condition is usually benign and resolves with the treatment of the underlying pathology.
- Corneal hydrops can have different clinical pictures in post-LASIK ectasia.
- Corneal dystrophies are relative contraindications for LASIK.
- Corneal neuralgia is a chronic complication of both LASIK and PRK. There is no cure for this condition and patients should be consulted about it preoperatively.

13 Complications of Smile Surgery

Soosan Jacob

Suction Loss

Case: (Fig. 13.1a, b) shows the laser pass interrupted after completion of lenticule cut, lenticule side cut, and cap cut. The caps side cut was not made. The software allows the cap side cut to be continued with by redocking the cone. An uncooperative patient however prevented the cap side cut also from forming in this case.

Management: Since the lenticule is completely dissected, a manual cut is made for the cap side cut (Fig. 13.1c). This is best done before dissipation of the cavitation bubbles in order to be able to place the incision at the correct site. Dissection of the lenticule is carried on as usual and the lenticule is extracted (Fig. 13.1d, e). The extracted lenticule is straightened and laid out flat to verify complete extraction (Fig. 13.1f).

Follow-up: (Fig. 13.2a) Slit-lamp image of the same patient as in the previous case. (Fig. 13.1) Showing a quiet, well-healed eye. (Fig. 13.2b) Topographic map shows a well centered lenticular extraction.

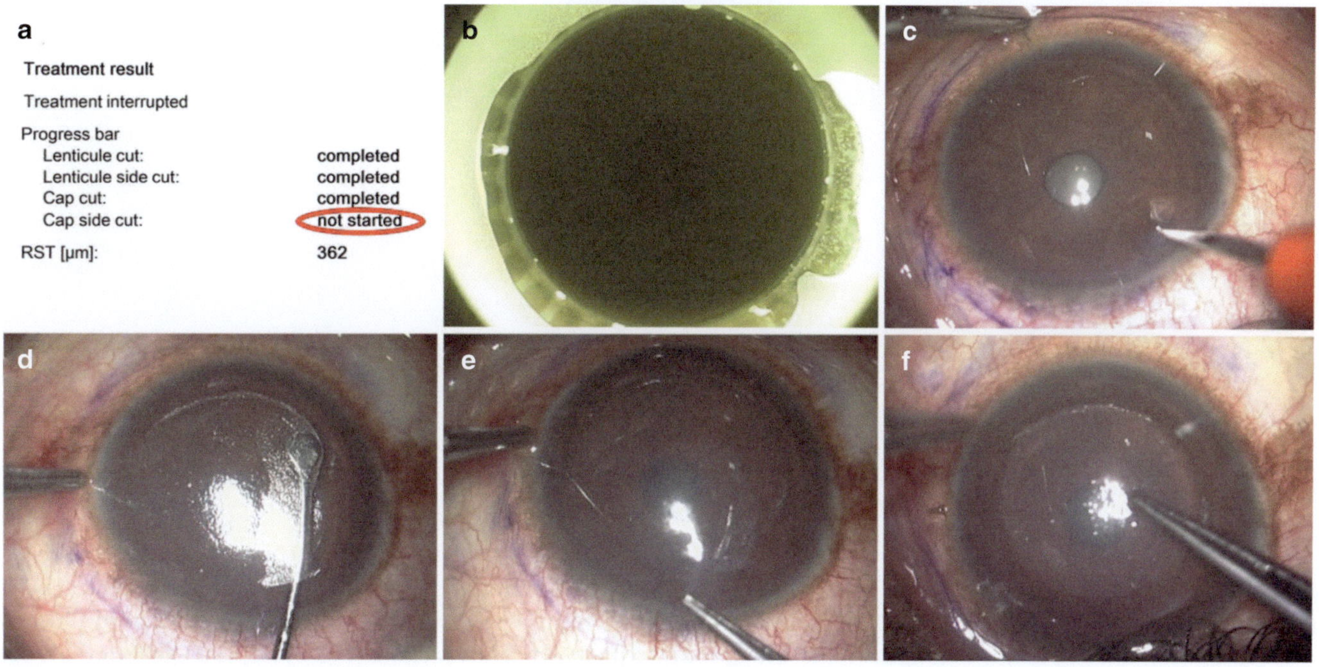

Fig. 13.1 Suction loss during cap side cut

S. Jacob (✉)
Dr. Agarwal's Refractive and Cornea Foundation, Cataract and Glaucoma Services, Dr. Agarwal's Group of Eye Hospital and Eye Research Centre, Chennai, India

S. A. Melki et al. (eds.), *Refractive Surgery Atlas*, https://doi.org/10.1007/978-3-031-60661-8_13

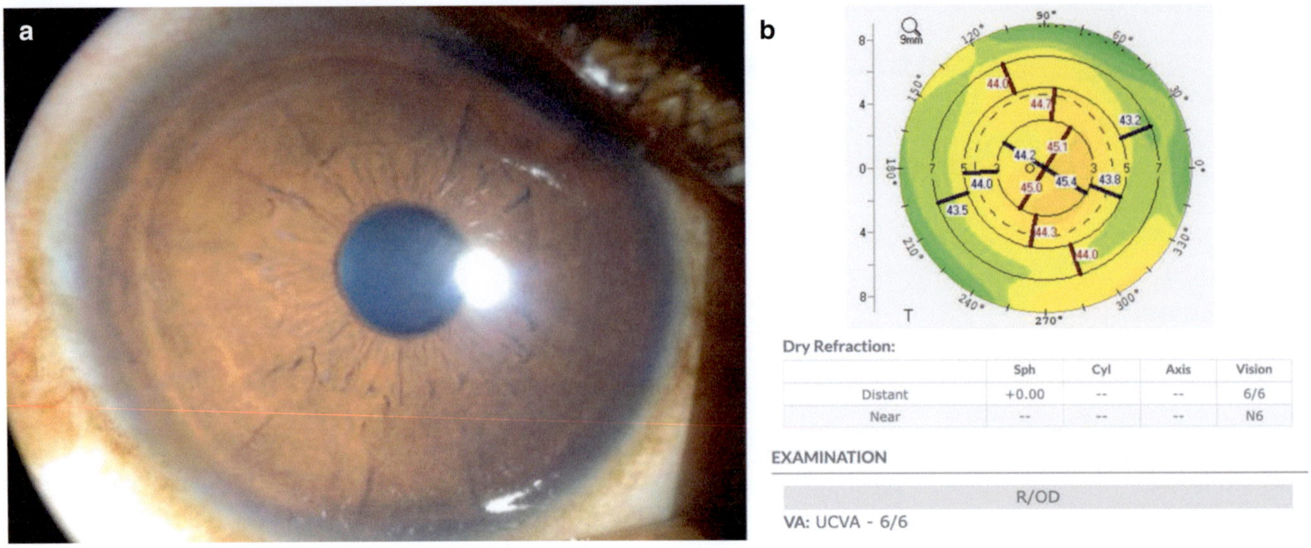

Fig. 13.2 Suction loss during cap side cut (Contd.)

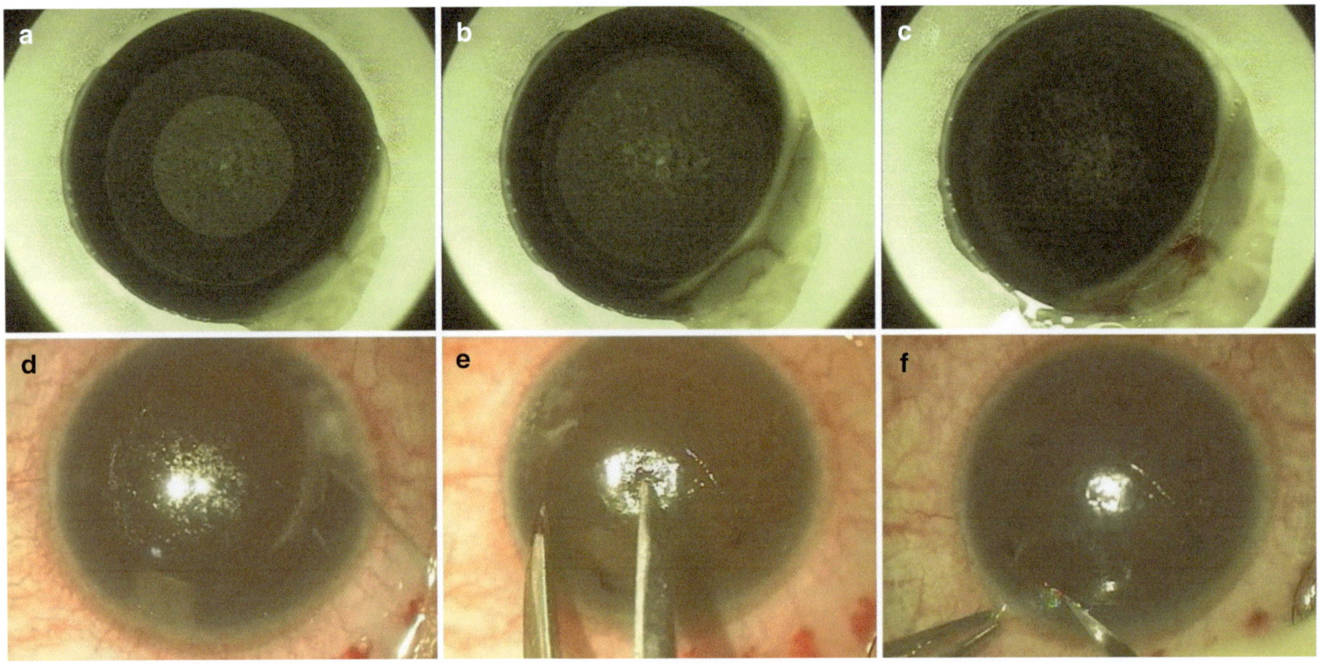

Fig. 13.3 Suction loss during cap cut

Case: (Fig. 13.3a–d) Lenticule cut and lenticule side cut are completed, cap cut is in progression when suction loss starts. Conjunctiva is however drawn into the applanating cone, creating pseudo-suction and all cuts are completed.

Management: (Fig. 13.3e) The completed margins of the cap cut are measured towards all sides to see the extent and size of the effective lenticule. Since an adequate optical zone was seen to be dissected, a decision was made to proceed with lenticular extraction. (Fig. 13.3f) A manual cap side cut is created within the cap cut margin.

Management (contd.): (Fig. 13.4a, b) The cap plane and the lenticular planes are identified and dissected. (Fig. 13.4c, d) The lenticule is extracted, laid out and checked.

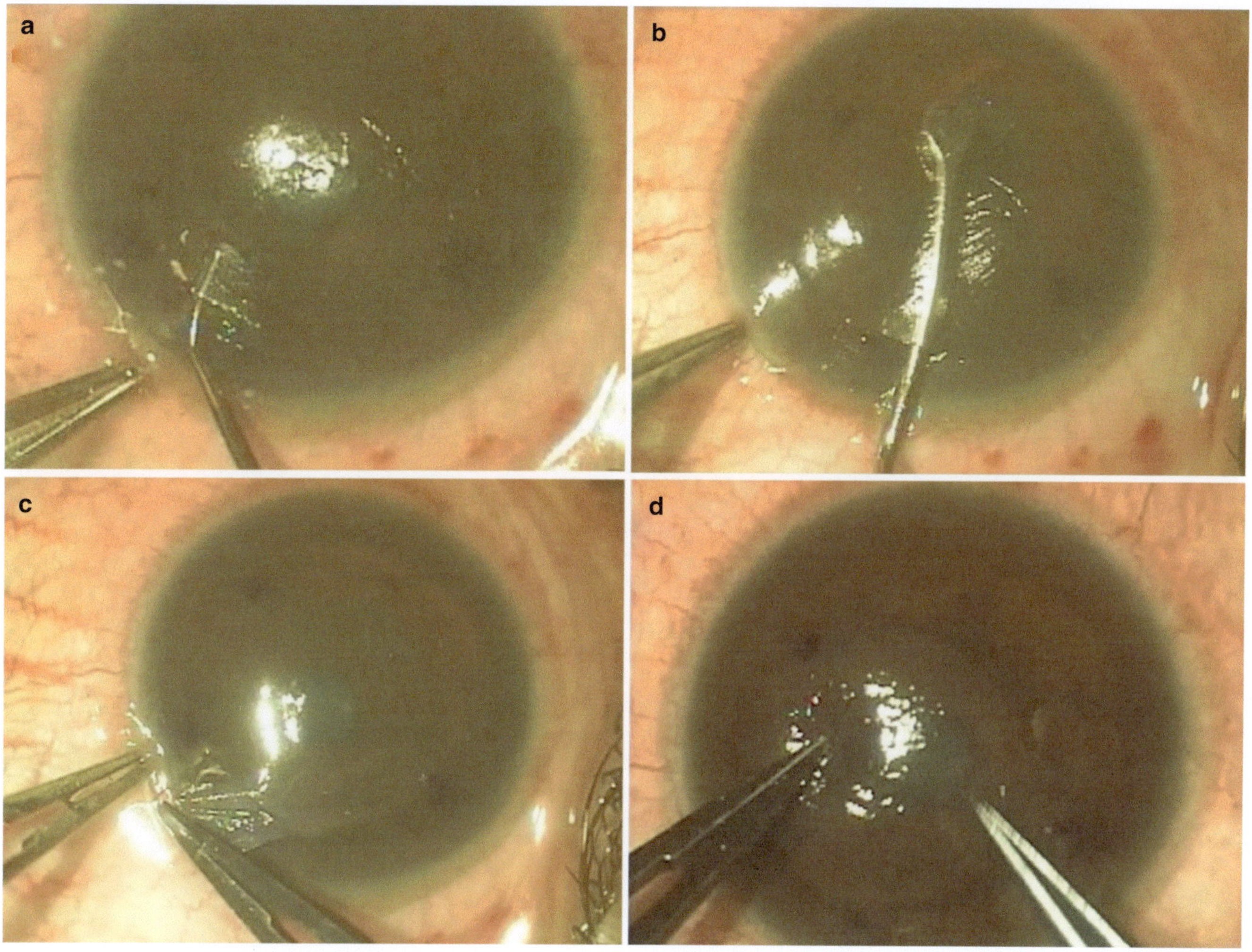

Fig. 13.4 Suction loss during cap cut (Contd.)

Follow-up: Postoperative visual and keratometric data of the affected eye (OD) described in Figs. 13.3 and 13.4 as compared to that of the left eye which underwent uneventful SMILE surgery. Satisfactory and comparable outcomes are seen in both eyes (Fig 13.5a, b).

Core Message: The manual cut should preferably be created before dissipation of the gas bubbles in order to be able to select the ideal location for the cut. In case of delay, it is wise to mark the extent of the lenticule and cap cuts with a surgical marker pen to assist in locating the cut accurately.

Case: (Fig 13.6a) Suction loss occurred after more than 10% of lenticule is cut.

Management: (Fig 13.6b) SMILE is abandoned and instead a femto-LASIK flap is cut at the same sitting. (Fig 13.6c) The femto-LASIK flap is lifted and excimer laser ablation is performed for refractive correction. (Fig 13.6d) Algorithm for suction loss after 10% lenticular or posterior plane cut.

Core Message: With suction loss greater than 10% of lenticule cut, it is advisable to convert to surface ablation or LASIK in the same sitting or at a later date.

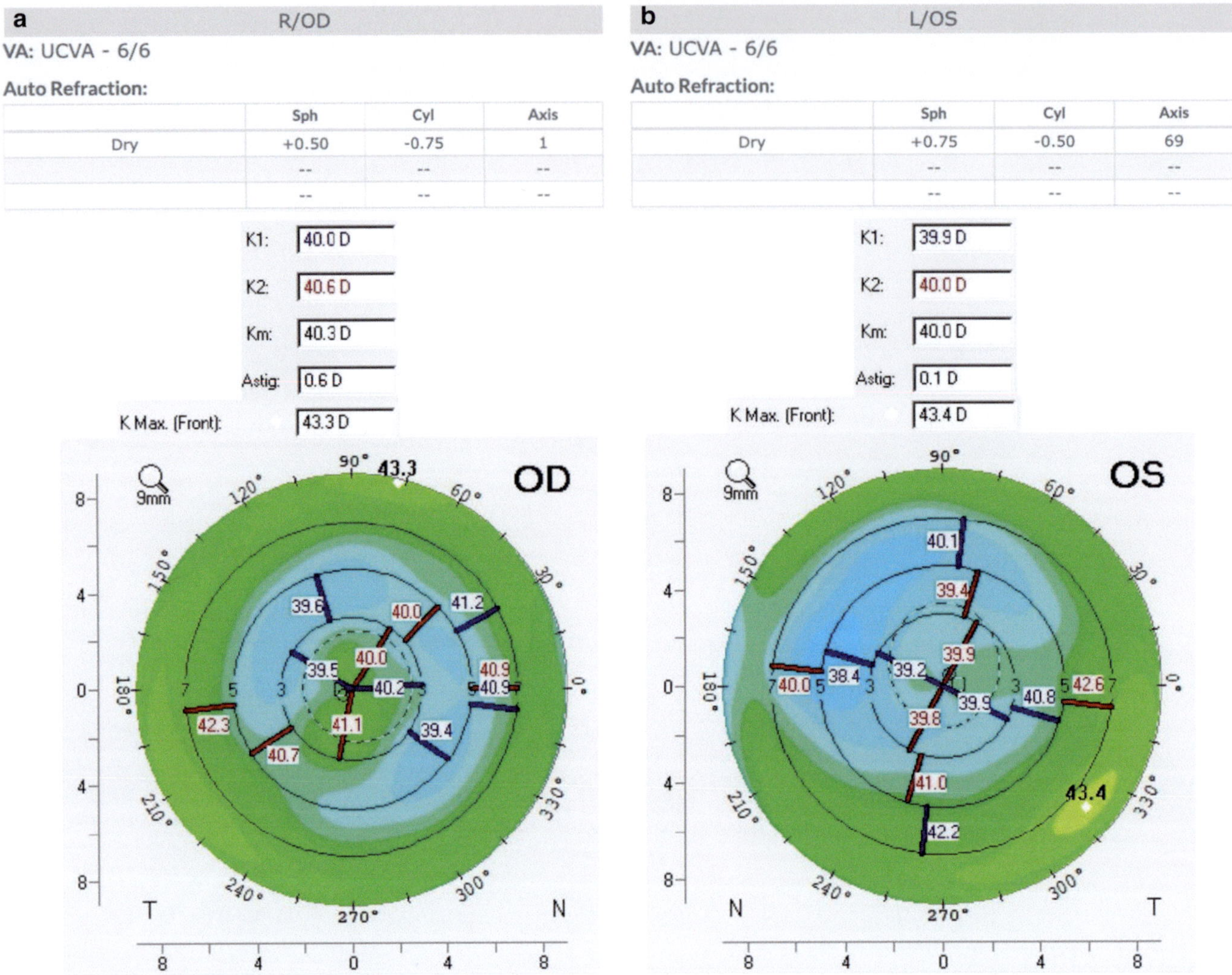

Fig. 13.5 Suction loss during cap cut (Contd.)

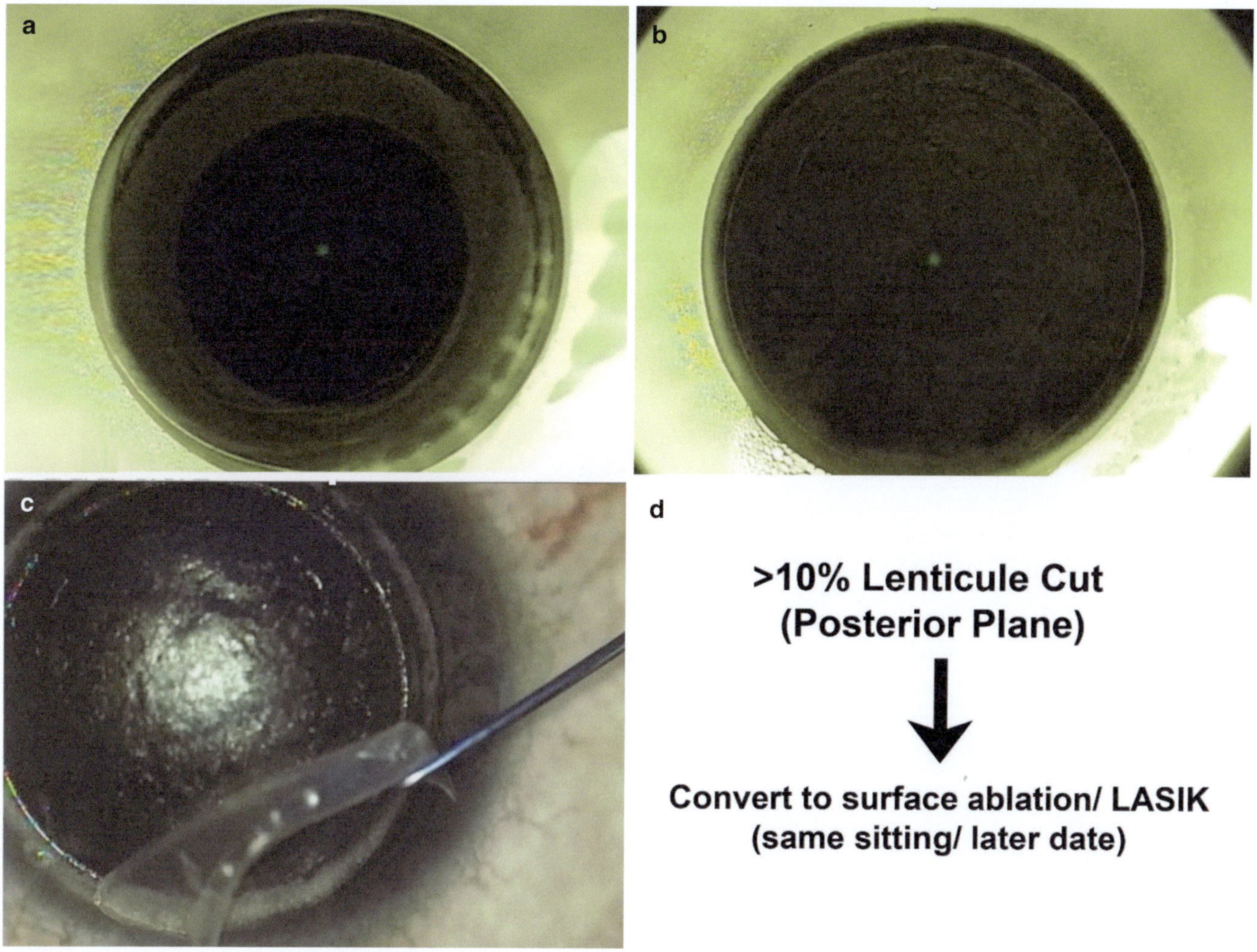

Fig. 13.6 Suction loss after more than 10% of lenticule cut

Laser Delivery Complications

Case: (Fig 13.7a, b) Right eye of a patient showing inadequate laser energy for all cuts. (Fig 13.7c, d) The energy was yet lower in the left eye and insufficient to create surgical planes.

Management: Surgery could however be completed in the right eye. Surgery was abandoned in the left eye and femto-LASIK was done at a later date.

Case: Black spots corresponding to undissected areas seen during the lenticular cut (Fig. 13.8a). The cap cut also leaves undissected area at the same locations (Fig. 13.8b).

Management: Black spots lead to difficult dissection and should be avoided. Extensive black spots over the visual axis may lead to poor or false plane dissection and irregular astigmatism. SMILE may be abandoned in this case and a femto-LASIK done at a later date.

Core message: Black spots may form due to debris under the cone such as water, meibomian secretions, mucus etc., and can result in difficult dissection in the involved areas.

Case: (Fig. 13.9a–c) Opaque bubble layer seen being formed. (Fig. 13.9d–f) show a normal cavitation pattern.

Management: Can proceed with lenticular dissection carefully.

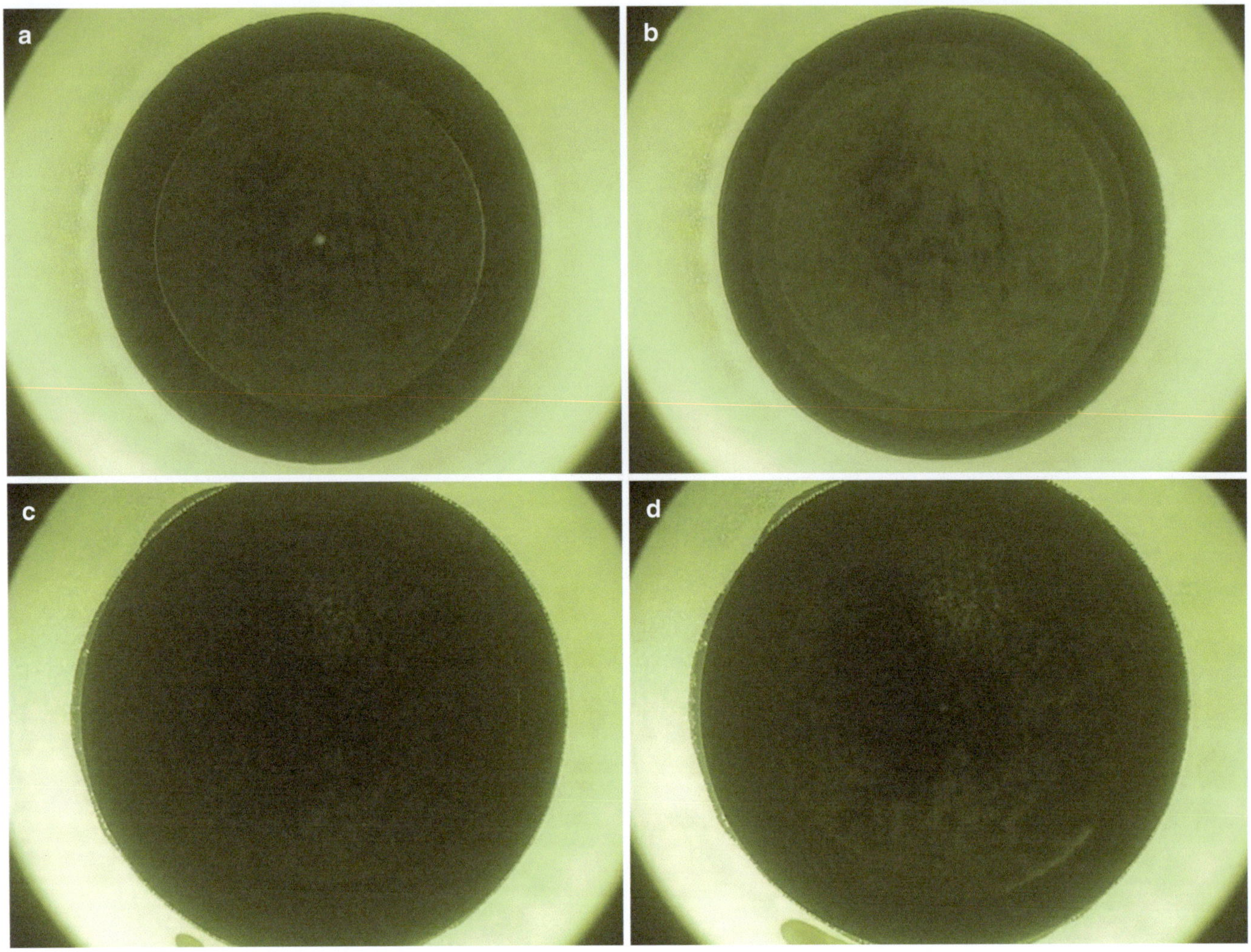

Fig. 13.7 Inadequate laser energy

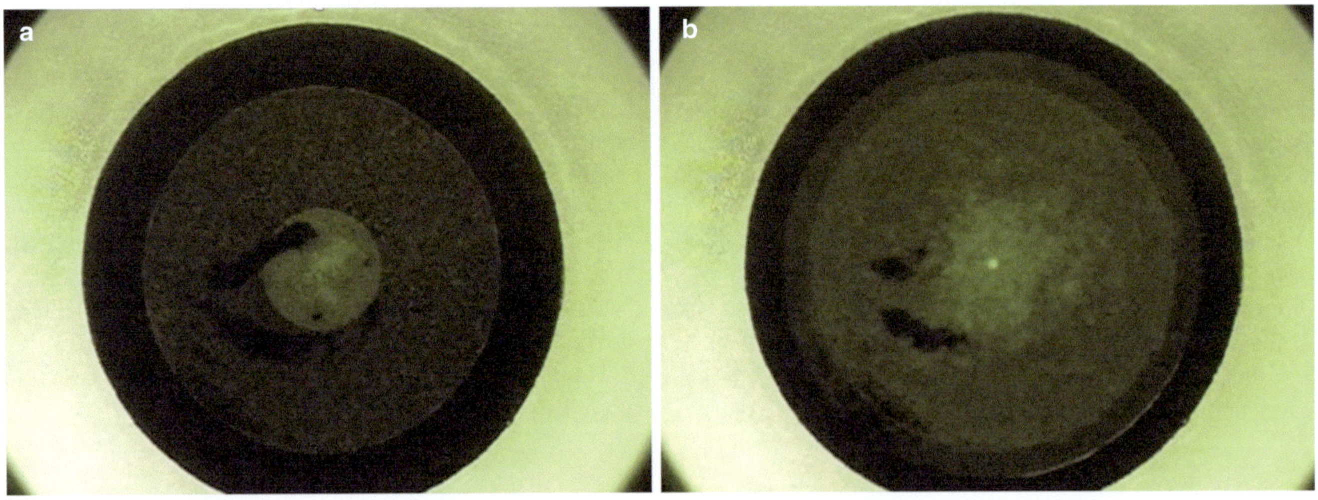

Fig. 13.8 Black spots

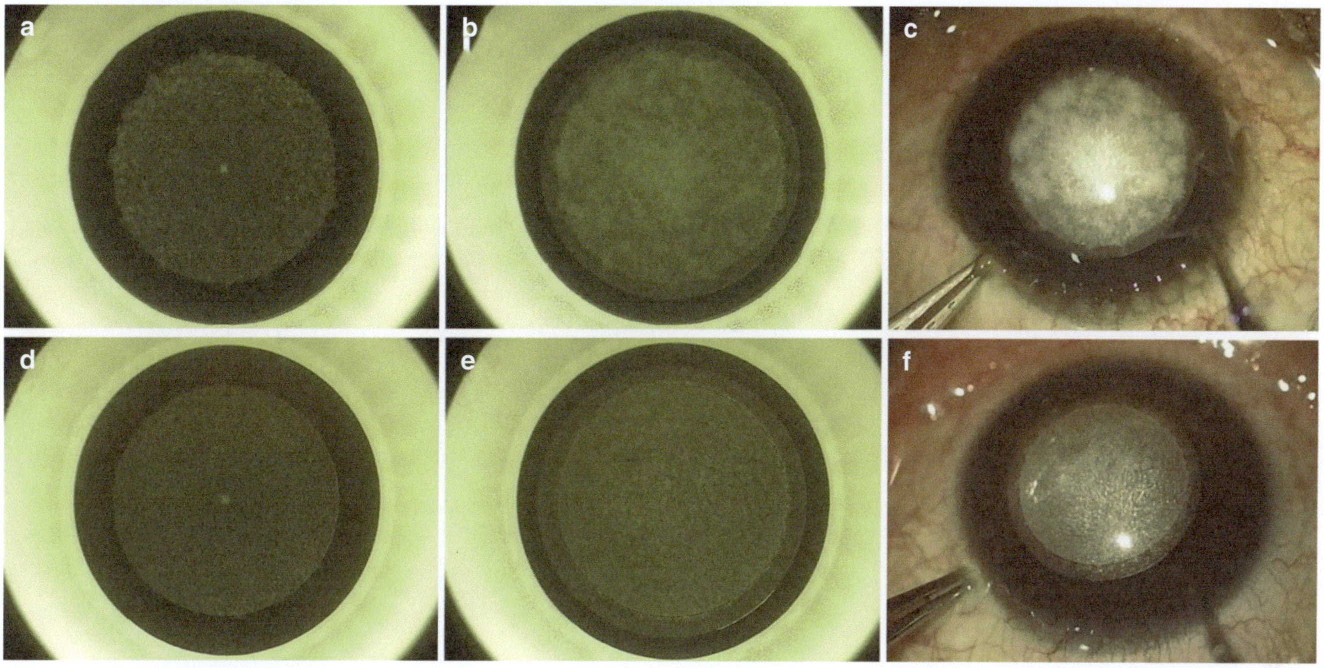

Fig. 13.9 Opaque bubble layer

Lenticular Dissection and Extraction Complications

Case: (Fig. 13.10a, b) The white ring refers to the lenticular side cut, the inner of the two circles. The relation of the instrument with the white ring is studied to determine whether the instrument is dissecting anterior or posterior to the lenticule. (Fig. 13.10c) Part of the white ring is hidden under the instrument indicating that the instrument is dissecting the anterior plane. (Fig. 13.10d) The white ring is seen over the instrument, indicating that the instrument is dissecting under the lenticule in the posterior plane. This sign is described by the author (SJ).

Case This sign helps to identify orientation of the dissecting instrument with respect to the lenticule. (Fig. 13.11a) The illustration shows the dissecting instrument lying above the white ring. (Fig. 13.11b) The white ring lies below the dissecting instrument.

Core Message: The white ring sign helps assure that the anterior plane dissection is completed before posterior plane. Reverse dissection can result in difficult dissection and cap tears.

Surgical technique: Described by the author (SJ).

This technique helps perform extraction of thin lenticules successfully and without complications. Sequential segmental dissection of the lenticular side cut is done after dissecting the posterior plane, leaving just the lenticular side cut undissected.

The sequential segmental terminal lenticular side cut dissection is then proceeded with following a specific order that allows the lenticule to remain immobile and in position till it is completely freed. This prevents excessive mobility and folding up of the lenticule edges (Fig. 13.12a, b). The lower edges are first dissected, followed by (Fig. 13.12c, d) the middle parts dissection on either side (Fig. 13.12e, f). The lenticular side cut on either side near the cap side cut are dissected last. The lenticule becomes free just before dissection of the very last segment (Fig. 13.12f). In case of any difficulty with this segment, a micro-forceps can be used to separate it.

Surgical technique:

(Fig. 13.13a, b) The parts near the cap side cut are freed last. (Fig. 13.13c, d) The lenticule is extracted and checked.

Surgical technique summary: Described by the author (SJ) (Fig. 13.14).

The lenticular side cut is freed in a particular order of dissection. The diagram shows this order of dissection of the lenticular side cut.

Core message: Dissection of the lenticular side cut following the correct order prevents premature mobility and folding up of the lenticule before it is completely dissected free.

Surgical technique:

(Fig. 13.15a, b) Posterior plane dissection is completed leaving the extreme edges of the lenticule still attached.

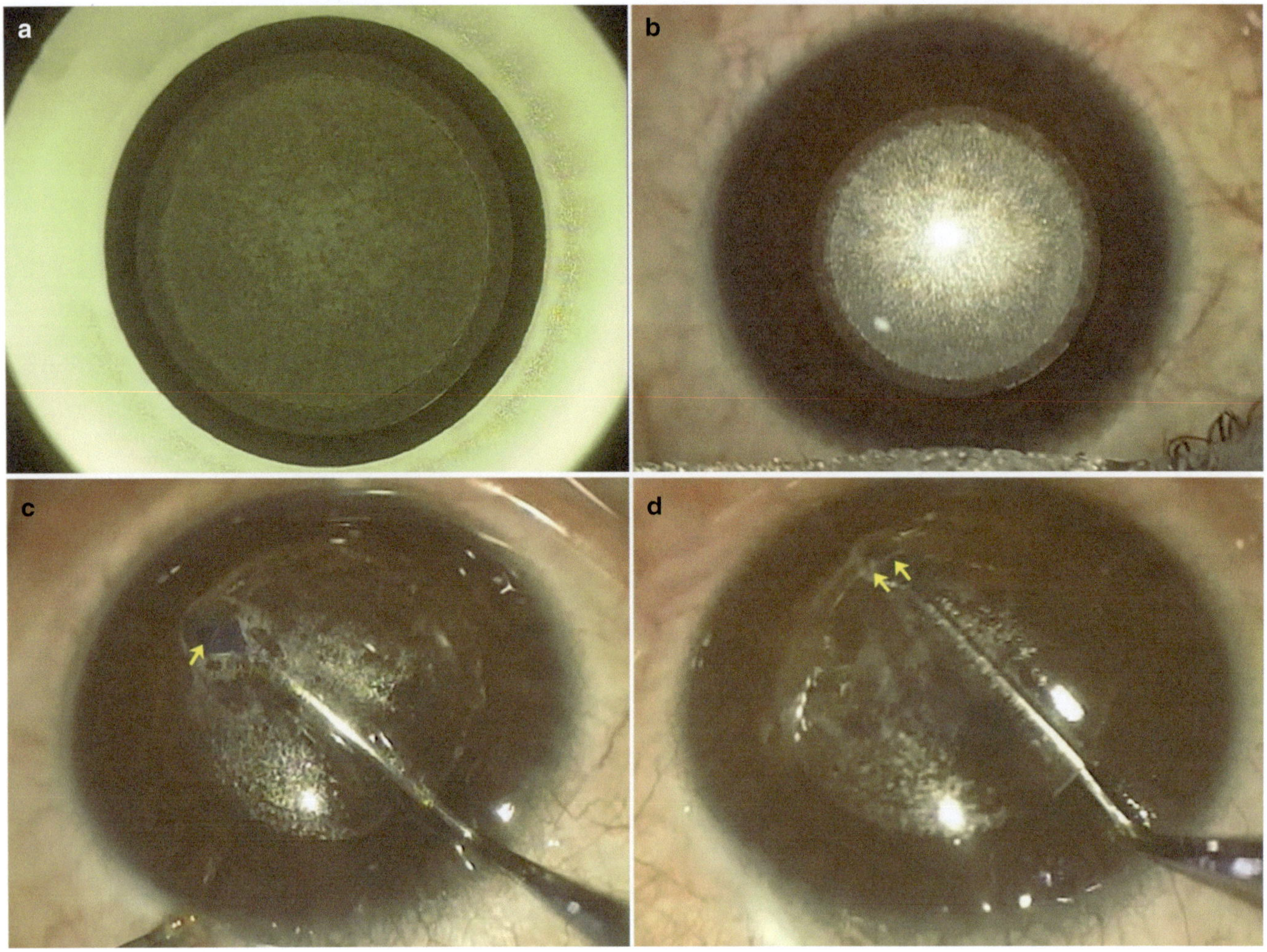

Fig. 13.10 White ring sign

Fig. 13.11 White ring sign (Contd.)

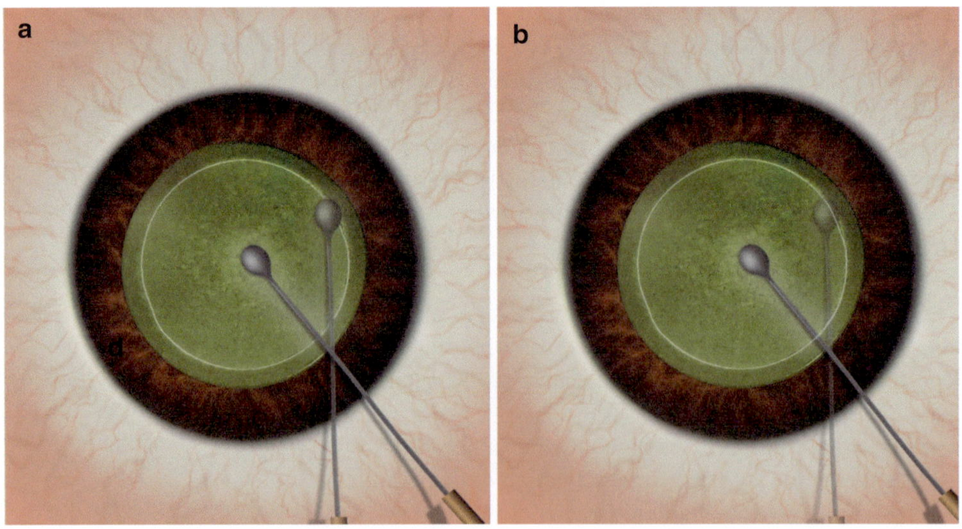

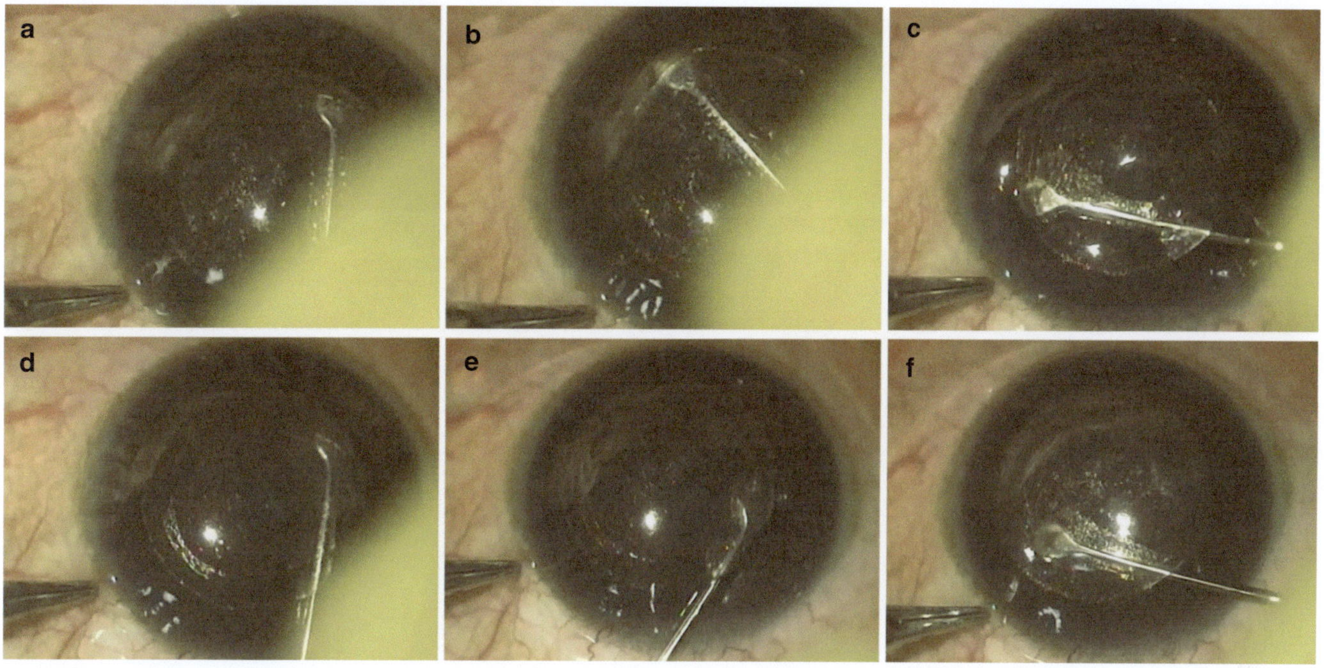

Fig. 13.12 Thin lenticule dissection—sequential segmental terminal lenticular side cut dissection

(Fig. 13.15c) A micro-forceps is carefully inserted and the lenticule grasped and extracted using a rhexis like maneuver.

(Fig. 13.15d) The extracted lenticule is examined.

Core message: A thin lenticule is more prone to tears and partial extraction. Care needs to be taken while extracting the lenticule. The central part of the lenticular attachments to the posterior stroma is dissected leaving the lenticular side cut undissected till last. This avoids the lenticule from folding up while dissecting.

Case: Posterior plane dissection was unintentionally performed first. (Fig. 13.16a) The lenticule is thus adherent to the cap and folds over when attempted to be dissected.

Management: (Fig. 13.16b, c) A micro-forceps is used to gently extract the lenticule. (Fig. 13.16d) The extracted lenticule is examined.

Core message: Lenticule adhesion should be avoided by ascertaining that the anterior plane dissection is completed before the posterior plane dissection.

Case:

Accidental dissection of the posterior plane before the anterior plane resulted in the lenticule being stuck to the cap.

(Fig. 13.17a) An instrument can be seen trying to separate the lenticule from the cap. A cap tear is seen secondary to excessive maneuvering. (Fig. 13.17b) The surgeon is seen trying to peel the lenticule from the cap. (Fig. 13.17c) The tear can be seen to further extend while attempting lenticular separation.

Management: (Fig. 13.17c) Micro-forceps is used to further peel and free the lenticule from the cap. (Fig. 13.17d) The lenticule has been extracted and the cap is replaced back. A bandage contact lens is placed. (Fig. 13.17e) The first post-operative day image shows a well healed cap. The tear is fortunately outside the visual axis. The UCVA recovers to 20/20 Fig. 13.17f.

Core message: The white ring sign helps identify and avoid this complication.

Case 1: (Fig. 13.18a, b) A cap tear is seen secondary to the micro-forceps getting caught on the cap side cut while peeling the lenticule.

Case 2: (Fig. 13.18c, d) A cap tear is seen secondary to the anteriorly lifted dissector tenting and causing excessive stretch of the cap side cut with resultant tear.

Core message: The cap can tear if excessive manipulation, maneuvering, or stretching of the cap side cut happens.

Case: (Fig. 13.19a) A micro-forceps being used to extract the lenticule. (Fig. 13.19b) Incomplete and torn lenticule seen extracted. (Fig. 13.19c) Margins of the remaining lenticule are seen marked in yellow.

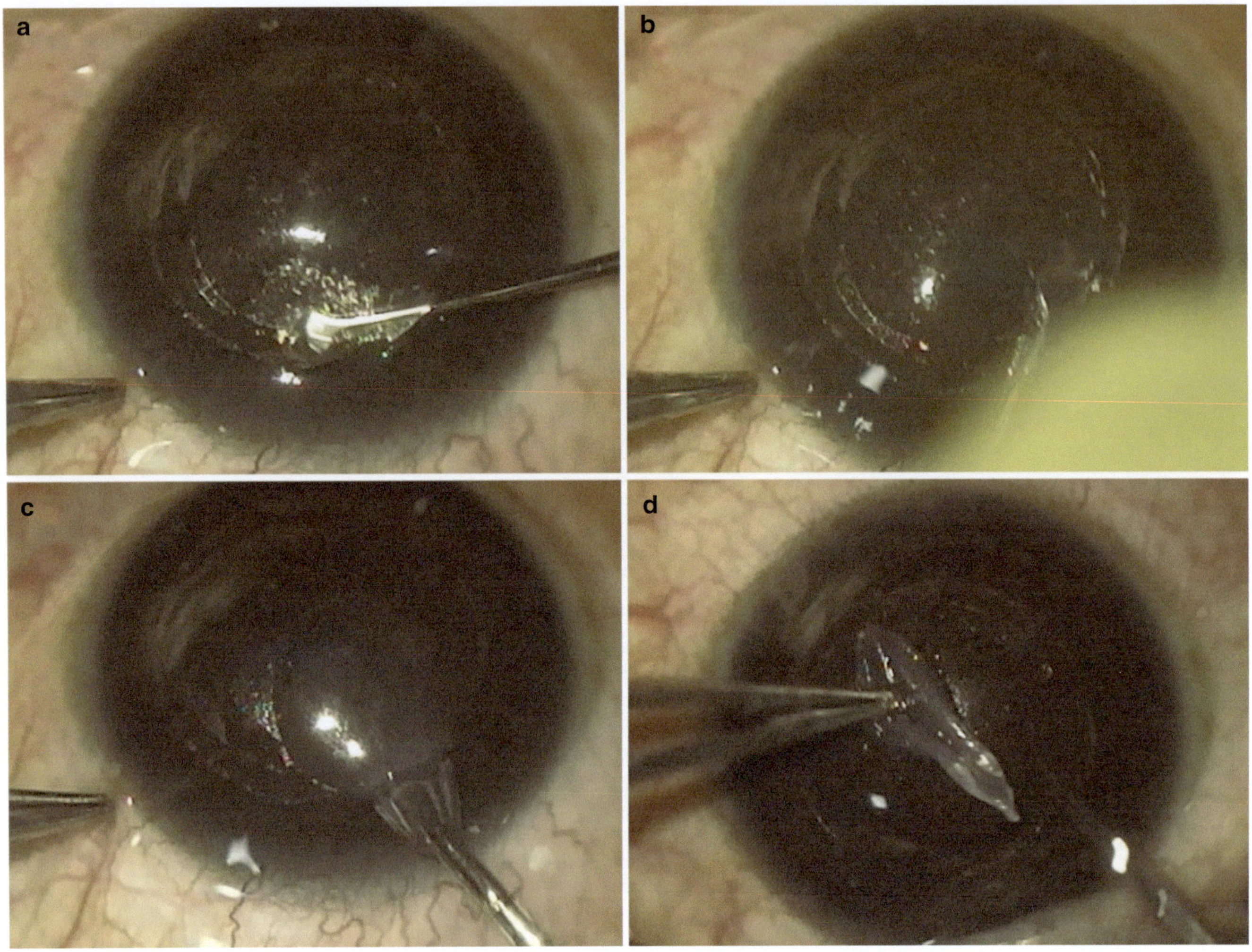

Fig. 13.13 Thin lenticule dissection—sequential segmental terminal lenticular side cut dissection (Contd.)

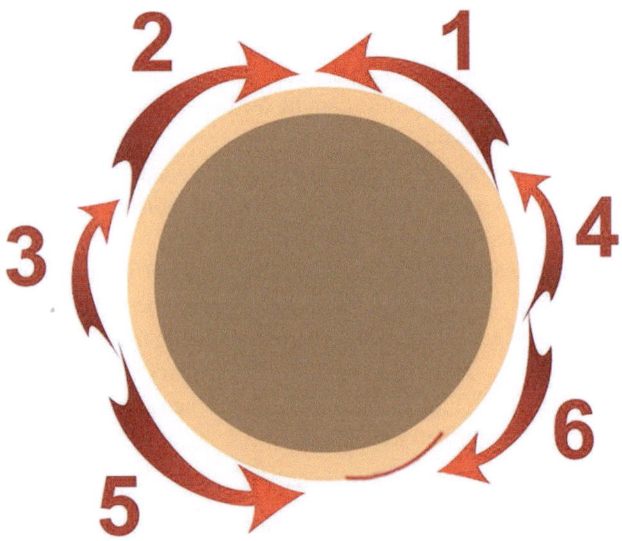

Fig. 13.14 Thin lenticule dissection—sequential segmental terminal lenticular side cut dissection. (Contd.)

Management: A micro-forceps is used to extract the remaining piece. (Fig. 13.19d) The two separately extracted lenticular pieces are seen to match and fit accurately with each other, thus ascertaining complete extraction.

Core message: Lenticular extraction should be done carefully and only after freeing the lenticule completely on both anterior and posterior sides. Gentle dissection and special techniques like the white ring sign and sequential segmental terminal lenticular side cut dissection help in preventing torn lenticules.

Case (Fig. 13.20a–c) The CIRCLE software is used for converting the SMILE cap into a flap. (Fig. 13.20d) The flap is dissected and lifted up. (Fig. 13.20e) The flap is replaced back. (Fig. 13.20f) The healed cap side cut is seen.

Core message: The CIRCLE software is useful as a backup technique to be able to convert the SMILE cap into a flap. This can be used to extract remnant lenticule, treat epithelial ingrowth, etc.

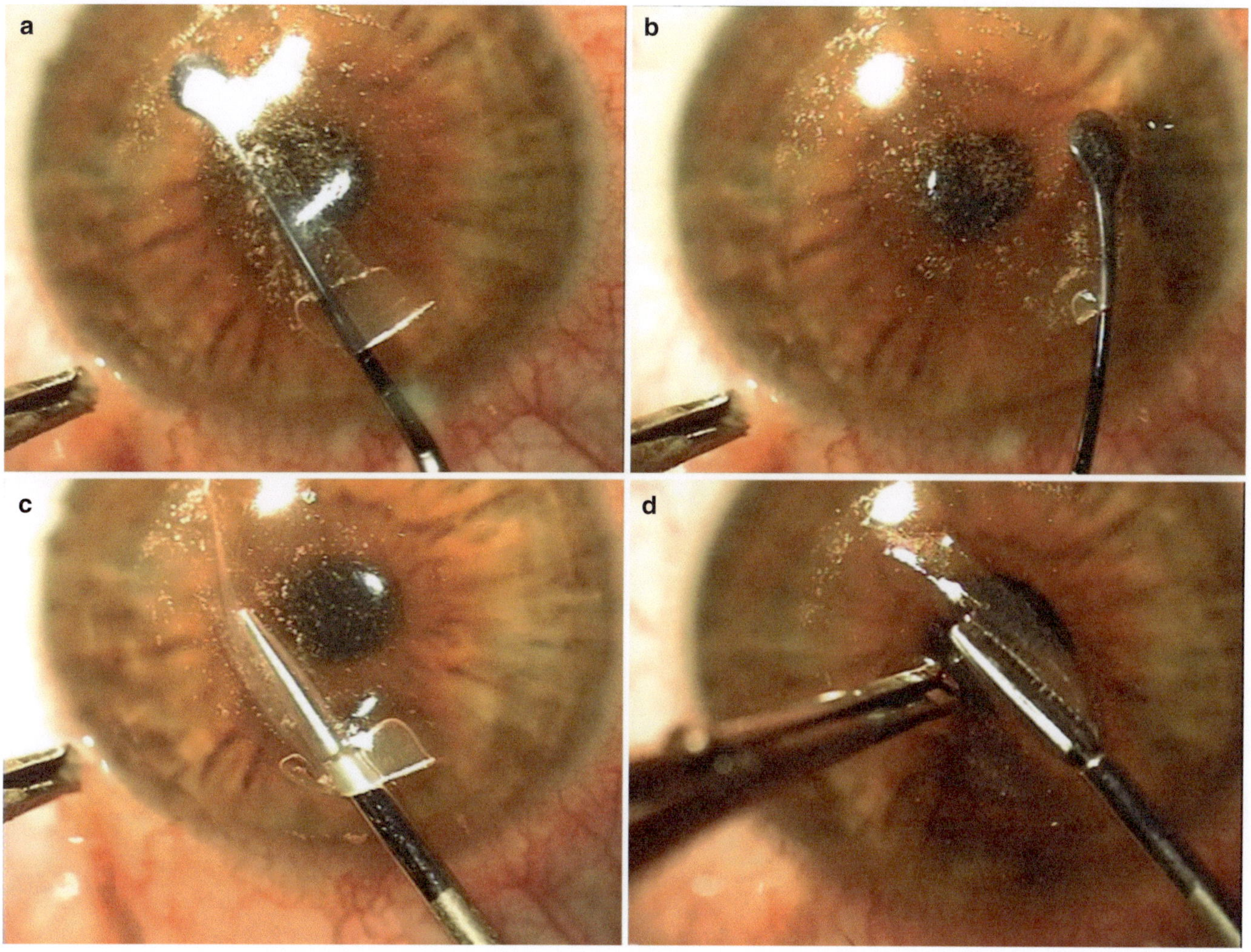

Fig. 13.15 Thin lenticule dissection—lenticulorhexis

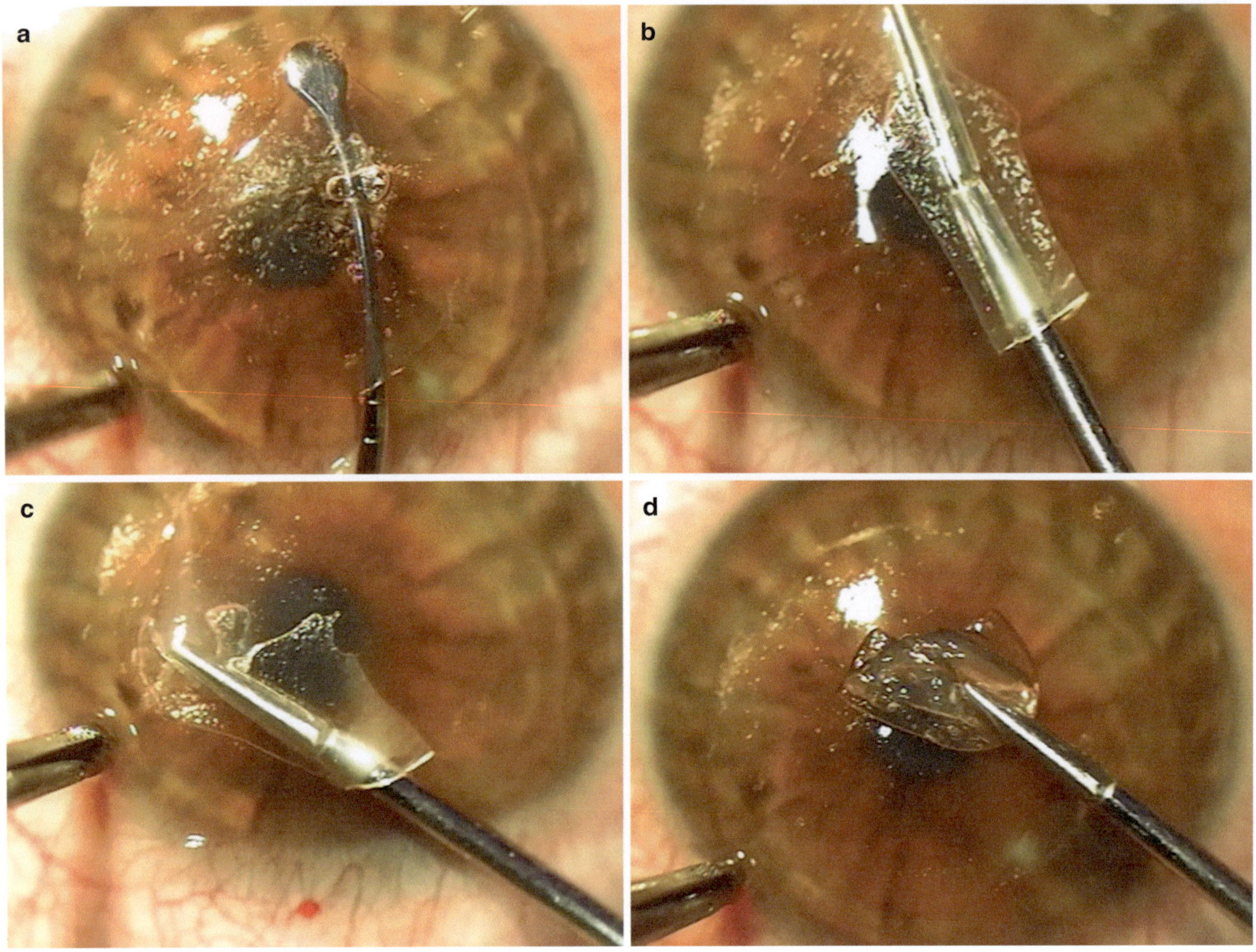

Fig. 13.16 Cap-lenticular adhesion

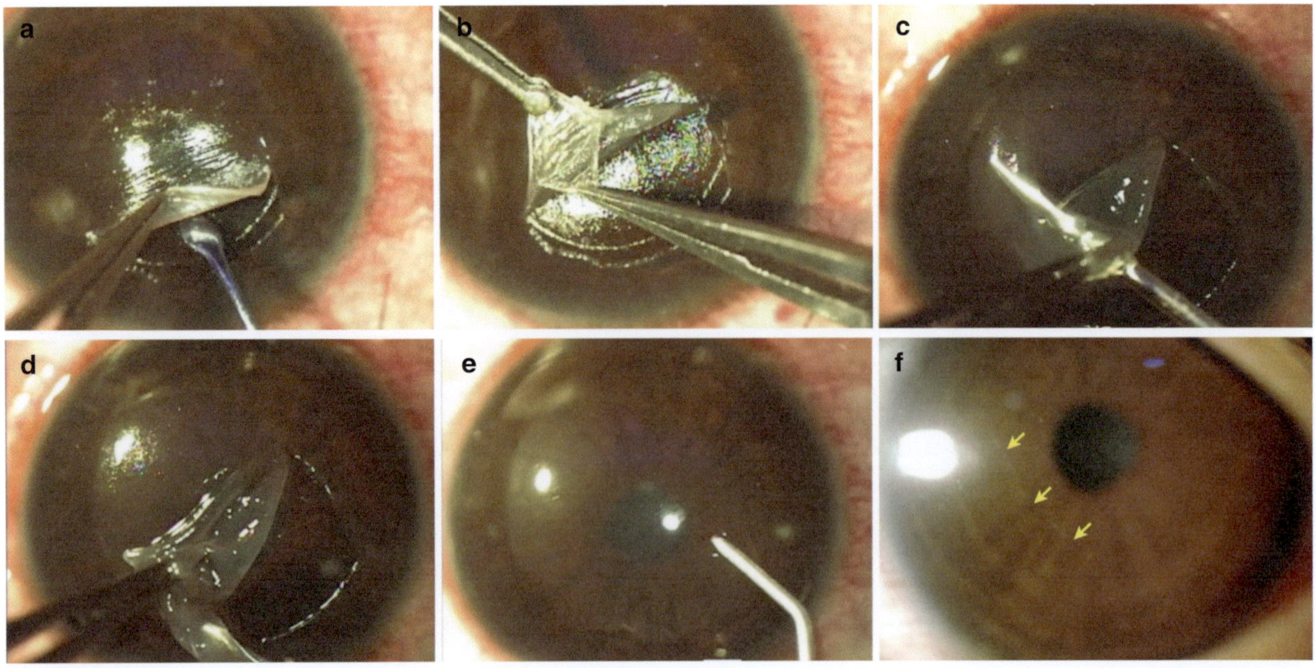

Fig. 13.17 Cap tear

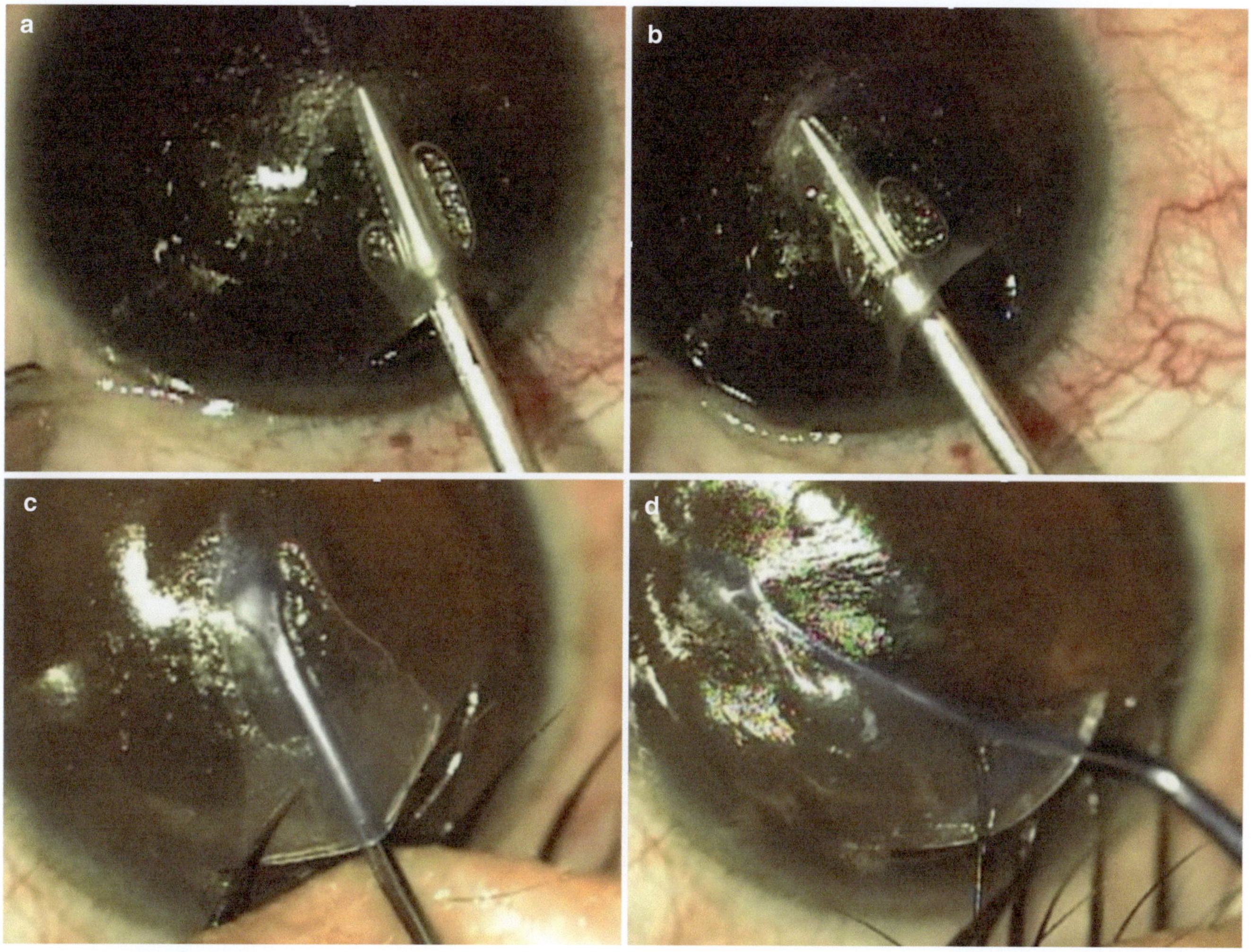

Fig. 13.18 Cap tear

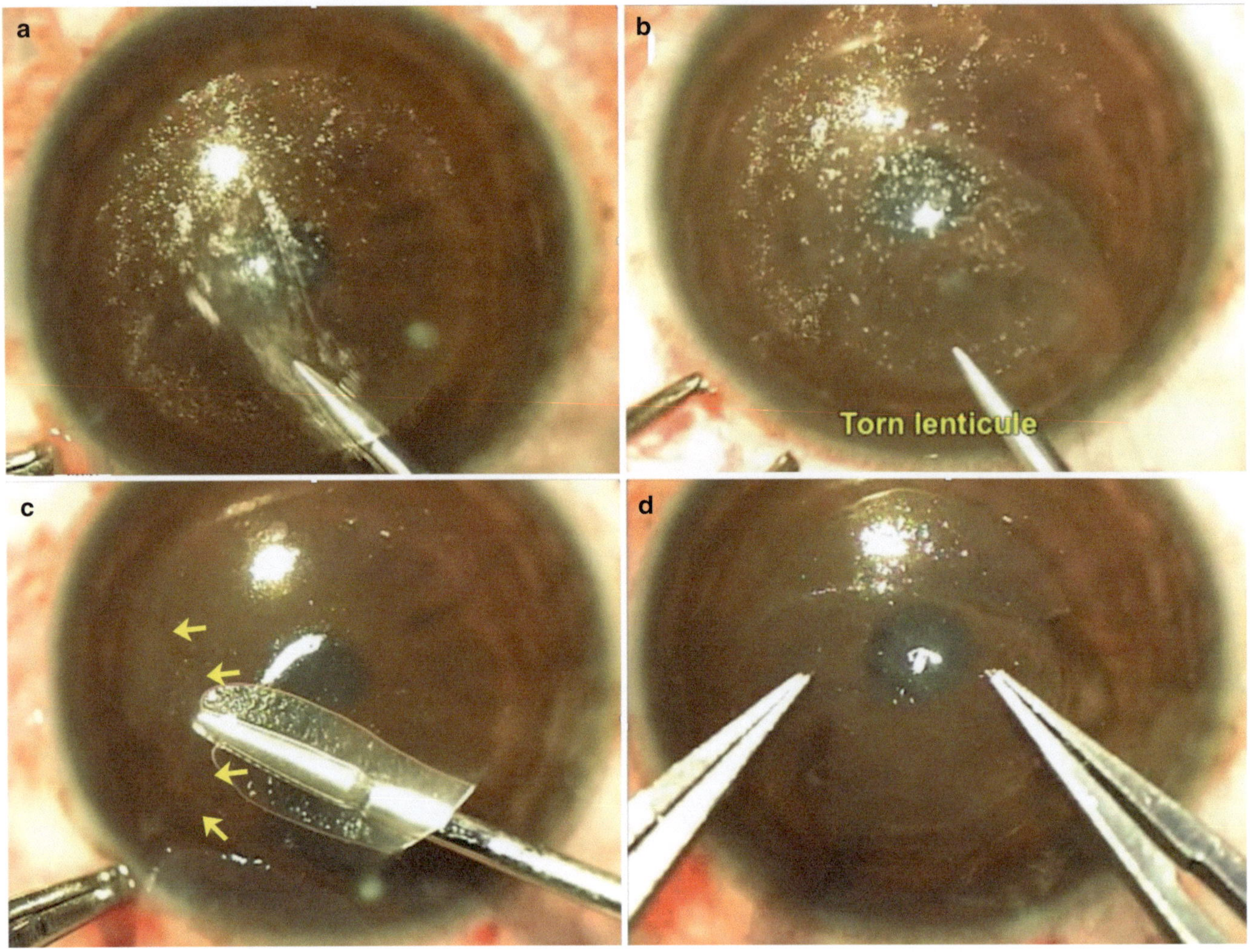

Fig. 13.19 Torn lenticule

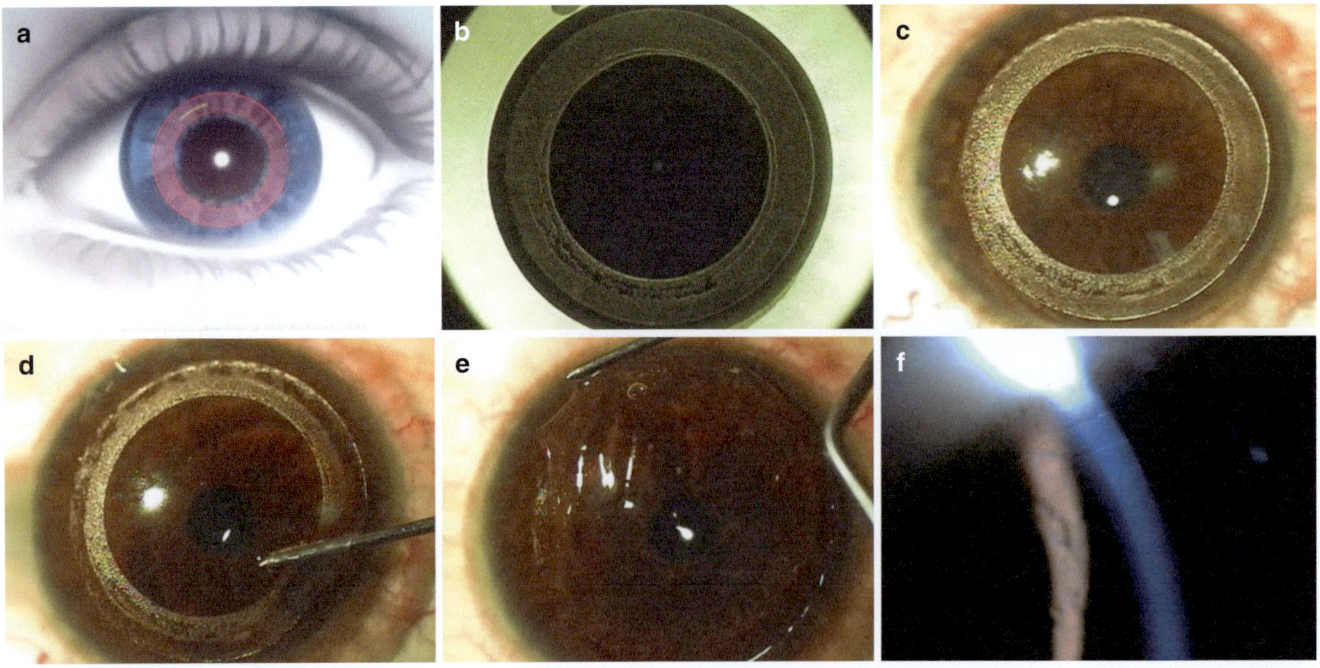

Fig. 13.20 Circle treatment

Post-Operative Complications

Case: A patient underwent interface flushing for an epithelial ingrowth post SMILE surgery for the first time, 1 year following surgery. Then he presented 10 months later with a second recurrence of the ingrowth (Fig. 13.21a). Patient underwent a second flushing of the interface (Fig. 13.21b) but he developed a third recurrence of ingrowth (Fig. 13.21c).

Exam: Stage 2, dense epithelial ingrowth noted at the interface extending from a supero-temporal incision (Fig. 13.21a). Stromal hydration can be noticed directly following interface flushing (Fig. 13.21b). Another stage 2 epithelial ingrowth recurrence is noted (Fig. 13.21c).

Management: Special instruments/spatula can be used to scrape the interface. Alternatively, corneal suture can be placed or conversion of the cap into a flap can be performed for a more thorough scraping of the interface.

Core message: Irrigation of the interface to remove epithelial ingrowth may have a high recurrence rate.

Case: (Fig. 13.22a) Epithelial ingrowth is seen extending from the lower edge of the cap side cut after SMILE surgery.

Management: (Fig. 13.22b) The CIRCLE software is used to convert the cap into a flap. (Fig. 13.22c) The flap is lifted up locally in the area of the ingrowth which is then scraped and washed. (Fig. 13.22d) Nine-month post-operative image shows a clear interface.

Core message: Epithelial ingrowth can occur after SMILE and all precautions taken to avoid this complication during LASIK should also be taken during SMILE.

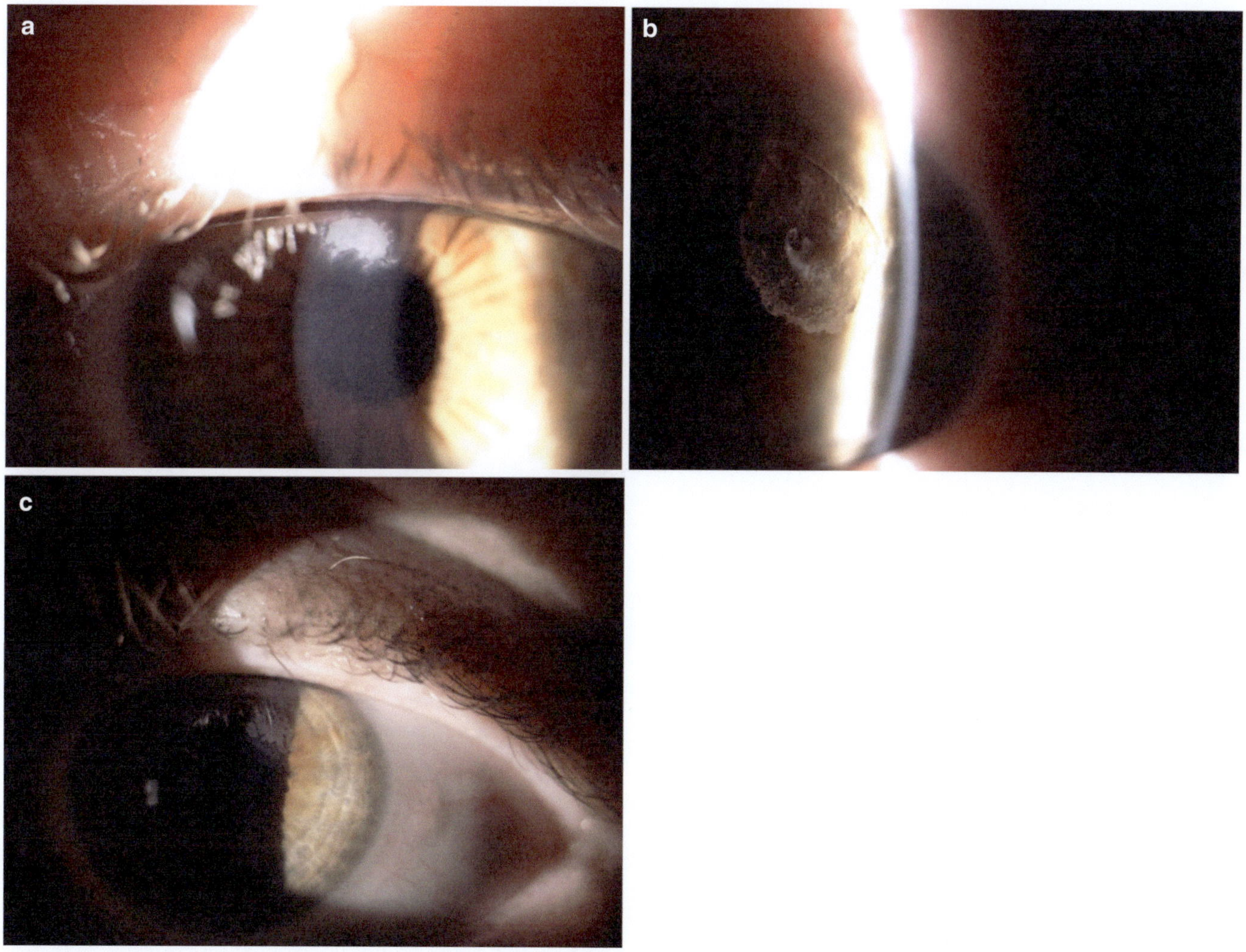

Fig. 13.21 Recurrence of epithelial ingrowth. (*Courtesy of Suphi Taneri MD. Augenzentrum am St. Franziskus Hospital Münster, Münster, Germany*)

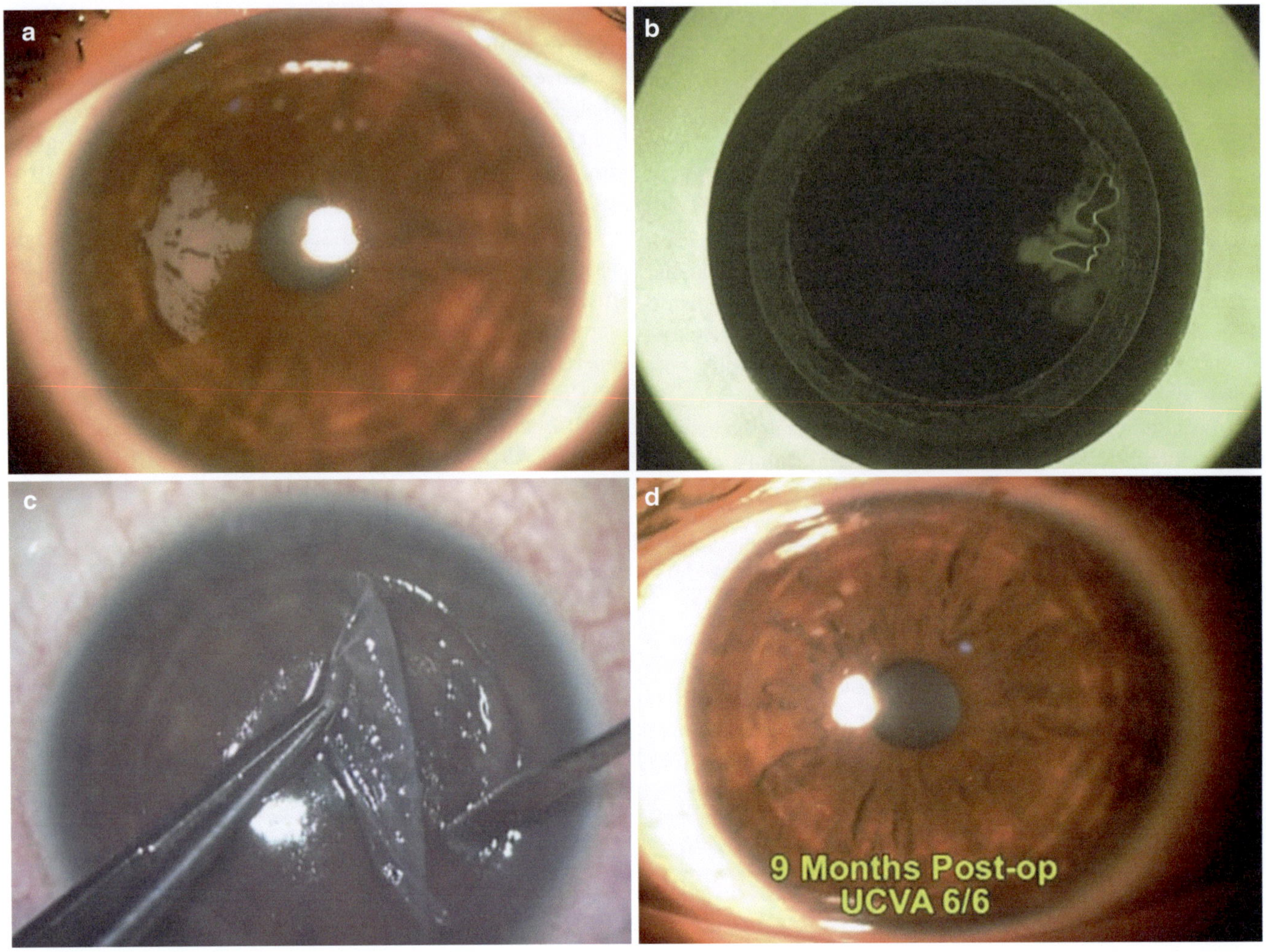

Fig. 13.22 Circle treatment for epithelial ingrowth

Other Post-Operative Complications after SMILE

These are similar to those after LASIK and include complications such as interface debris, residual refractive error, higher order aberrations, dry eyes, diffuser lamellar keratitis, transient light sensitivity, infectious keratitis, pressure induced stromal keratitis, corneal ectasia, etc.

Take-Home Message

- With adequately created lenticule, if the cap side cut is not formed even after redocking and restarting the procedure, a manual cut can help gain access to the dissection planes in order to continue with lenticular extraction.
- With suction loss at any point other than at a lenticular cut more than 10%, it is possible to redock and restart the procedure to continue as SMILE surgery.
- The risk of suction loss is increased with a narrow palpebral fissure, squeezing of the eyelids, uncooperative patient, surgeon inexperience, small cornea, conjunctival chemosis, large cap, excessive fluid in the conjunctival sac, high astigmatism, etc. Most suction loss occur during the cap cut.
- Suction loss can be avoided in many cases by explaining to the patient the need to be still and what is to be expected during the laser pass, together with careful preparation of the eye prior to docking. The new faster SMILE machines can decrease the incidence of suction loss still further.
- Black spots should be avoided by ensuring a clear interface between the cornea and the applanating cone. Large undissected areas (black islands), especially over the visual axis can result in false plane dissection and irregular astigmatism. The procedure may be aborted in this case and femto-LASIK or surface ablation done at a later date.

- Thick cornea, stiff cornea, thin lenticule, higher laser energy setting, and increased line spacing are risk factors for OBL. OBL can interfere with identification of lenticular edge and thereby result in false planes.
- Careful identification of lenticule edge through the OBL can prevent false planes. A thicker cap may decrease the incidence of OBL.
- The transparent lenticule makes the identification of planes difficult. The white ring sign described by the author (SJ) confirms placement of the dissecting instrument with respect to the anterior or posterior plane of dissection.
- The lower edges of the lenticular side cut hold the lenticule in place till dissection is completed.
- A thin lenticule needs special care to avoid tears. The author has described the sequential segmental terminal lenticular side cut dissection for ensuring uneventful extraction.
- Maneuvers for lenticular dissection and extraction should be gentle, follow the curve of the cornea and not tent up or stretch the cap side cut. Instruments should swivel within the cap side cut to decrease distortion and stretching. During the learning curve, a larger cap side cut can be used and with more surgical experience, it's length can be decreased to 2 mm.
- Any tears in the lenticule should always be looked for and if large and visually significant, the remnant lenticule should be searched for and removed. Remnant lenticule may be identified by retro-illumination with dilated pupil, intra-operative OCT, or by staining with triamcinolone acetonide. It can be removed using a micro-forceps. If unsuccessful, it can be extracted after using the CIRCLE software to convert the cap into a flap.
- CIRCLE software is a rescue technique in certain situations where access is needed into the pocket under the SMILE cap or to the residual stroma bed.
- The CIRCLE software can be useful to treat clinically significant and recurrent epithelial ingrowth.

Corneal Implants

14

Reeda Bou Said, Samir A. Melki, Jason Brenner, and Wassef Chanbour

Intrastromal Corneal Ring Segments (ICRS)

See Table 14.1.

Case: A 42-year-old woman with keratoconus managed with polymethyl-methacrylate (PMMA) ring segments for both eyes 5 years ago presented with left eye pain and foreign body sensation. She denied frequent eye rubbing (Fig. 14.1).

Exam: An epithelial defect can be seen on the slit lamp (Fig. 14.1a) while the OCT section shows a translucent area extending from the surface to the PMMA segment denoting acute stromal necrosis (ASN) **(white arrow)** (Fig. 14.1b).

Management: The condition was managed by removal of the ring segment, which was followed by epithelial down growth in place of the necrosis all the way to the tunnel floor **(black arrow)** (Fig. 14.1c) with improvement in vision.

Table 14.1 Characteristics of intrastromal corneal ring segments

Material	PMMA ring segments or biologic corneal inlay (keranatural or corneal allogenic intrastromal ring segments (CAIRS))
History	• INTACS (CorneaGen, Seattle, WA) received FDA approval in 2004 for patients who are 21 years or older, no longer tolerant to contact lenses or spectacles with visual deterioration, with clear central corneas and at least 450 microns thickness at the incision site [1] • Ferrara ring (Ferrara Ophthalmics, Belo Horizonte, Brazil) and Keraring (Mediphacos, Belo Horizonte, Brazil) are still not FDA approved for use in the USA • Keranatural (lions vision gift) is an allograft corneal ring segment that is produced from donor corneas and currently available in the US
Principle	• Potentially reversible • Placed in mid-peripheral cornea at 2/third depth for PMMA and 200 microns in keranatural • Spacer between collagen fibers leading to central flattening. • 1 or 2 segments depending on location of cone
Characteristics	• The thicker the segment, and the closer it is to the center, the greater the flattening effect • The shorter the segment, the greater the skewing effect
Surgical technique	• Vertical incision using diamond blade or femtosecond laser • Tunnel formation either manually or using femtosecond laser (more precise), diameter varies according to type of ring used • Placement of the ring segment in the tunnel and manipulation through holes located at its tip • Placement of 10–0 buried suture to close the incision (prevents migration). (Chap. 1)

(continued)

R. B. Said
Department of Ophthalmology, Mayo Clinic, Rochester, MN, USA

S. A. Melki (✉) · J. Brenner
Boston Vision, Department of Ophthalmology, Harvard Medical School, Boston, MA, USA
e-mail: Melki@bostonvision.com; brenner@bostonvision.com

W. Chanbour
Department of Ophthalmology and Visual Neurosciences, University of Minnesota, Minneapolis, MN, USA

S. A. Melki et al. (eds.), *Refractive Surgery Atlas*, https://doi.org/10.1007/978-3-031-60661-8_14

Table 14.1 (continued)

Complications	• Visual complaints: Halos, blurring • Infectious keratitis, migration, melting, extrusion, channel deposits, neovascularization
Monitoring	Slit lamp examination, topography
Explantation	Rate: Range of 0.5–83.3%, in large studies: 0–1.4% [2] (for PMMA rings) Indications: Poor vision, keratitis, stromal melting, extrusion, neovascularization

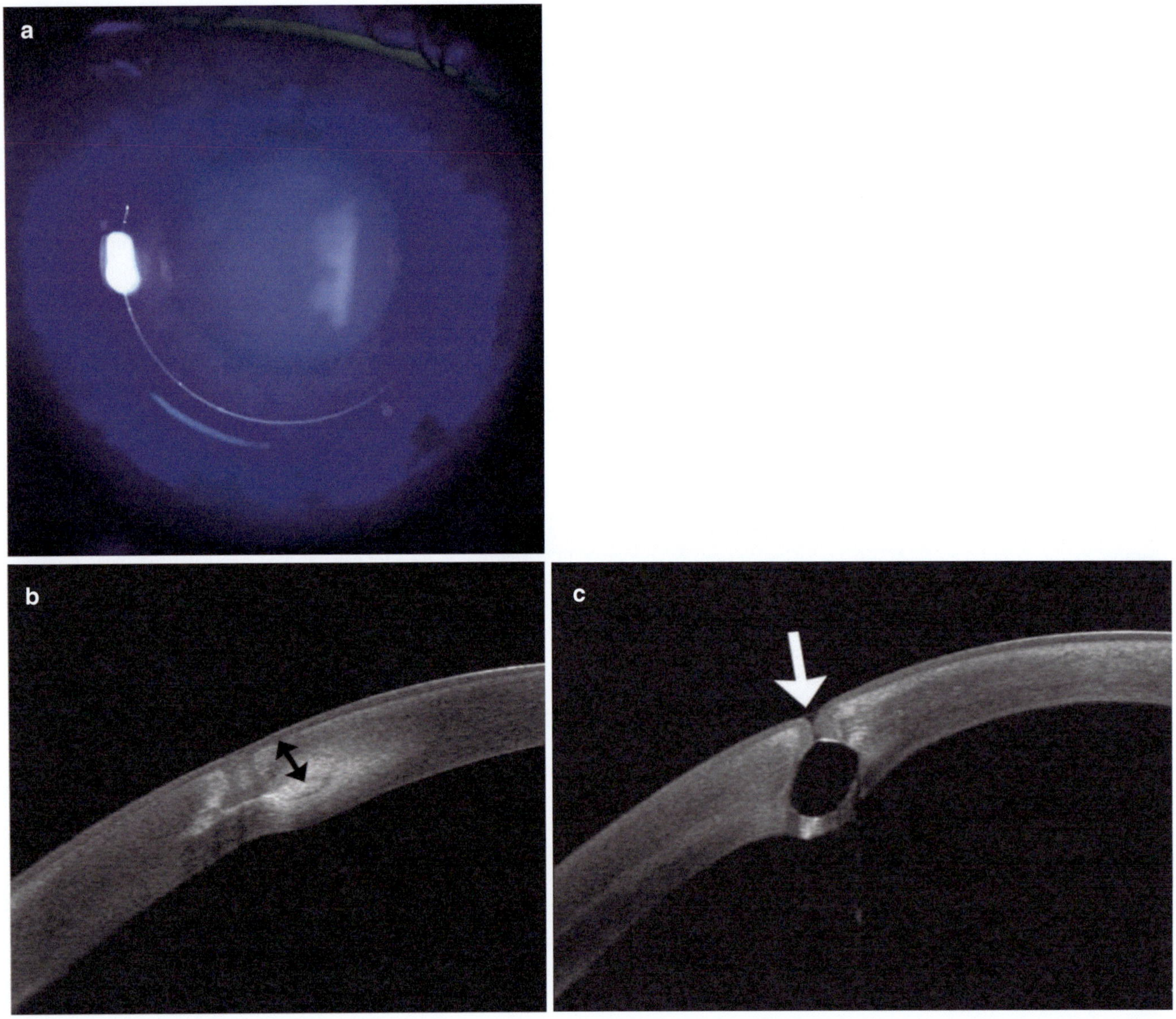

Fig. 14.1 Epithelial downgrowth following ring explantation. (*Courtesy of Shady T. Awwad, MD. American University of Beirut Medical Center, Beirut, Lebanon*)

Core message: ASN can sometimes present simply as an epithelial defect, but OCT shows that this narrow defect is actually a stromal melt extending to the PMMA.

Case 1: 5 years following ICRS implantation a patient presented with foreign body sensation (Fig. 14.2a, b).

Case 2: 2 years after implantation of a single INTACS ICRS segment, patient presented with foreign body sensation (Fig. 14.2c, d).

Exam:

Patient 1: Implant extrusion surrounded by areal of melted cornea (Fig. 14.2a, b).

Patient 2: Melting at the insertion site with extrusion of the edge of the ring, and neovascularization (Fig. 14.2c).

Management: Amniotic membrane was glued to the area of melting in patient 2 (Fig. 14.2d); however, corneal melting reoccurred and explantation was therapeutic.

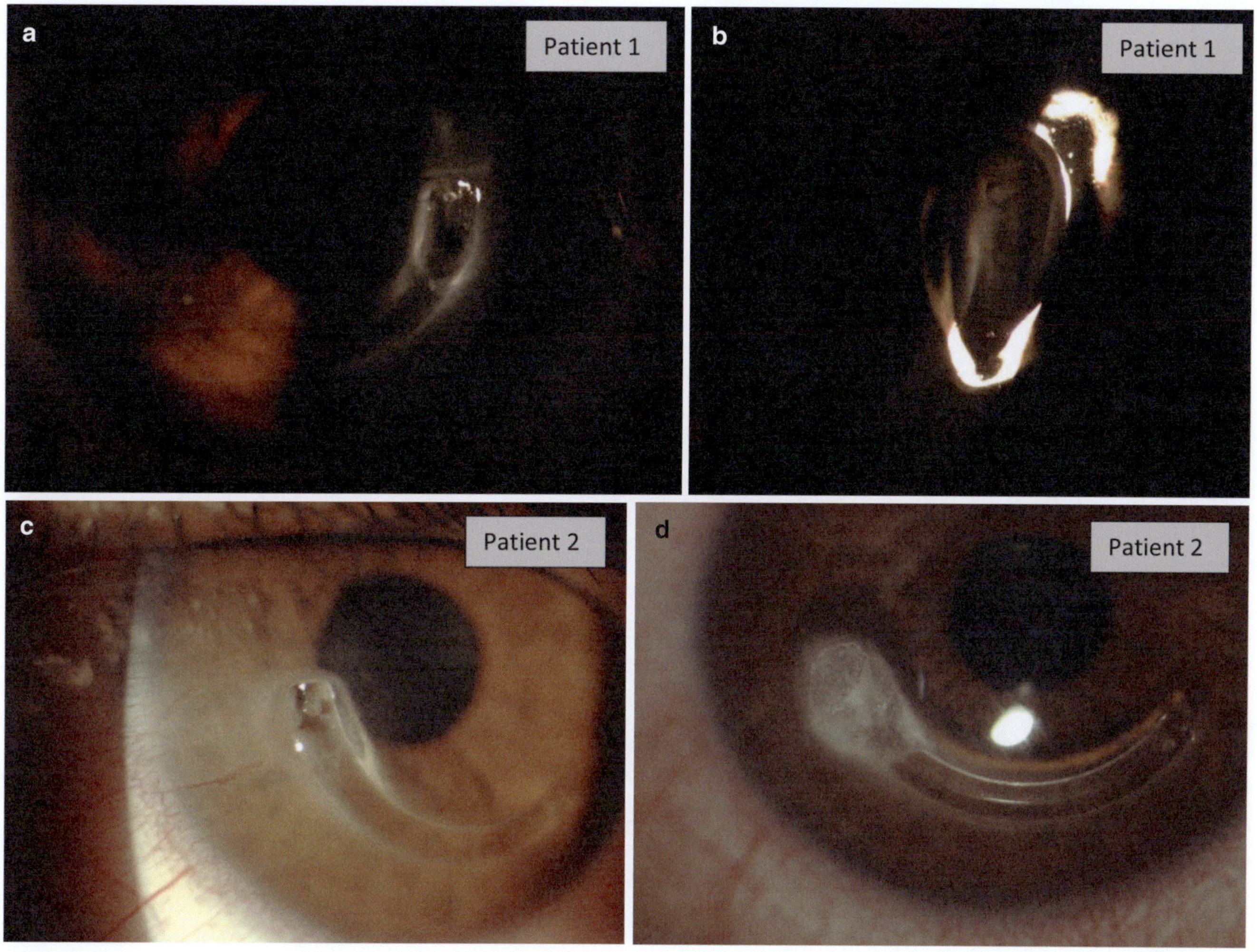

Fig. 14.2 Corneal melting following ICRS

Implant should be explanted as soon as the melting is identified and possibly replaced by a biocompatible corneal segment.

Core message: Thinning, melting, and subsequent extrusion is an important complication post ICRS that requires explantation. Amniotic membrane is usually ineffective in reversing the melting.

Case: Following the implantation of 2 ICRS, two asymptomatic patients presented for follow up (Fig. 14.3).

Exam: Migration of the ring segments touching their distant end (Fig. 14.3a, b) in one patient and dissecting laterally inside the cornea (Fig. 14.3c, d) in the second patient.

Management: Observation if patients are asymptomatic and the cornea does not show any melting. Repositioning can be attempted if there are signs of melting, inflammation, or topographic changes.

Core message: Corneal 10–0 suturing at the incision location deep inside the cornea creates a scar and prevents the ICRS migration.

Case: 2 years after ICRS implantation, a patient presented for a follow up (Fig. 14.4).

Exam: Corneal neovascularization was noted in the channels around the ring segments (Fig. 14.4a–c).

Management: Close monitoring and explantation if there are signs of corneal thinning or melting.

Case: Asymptomatic patients were seen in clinic for follow up (Fig. 14.1).

Exam: Dense white deposits around the ICRS along the corneal channel (Fig. 14.5a, c). Deposits are minimal and located at the border of the ICRS (Fig. 14.5d, e).

Management: Close observation is advised.

Core message: Non-inflammatory deposits in the corneal tunnels are not visually significant and do not cause melting.

Case: Patient presenting with photophobia, redness, pain, and blurry vision few days following ICRS implantation (Fig. 14.6).

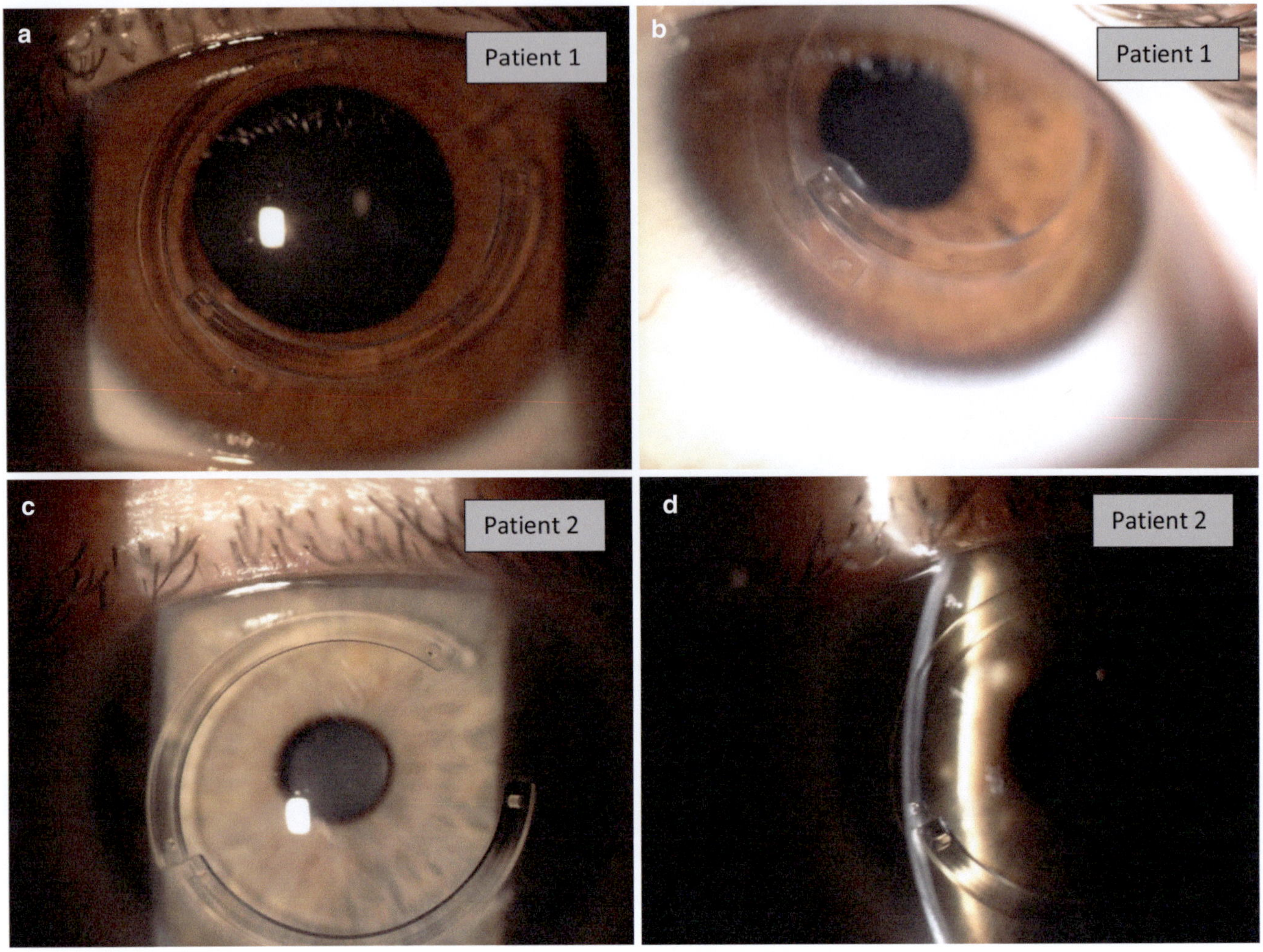

Fig. 14.3 ICRS migration

Exam: Crystalline keratopathy, infiltrates can be seen around the ring with associated corneal edema.

Management: Implant should be explanted and topical fortified antibiotics started.

Case: A patient with keratoconus S/P ICRS implantation 4 years ago presented with sudden onset of blurry vision. Patient was referred to us after failure of antibiotic treatment and ICRS was explanted due to suspicion of infectious keratitis (Fig. 14.7).

Exam: Inferior corneal stromal edema, scarred ring tunnels and peripheral corneal neovascularization (Fig. 14.7a).

Management: Corneal hydrops was suspected, patient was given topical steroids, aqueous suppressors, and his condition improved over a month with residual scarring in the ring tunnel (Fig. 14.7b).

Core Message: Corneal hydrops can occur in the early or late postoperative period following ICRS implantation.

Case: Broken ICRS noted postoperatively (Fig. 14.8).

Management: Observation if the best corrected visual acuity was stable or improved following implantation.

Case: Patient with previous ICRS melting had a CAIRS replacement (Fig. 14.9).

Exam: Slit lamp showing a well centered intrastromal allogenic implant (Fig. 14.9a). The implant segments were shaped manually from a corneal graft (Fig. 14.9b). Corneal OCT shows the allogenic stomal implants with hyperreflective filling ***(white arrow)*** (Fig. 14.9c) compared to the ICRS implant, which is hypo reflective ***(Asterix)*** (Fig. 14.9d).

Core message: CAIRS implants can safely relace ICRS when there is a corneal melting. It can be prepared manually, or via femtosecond.

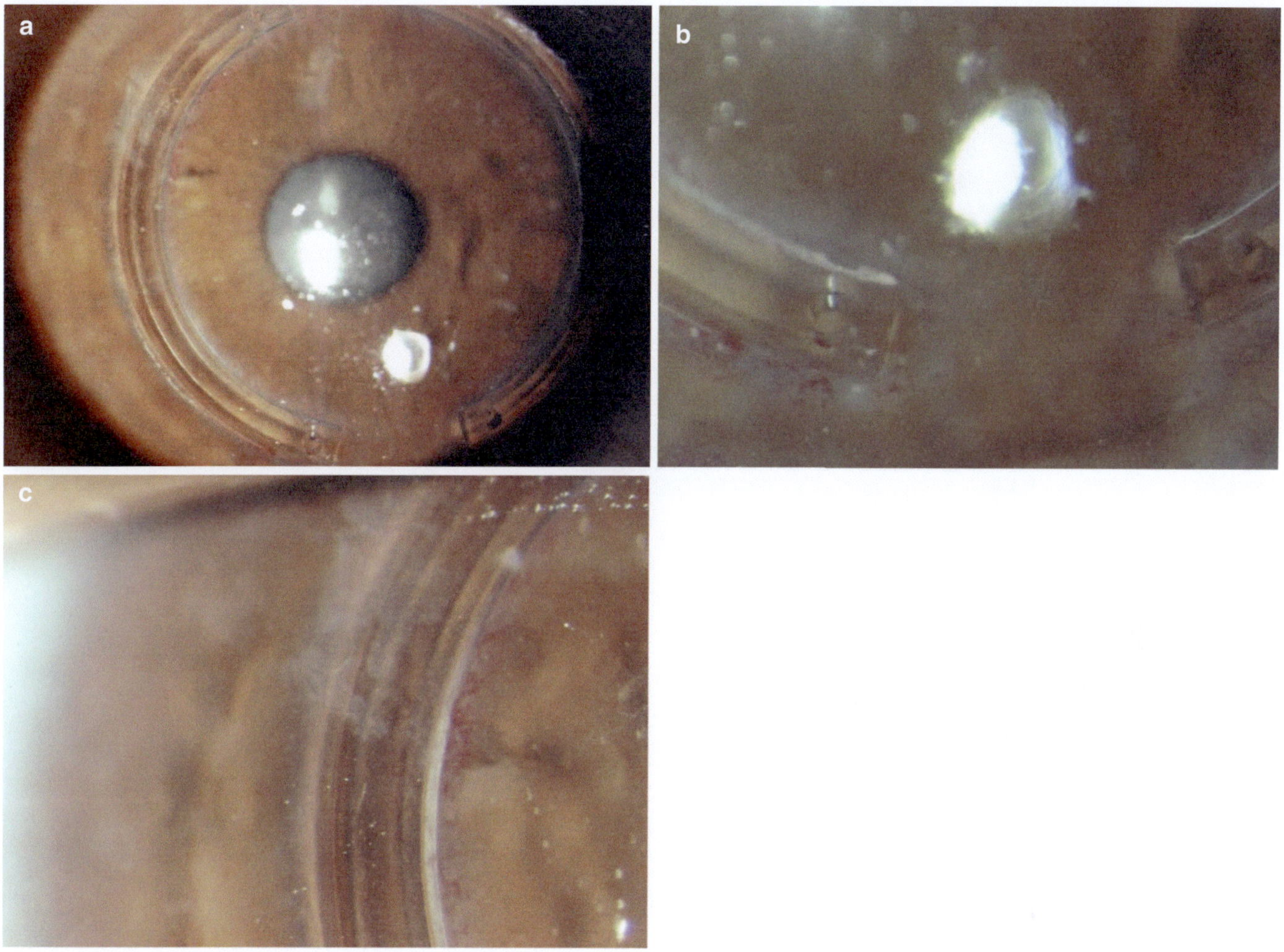

Fig. 14.4 ICRS neovascularization

Case: Follow up exam 3 months s/p keranatural implantation in a patient with keratoconus, UCVA improved from 20/400 to 20/80 (Fig. 14.10).

Exam: Intrastromal transparent and smooth shape corneal ring segment without complications (Fig. 14.10a, b).

Core message: Keranatural is a biocompatible implant, it is made in the lab as compared to CAIRS, which is usually shaped by the surgeons.

Case: Patient presented several years following penetrating keratoplasty with irritation and pain (Fig. 14.11).

Exam: A titanium ring can be seen at the junction graft-host (Fig. 14.11a); fluorescein staining shows a nasal extrusion of the implant (Fig. 14.11b).

Management: Implant explantation was performed urgently.

Core message: Titanium ring is discontinued now. It was used in the past to reduce post-penetrating keratoplasty astigmatism. It should be removed whenever extruded from the cornea.

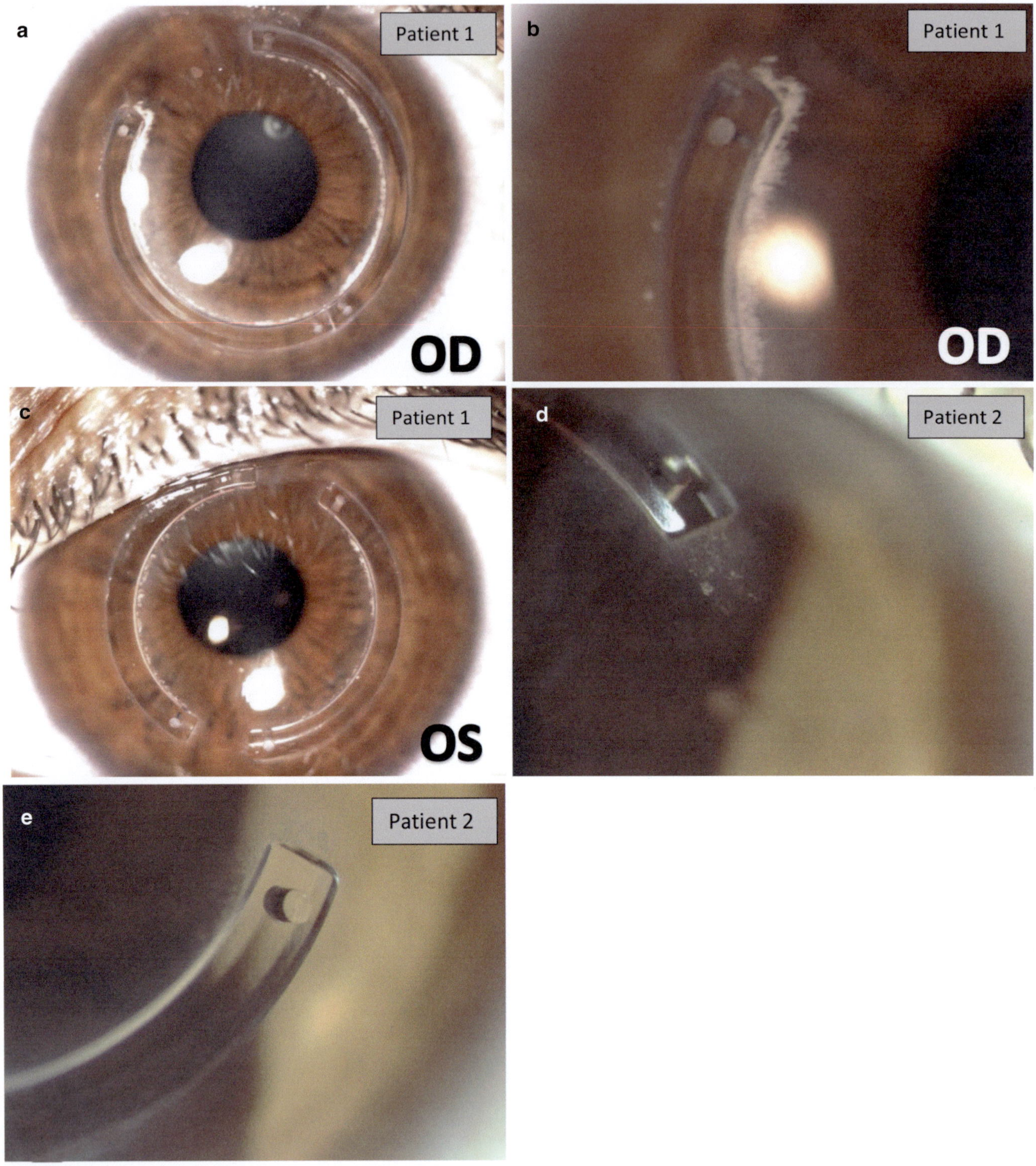

Fig. 14.5 Intrastromal tunnel deposits

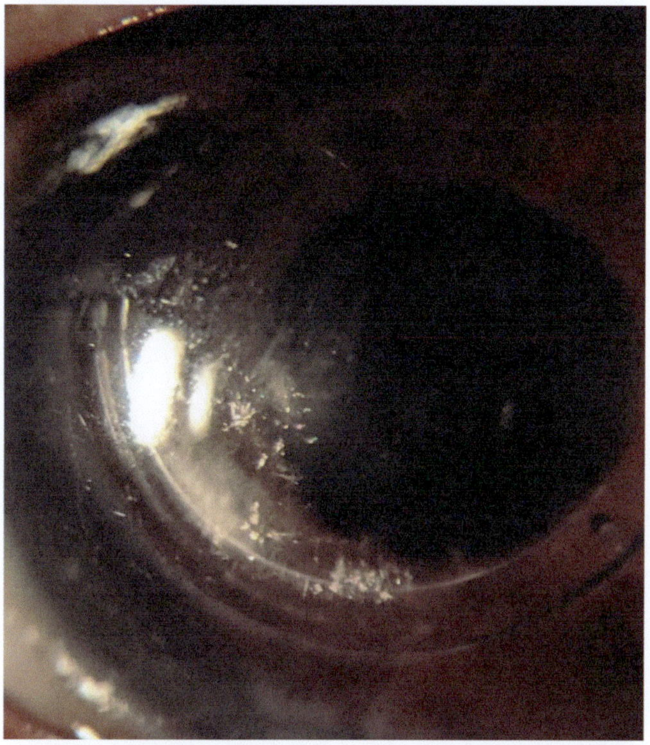

Fig. 14.6 Cristalline keratopathy. (*Courtesy of Jimmy Hu, MD. New York Eye and Ear Infirmary at Mt. Sinai, New York, USA*)

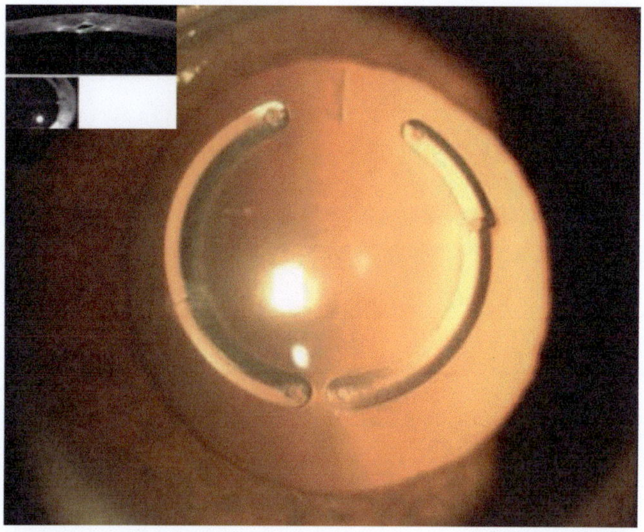

Fig. 14.8 Broken ICRS. (*Courtesy of Arun Gulani, MD. Gulani Vision Institute, Florida, USA*)

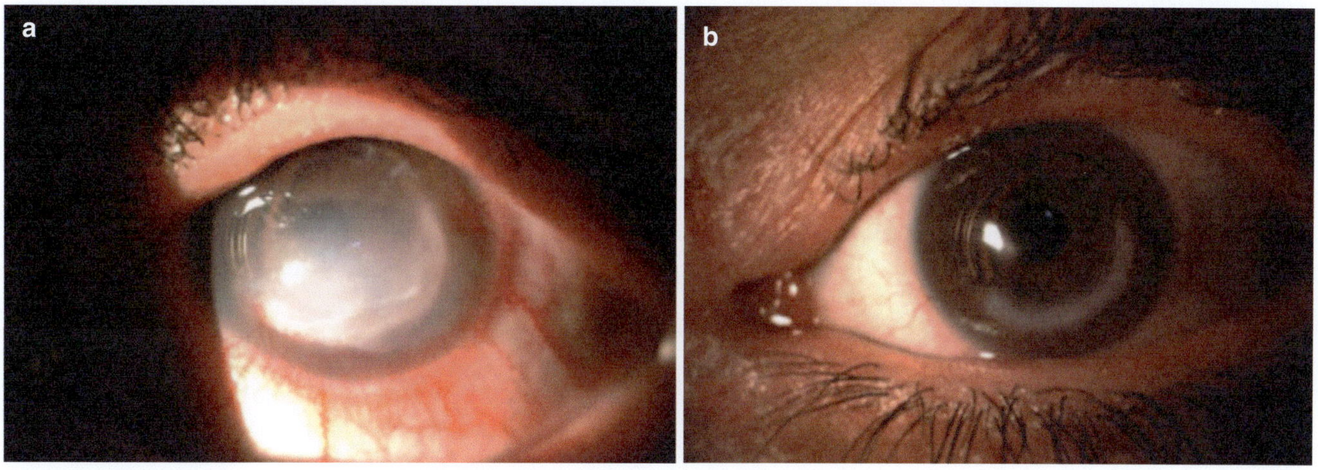

Fig. 14.7 Corneal hydrops following ICRS. (*Courtesy of Johnny Khoury, MD*)

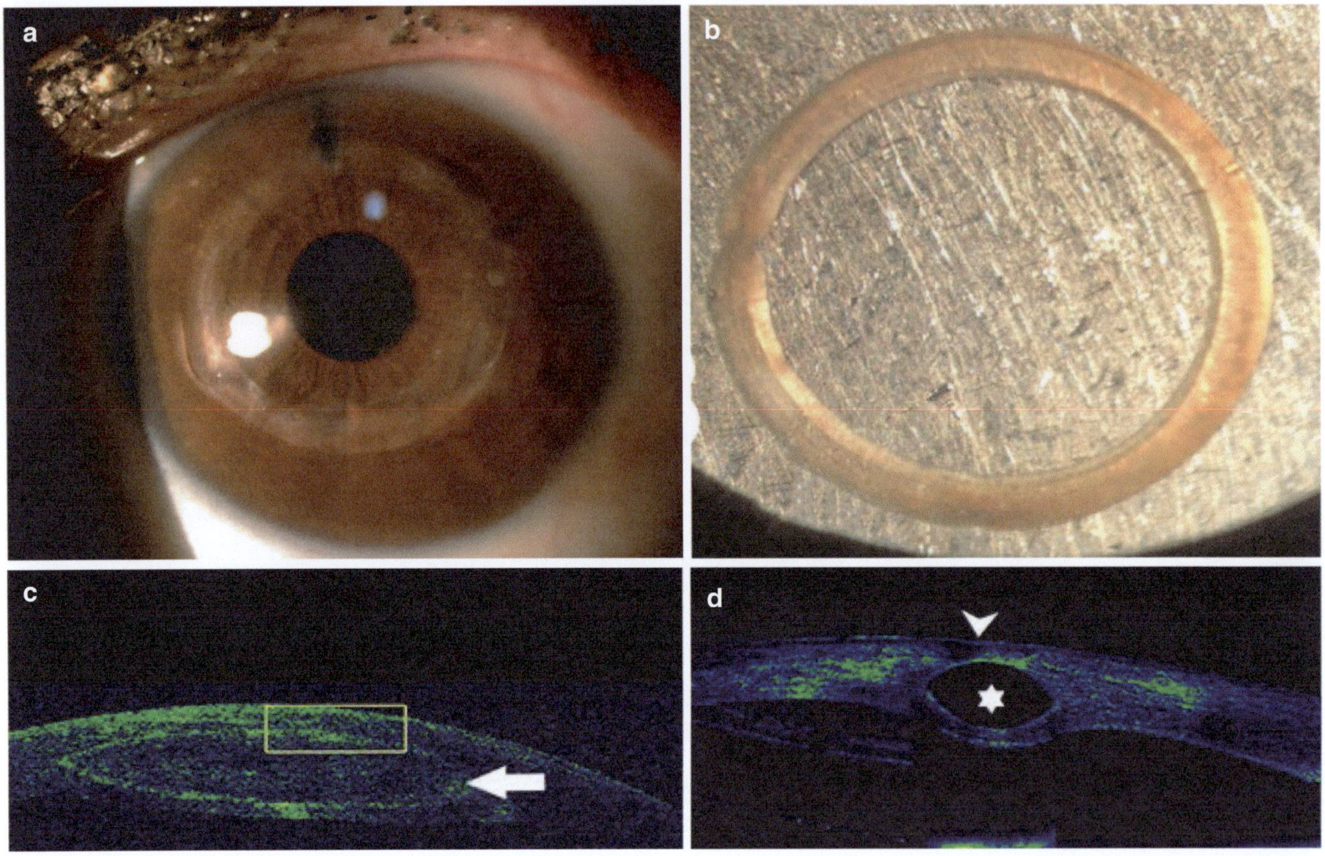

Fig. 14.9 CAIRS. (*From "Biologic stromal ring to manage stromal melting after intrastromal corneal ring segment implantation" by Jarade E, Issa M, Chanbour W, Warhekar P., 2019, J Cataract Refract Surg. 2019 Sep;45* (9)*:1222–1225. Reprinted with permission from Wolters Kluwer Health, Inc. License: 5471601266461*)

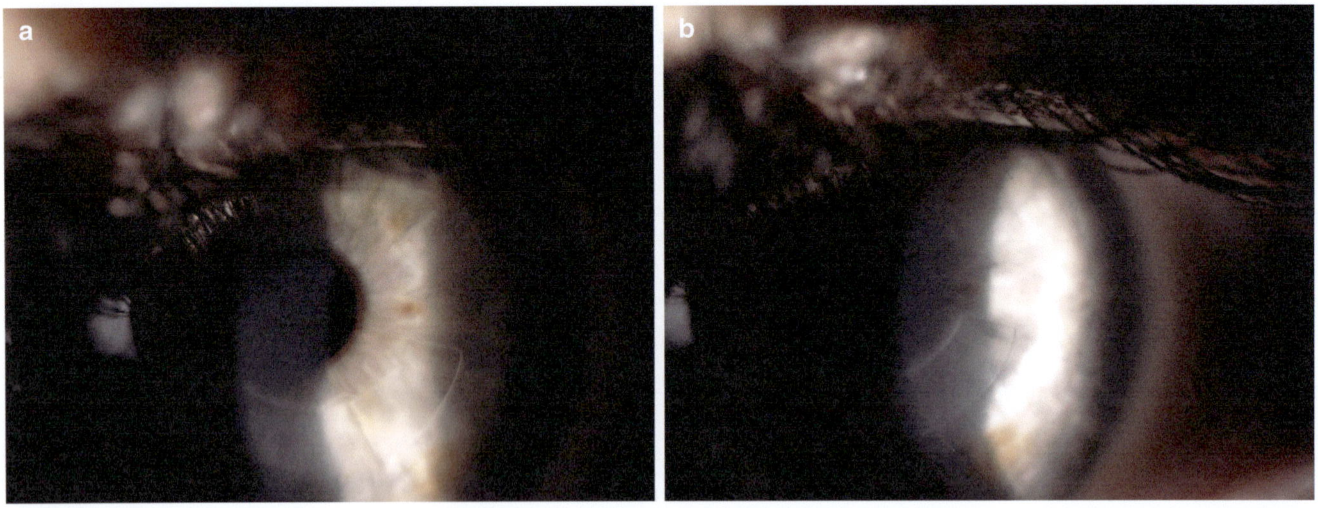

Fig. 14.10 Keranatural. (*Courtesy of Suphi Taneri. MD. Augenzentrum am St. Franziskus Hospital Münster, Münster, Germany*)

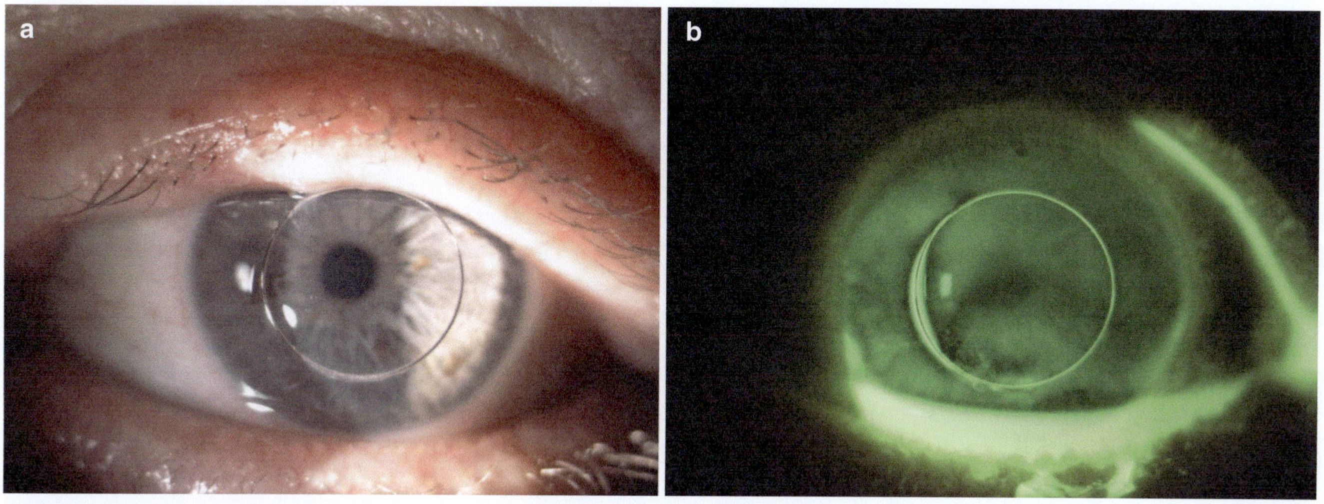

Fig. 14.11 Titan ring. (*Courtesy of Suphi Taneri MD. Augenzentrum am St. Franziskus Hospital Münster, Münster, Germany*)

Raindrop Implant

See Table 14.2.

Cases and respective exam:

Fig. 14.12A1, 2: Grade 1 haze 1 month following uneventful Raindrop insertion.

Fig. 14.12B1, 2: Grade 2 haze 1 year following Raindrop implantation.

Fig. 14.12C1, 2, 3, 4: Grade 3 haze 2 years after non-complicated implantation.

Fig. 14.12d Grade 2 haze in the left eye of a 50-year-old female 1 year after inlay placement **(1)**, and 1-month postoperative appearance after explantation showing persistent central stromal scarring **(2)**

Management: Explantation followed by steroid and antibiotic drops.

Core message: Explantation and corneal scraping should be performed for all patients who had a Raindrop implanted.

Case: 1 month post Raindrop inlay implantation in the left eye of a 50-year-old female patient (Fig. 14.13).

Exam: Mild temporal decentration, early grade 1 haze, and superficial punctate keratopathy.

Management: Explantation.

Table 14.2 Characteristics and complications of raindrop implant

Description	2 mm diameter, hydrogel, 80% water content
History	Approved by the FDA in June 2016 for presbyopia, then recalled in October 2018 due to corneal haze
Principle	Similar refractive index to the cornea Increases diameter of central overlying cornea, increasing its steepness
Surgical technique	• Placed in non-dominant eye, over light-constricted pupil • Under a flap/intracorneal pocket of 120–200 microns [3] • Some advocated use of mitomycin which delays, but does not eliminate the appearance of corneal haze
Complications	• Visual complaints: Halos, blurring • Haze, can be graded based on extent: Grade 0 (no haze), grade 1 (mild peripheral edge haze), grade 2 (prominent peripheral edge haze), or grade 3 (central haze) [4] • Infectious keratitis, decentration, melting, extrusion
Recommendation	Notification of patients and explantation is recommended due to the haze

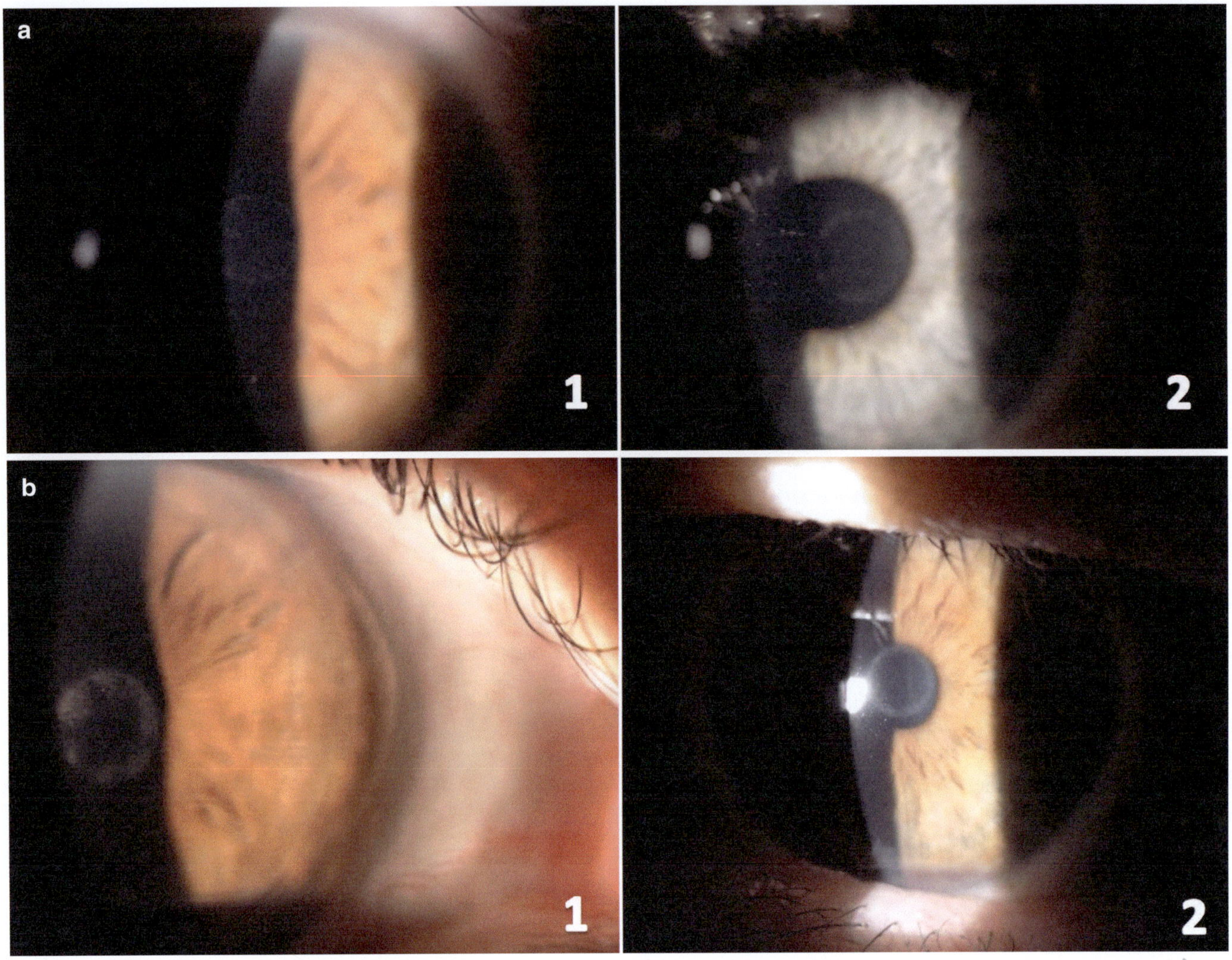

Fig. 14.12 Corneal haze following Raindrop implants

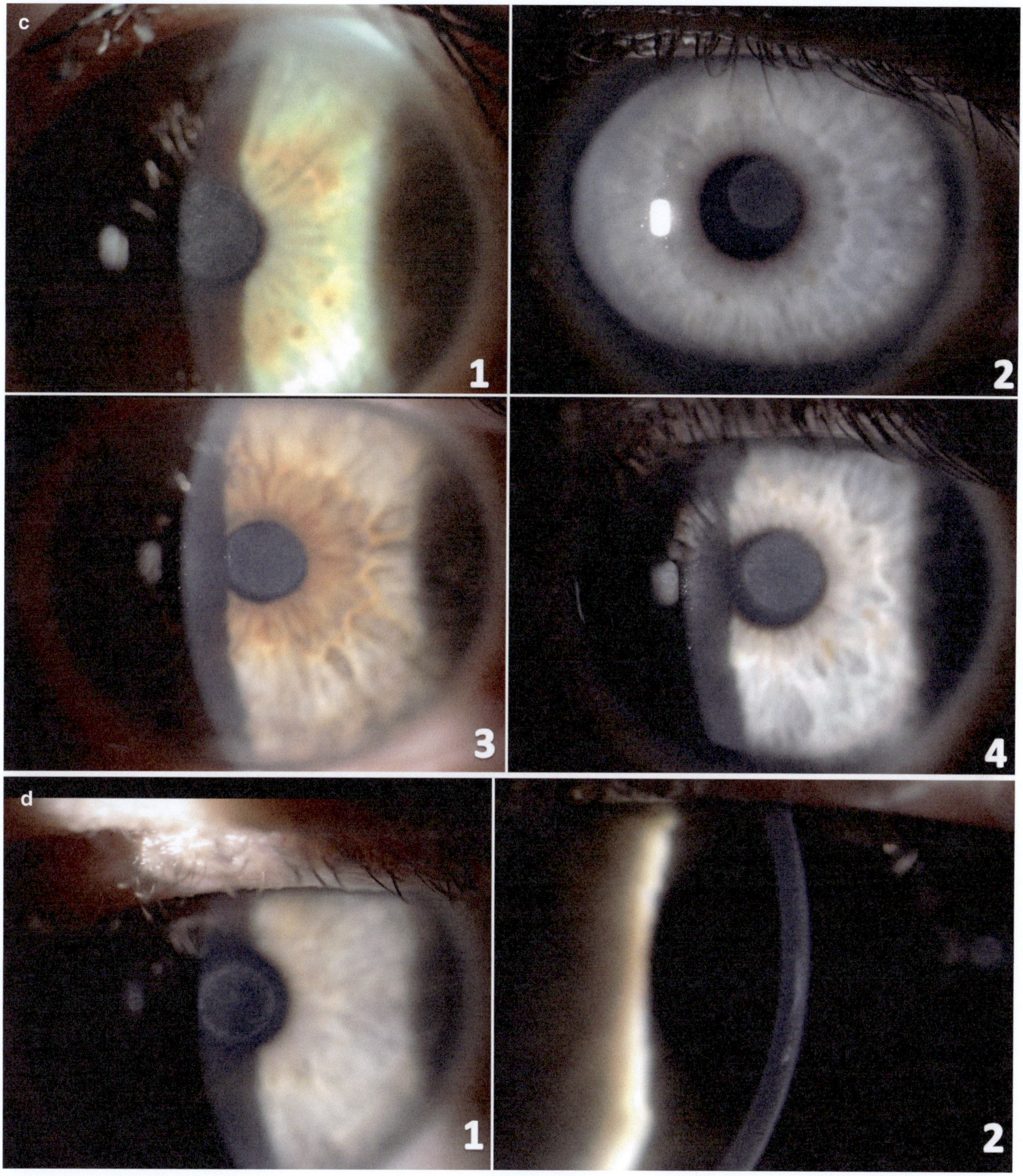

Fig. 14.12 (continued)

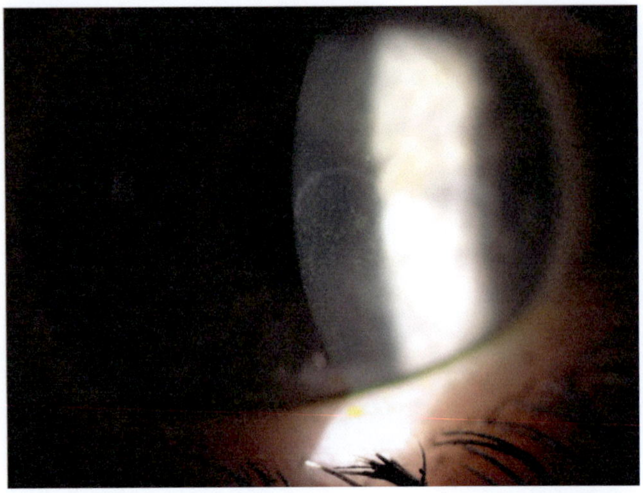

Fig. 14.13 Raindrop implant migration

Epikeratophakia

See Table 14.3.

Case: 22 years following Lenticule implantation to treat refractive error in a patient with keratoconus (Fig. 14.14).

Exam: Slit lamp exam showed a hazy interface between the anterior epikeratophakia lenticule and the posterior host cornea.

Management: Implant should be explanted. CXL should be considered in case of documented keratoconus progression.

Case: A young high hyperopic patient with shallow anterior chamber presented for refractive surgery (Fig. 14.15).

Management: LASIK flap was created followed by an allogenic lenticule transplantation onto the stromal bed. Surgery was followed with a re-lift and customized ablation of the lenticule 4 weeks later to correct residual refractive error.

Table 14.3 Characteristics, indications and complications of epikeratophakia [5]

Description	Allogenic lenticule implantation in the cornea. Implantation of an allogenic corneal lenticule to correct refractive error or reinforce the cornea
History	• Introduction by Kaufman in 1979 • Fallen out of favor after the introduction of PRK/LASIK • Reintroduced in Europe as Lenticule intrastromal keratoplasty (LIKE)
Indications	• Correct high refractive error in aphakic patients or high hyperopes • Correct myopia • Reinforce the cornea in keratoconus patient
Surgical technique	• Freeze dried lenticules prepared • Lenticule is then inserted in the cornea through a trephination, a Lasik flap, or a pocket
Complications	• Not accurate • Not predictable • Corneal haze/scar • Loss of BCVA

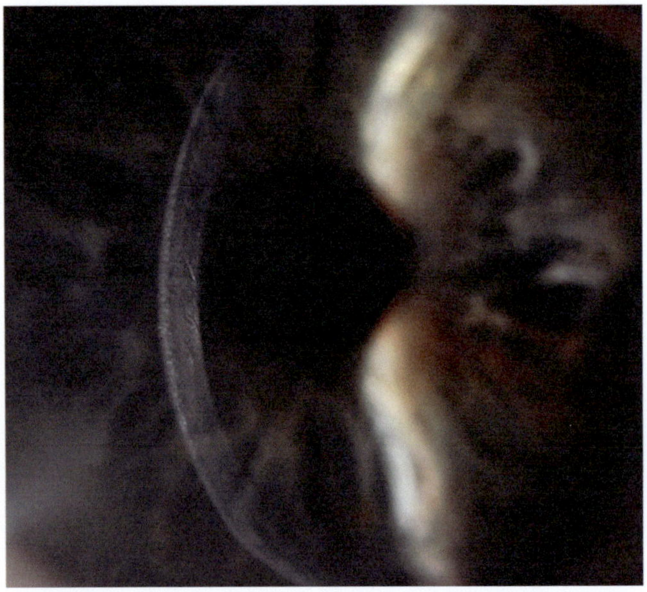

Fig. 14.14 Epikratophakia for keratoconus. (*Courtesy of Roy Rubinfield, MD. Georgetown University, Washington, DC, USA*)

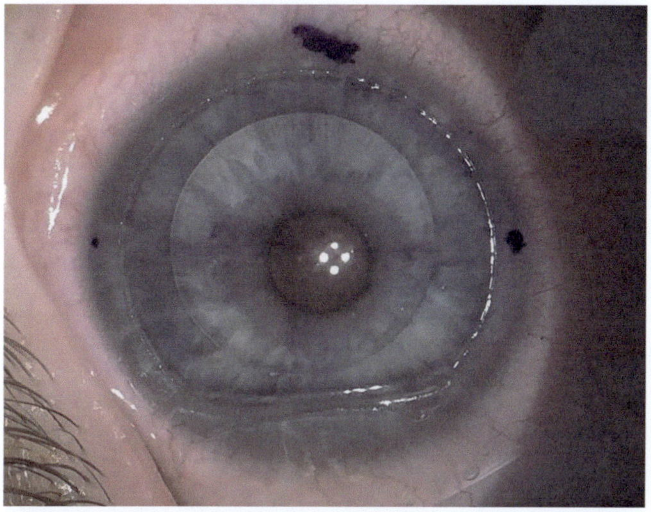

Fig. 14.15 Lenticule intrastromal keratoplasty (LIKE) . (*Courtesy of Bogdan Spiru, MD. The Institute for Refractive and Ophthalmic Surgery (IROC), Zurich, Switzerland*)

KAMRA Inlay

See Table 14.4.

Case: Slit lamp photo showing a corneal inlay in place. This 3.8-mm diameter disk with a 1.6-mm aperture and an opaque rim is placed through a 250-µm stromal pocket between the center of the pupil and the first light reflex (corneal vertex) (Fig. 14.16a).

AS-OCT section showing the inlay in place. The OCT signal is thus blocked in two distinct areas as shown by the complete opacity at each side of the aperture. The smaller pupil created focuses central light rays and blocks peripheral scattered rays to achieve a better depth of focus (Fig. 14.16b).

Case: Slit lamp photo of a well centered KAMRA inlay (Fig. 14.17a) compared to an Acufocus IC-8 IOL in the posterior chamber (Fig. 14.17b).

Case: 53-year-old female patient presented with progressive blurry vision following KAMRA implantation (Fig. 14.18).

Table 14.4 Characteristics, indications, and complications of KAMRA inlay

Description	3.8 mm in diameter, 6 microns in thickness, opaque microperforated disk, made of polyvinylidene fluoride and carbon, with a small opening (1.6 mm in diameter) in the center
History	FDA approved [6] in April 2015 for intrastromal placement in the nondominant eye in phakic patients between 45 and 60 years of age with a cycloplegic spherical equivalent between +0.50 and – 0.75 D
Principle	• Pinhole effect, obscures more peripheral rays • Increases depth of focus (small-aperture optics) [7] • Can be combined with refractive surgery in ametropic eyes [8]
Surgical technique	• Use pilocarpine drops to induce miosis to position the inlay over the pupil • Mark the first purkinje image if the distance between this image and the pupil center is less than 300 microns, otherwise mark the mid-distance between the two [9] • With the aid of femtosecond LASIK, a pocket is created at 200–250 microns depth • Dissect the pocket then place the inlay
Complications	• Visual complaints: Halos, blurring, double vision • Hyperopic shift [9], decreased contrast sensitivity, infectious keratitis [10], epithelial ingrowth, diffuse lamellar keratitis (DLK), decentration, melting, extrusion, haze [11]
Monitoring	Slit map examination, topography
Explantation	• Recurrent epithelial ingrowth, thinning or loss of 25% of corneal thickness, non-resolving DLK • May be needed before retina surgeries or laser procedures

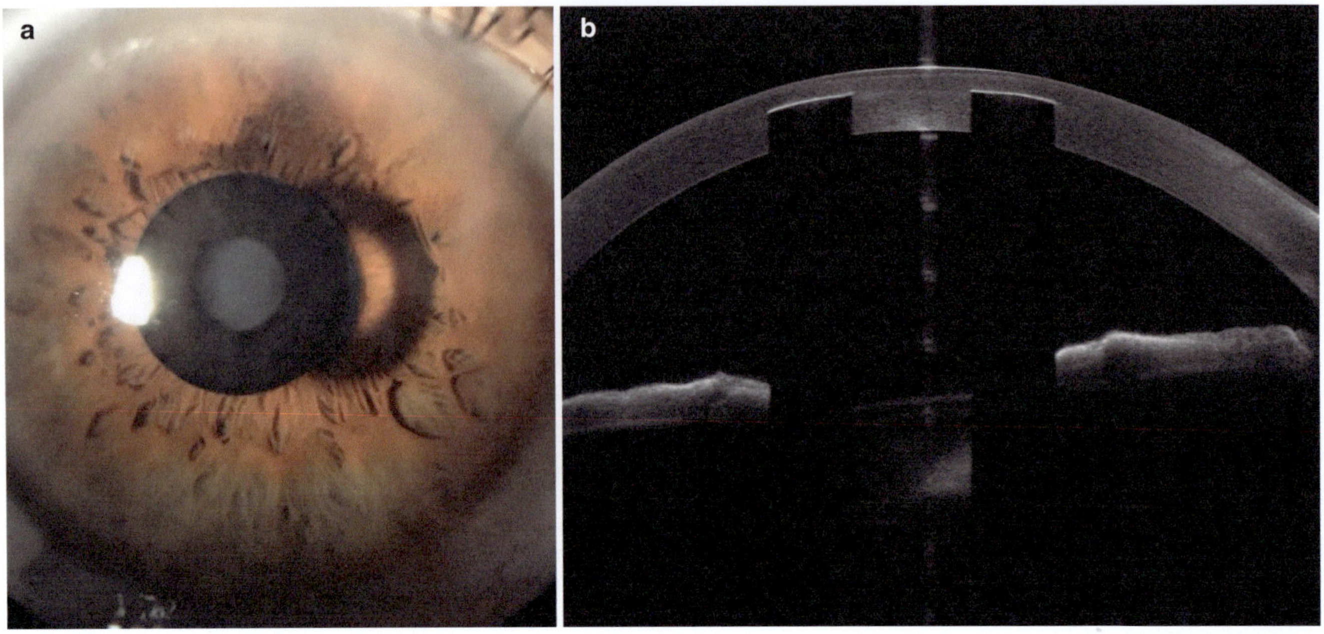

Fig. 14.16 KAMRA inlay AS-OCT. (*Courtesy of Shady T. Awwad, MD. American University of Beirut Medical Center, Beirut, Lebanon*)

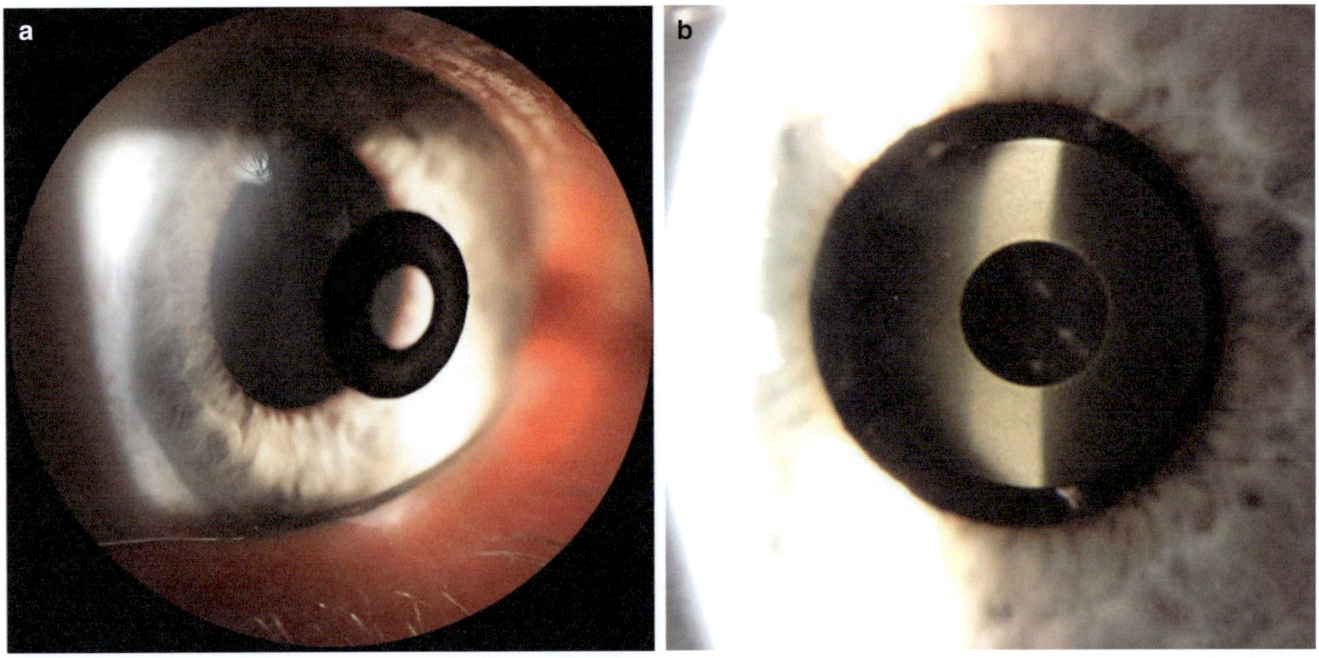

Fig. 14.17 Different pinhole implants. (*Courtesy of Majid Moshirfar, MD Moran Eye Center, Department of Ophthalmology and Visual Sciences, University of Utah School of Medicine, Utah, USA*)

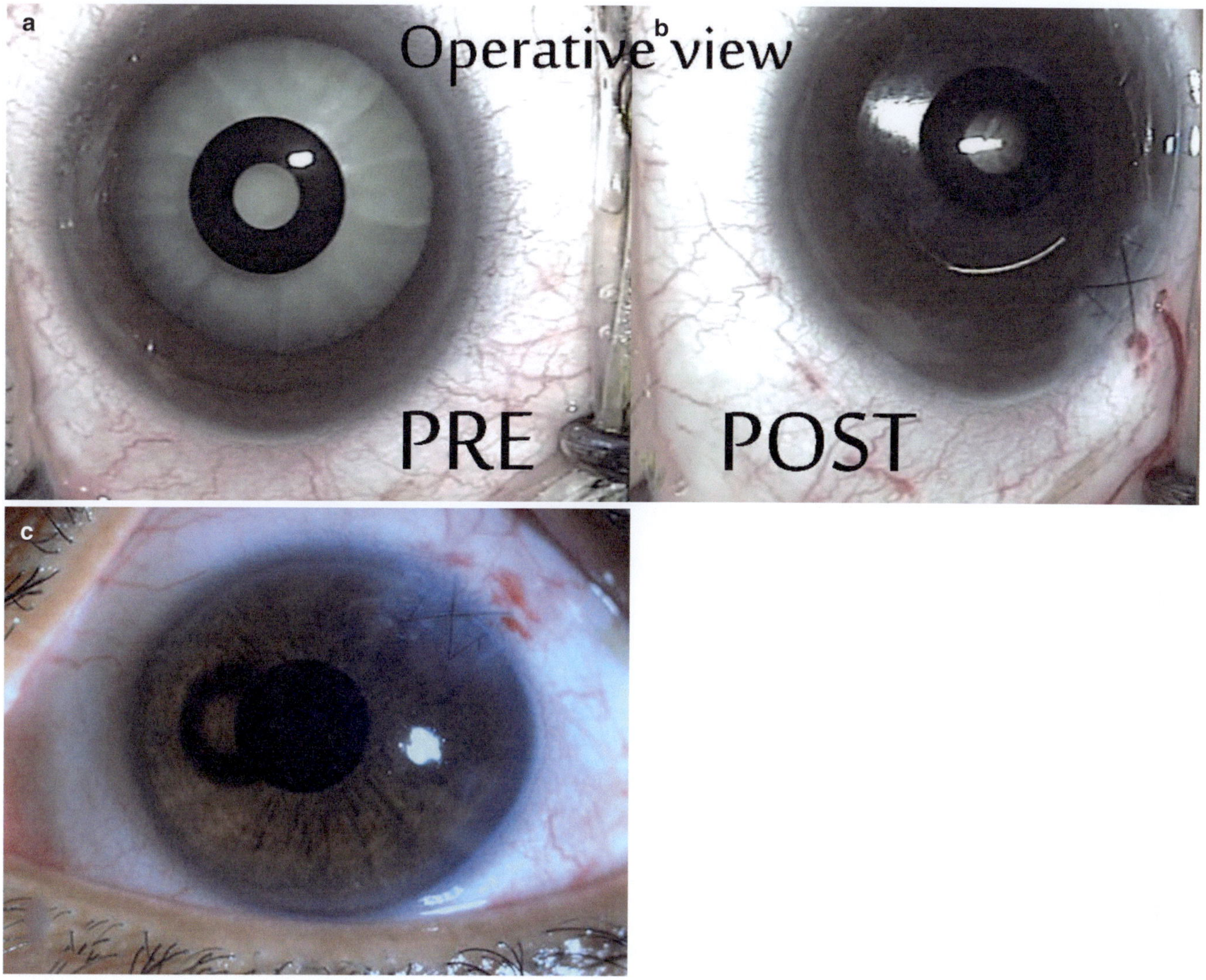

Fig. 14.18 Cataract following KAMRA

Exam: Intraoperative view of the centered KAMRA implant with a white cataract (Fig. 14.18a).

Management: Phacoemulsification and IOL implantation was performed with the KAMRA in place without complications (Fig. 14.18b). Slit lamp front view showing a well centered KAMRA next day (Fig. 14.18c). The patient near vision improved to J2.

Core message: Phacoemulsification is possible without removing the KAMRA implant.

Case: Patient presented few weeks following KAMRA implantation under a LASIK flap with monocular double vision (Fig. 14.19).

Exam: AcuTarget® Optical Quality Analysis System measurement showed well centered implant in the early post operative period (Fig. 14.19a) and a decentered implant noted at presentation (Fig. 14.19b).

Management: Flap lift and reposition was performed and the implant was recentered (Fig. 14.19c).

Core message: Pocket creation with femtosecond laser is better used when KAMRA is implanted as a solo procedure to decrease the risk of decentration under a full flap.

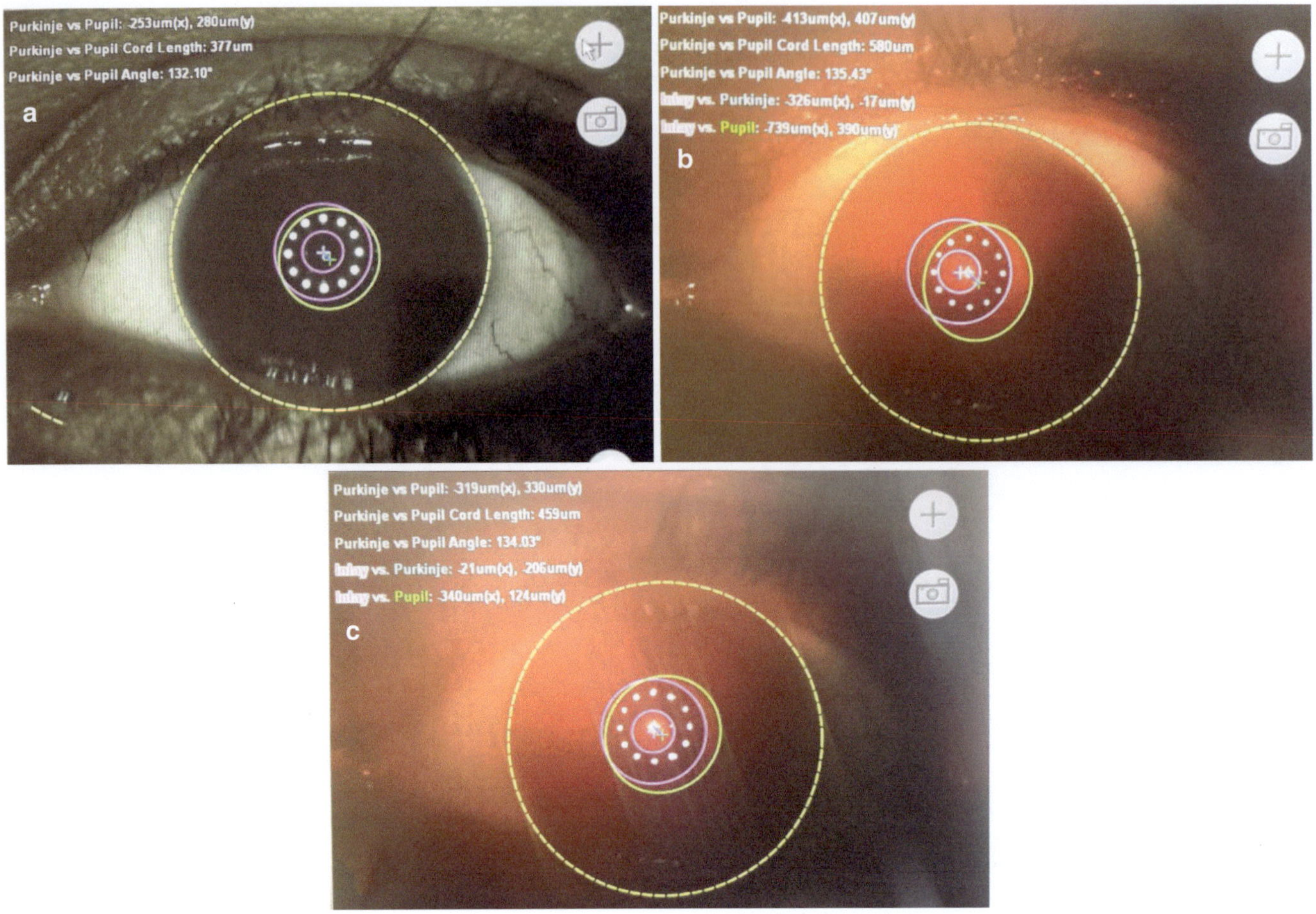

Fig. 14.19 Decentered KAMRA

Take-Home Message

- ICRS are a potentially reversible, refractive solution in keratoconus patients with contact lens intolerance and low BCVA.
- When there is an acute stromal necrosis over an intra-stromal ring segment, early intervention by removal of the ring segment is crucial before expansion of the necrosis. If the patient had good visual outcomes before melting, an allogenic corneal ring segment can be used to maintain the shape of the cornea.
- Corneal inlays should be monitored postoperatively with possible need for readjustment or explantation.
- Raindrop inlays for presbyopia have been recalled due to high potential of corneal haze. Inlays developing haze should be removed.
- KAMRA implants enhance near vision but are not without short- and long-term complications.
- Cataract surgery is safe following KAMRA implantation. Intraoperative ocular rotation with forceps may be necessary to improve visualization.

References

1. U.S. Food and Drug Administration, Center for Drug Evaluation and Research. Summary of Safety and Probable Benefit for H040002 INTACS® Prescription Inserts for Keratoconus. https://www.accessdata.fda.gov/cdrh_docs/pdf4/h040002b.pdf.
2. Bautista-Llamas MJ, Sánchez-González MC, López-Izquierdo I, et al. Complications and Explantation reasons in Intracorneal ring segments (ICRS) implantation: a systematic review. J Refract Surg. 2019;35(11):740–7.
3. Moarefi MA, Bafna S, Wiley W. A review of presbyopia treatment with corneal inlays. Ophthalmol Ther. 2017;6(1):55–65.
4. Fenner BJ, Liu YC, Koh SK, et al. Mediators of corneal haze following implantation of Presbyopic corneal inlays. Invest Ophthalmol Vis Sci. 2019;60(4):868–76.
5. Cahill M, Condon P, O'Keefe M. Long-term outcome of epikeratophakia. J Cataract Refract Surg. 1999;25(4):500–7.
6. Premarket Approval (PMA). https://www.accessdata.fda.gov/scripts/cdrh/cfdocs/cfpma/pma.cfm?ID=P120023. Accessed 27 Mar 2022.
7. Yılmaz OF, Alagöz N, Pekel G, et al. Intracorneal inlay to correct presbyopia: long-term results. J Cataract Refract Surg. 2011;37(7):1275–81.
8. Wallace MM, Ryan T. The KAMRA corneal inlay in practice. https://www.reviewofophthalmology.com/article/the-kamra-corneal-inlay-in-practice. Accessed 3 Apr 2022.

9. Moshirfar M, Desautels JD, Walker BD, et al. Long-term changes in keratometry and refraction after small aperture corneal inlay implantation. Clin Ophthalmol. 2018;12:1931–8.
10. Duignan ES, Farrell S, Treacy MP, et al. Corneal inlay implantation complicated by infectious keratitis. Br J Ophthalmol. 2016;100(2):269–73.
11. Paley GL, Harocopos GJ. Histopathologic analysis of explanted KAMRA corneal inlays demonstrating adherent Fibroconnective tissue scar formation. Ocul Oncol Pathol. 2019;5(6):440–4.

15 Phakic Intraocular Lens Implants

Francesca Kahale, Samir A. Melki, Jason Brenner, and Wassef Chanbour

See Table 15.1.

Table 15.1 Different types of phakic intraocular lens implants

<table>
<tr><th>Phakic lens</th><th>Lens type</th><th>Dioptric power for myopia</th><th>Dioptric power for hyperopia</th><th>Toric lens</th><th>Complications[a]</th><th>Contraindications</th></tr>
<tr><td>Posterior chamber</td><td>ICL[b]
STAAR surgical (Monrovia, CA, USA)</td><td>USA: −3 to -16D
Worldwide: −3 to −18</td><td>USA: Not available
Worldwide: +3 to +10</td><td>USA: Up to 4D
Worldwide up to 6D</td><td>– Cataract
– Glaucoma, IOP elevation
– Aqueous misdirection
– Pupillary block
– Malrotation, dislocation, decentration</td><td rowspan="5">– Active anterior segment disease
– Recurrent or chronic uveitis
– Cataracts
– Previous ocular surgery
– Glaucoma or IOP >21 mmHg
– Preexisting macular pathology or retinal disease
– Anomalous irises or pupils
– Systemic diseases associated with poor healing (e.g., diabetes mellitus, connective tissue disease, autoimmune disease)</td></tr>
<tr><td rowspan="3">Iris-fixated</td><td rowspan="2">Artisan
Or Verisyse</td><td>Size: 5/8.5 mm, power: −1.0 to −23.5 D</td><td rowspan="2">+1.0 to +12.0 D</td><td rowspan="2">Up to 7D</td><td rowspan="3">– Cataract
– Pupillary block
– Dislocation, decentration
– Uveitis
– Hyphema</td></tr>
<tr><td>Size:6/8.5 mm powers: −1.0 to −15.5 D</td></tr>
<tr><td>Artiflex
Or Veriflex
(foldable lens)</td><td>−2.0 D to −14.5 D</td><td>x</td><td>1.0 to 5.0D</td></tr>
<tr><td>Anterior chamber</td><td>Not currently available (removed from the market)</td><td>x</td><td>x</td><td>x</td><td>Endothelial cell loss, pupil ovalization, cataract</td></tr>
</table>

[a]All lenses are associated with pigment dispersion, glare, starburst, halos
[b] FDA approval for ICL: 21 to 45 years old, AC depth > 3 mm, AC angle grade 3 and up

F. Kahale
Mass Eye and Ear infirmary, Boston, MA, USA

S. A. Melki (✉) · J. Brenner
Boston Vision, Department of Ophthalmology, Harvard Medical School, Boston, MA, USA
e-mail: Melki@bostonvision.com; brenner@bostonvision.com

W. Chanbour
Department of Ophthalmology and Visual Neurosciences, University of Minnesota, Minneapolis, MN, USA

S. A. Melki et al. (eds.), *Refractive Surgery Atlas*, https://doi.org/10.1007/978-3-031-60661-8_15

Posterior Chamber IOL

Case: Post operative slit lamp view of a non-complicated ICL. Anterior ICL surface **(arrow)**, anterior lens capsule **(arrowhead)**, vault **(double arrow)** (Figs. 15.1 and 15.2).

Core Message: ICL vault should be between 250 and 750 μm (minimum of a half thickness of the cornea).

Case: 27-year-old female seen day 1 following Visian Toric ICL implantation. Patient had pain, nausea, vomiting, and decreased vision. IOP to >60 mmHg with a fixed, dilated pupil. Multiple peripheral iridotomies were attempted but the pupillary block did not resolve (Fig. 15.3).

Exam: The entire perimeter of the ICL can be visualized with transillumination defects. There are multiple patent peripheral iridotomies (Fig. 15.3a). The UBM demonstrates posterior vaulting of the ICL indicating that the implant is upside down (Fig. 15.3b).

Management: The patient was brought back to the OR and the implant was removed, rinsed, and replaced in the correct orientation. She maintains normal intraocular pressures and 20/15 uncorrected vision.

Core message: Correct ICL positioning can be identified during implantation, the hole located inside the leading haptic should be on the right-side during implantation (Fig. 15.3c).

Case: Two patients seen following ICL implantation (Fig. 15.4).

Exam:

Patient 1 A very shallow ICL V4c was noted with a shallow vault and Lens-ICL touch. The central ICL hole can be seen in the pupillary axis ***(red arrow)*** (Fig. 15.4a).

Patient 2: Ultrasound biomicroscopy showed a vault <175 microns (Fig. 15.4b, c).

Management: Exchange of ICL with a larger diameter is advised to avoid early cataract.

Core Message: Lens-ICL touch is an indication for ICL exchange. ICL is available with the following sizes: 12.1 mm, 12.6 mm, 13.2 mm, and 13.7 mm.

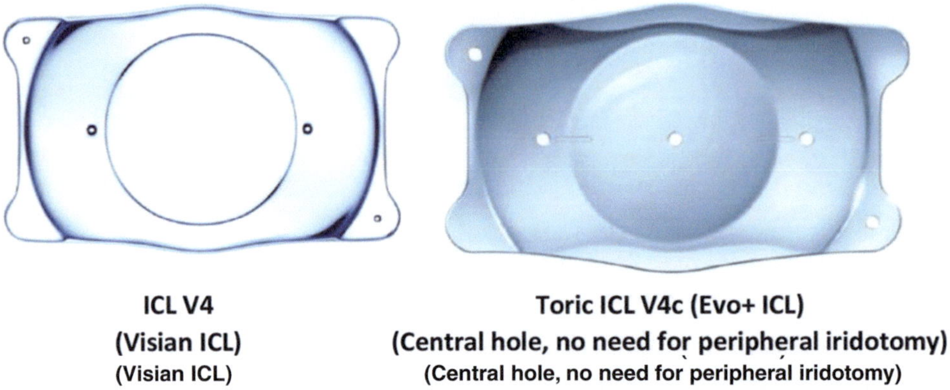

Fig. 15.1 Currently available ICL subtypes in the US. (**a**) ICL V4 (Visian ICL). (**b**) Toric ICL V4c (Evo + ICL) (Central hole, no need for peripheral iridotomy)

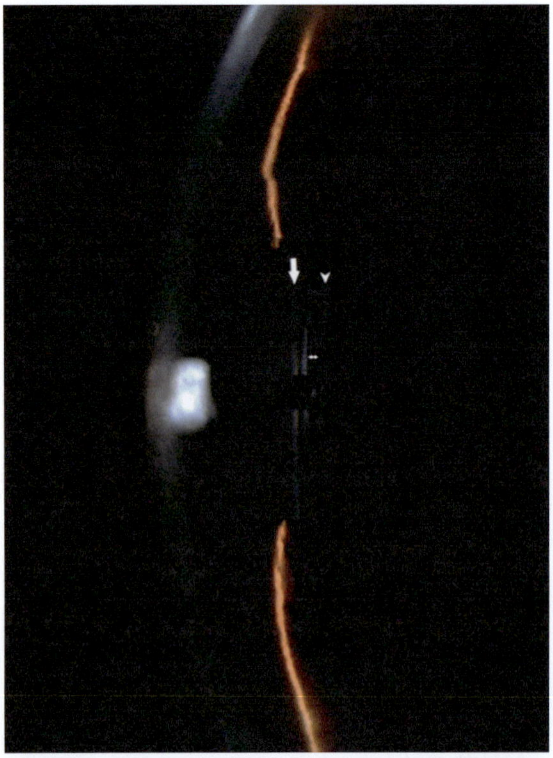

Fig. 15.2 Normal ICL positioning

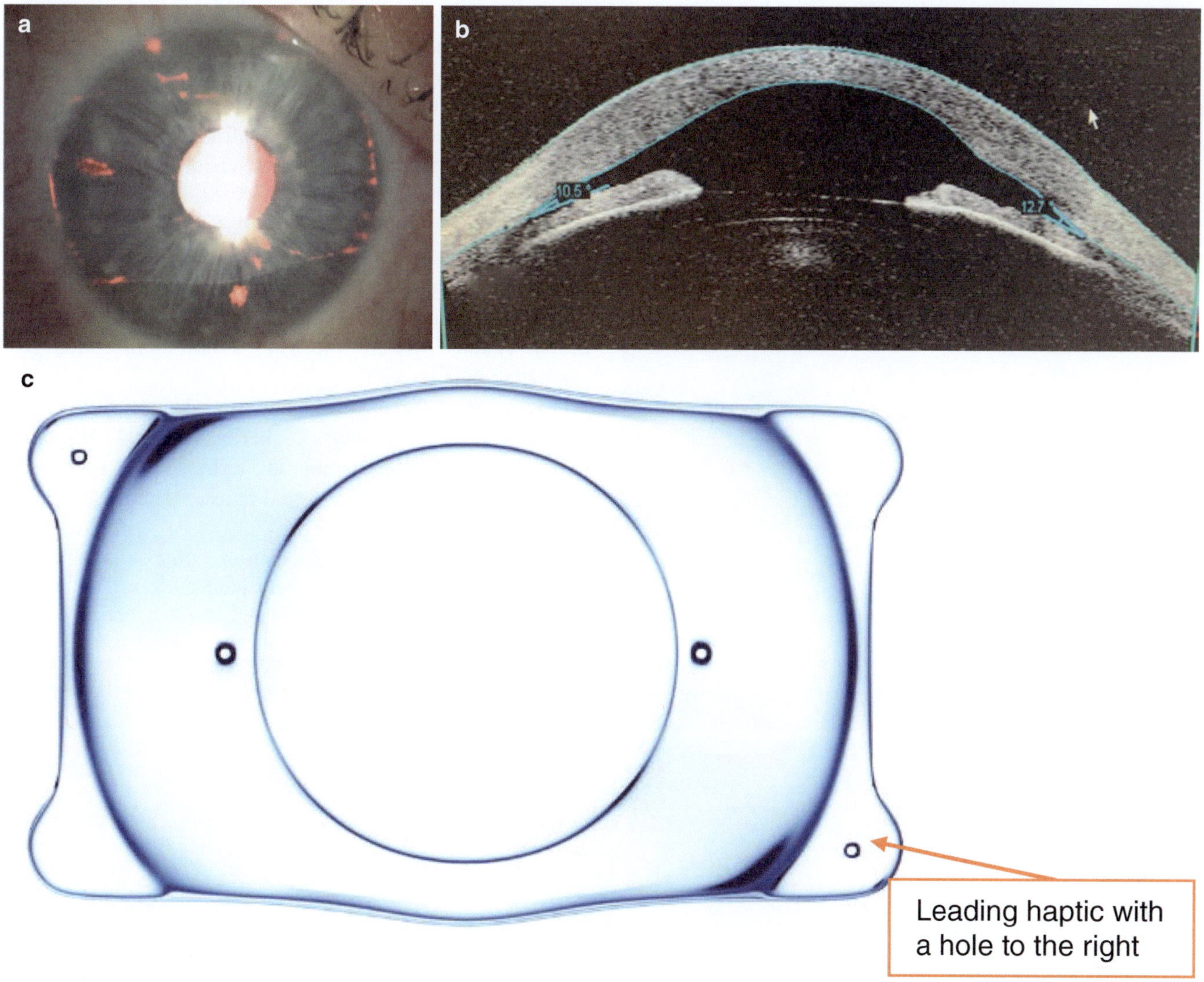

Fig. 15.3 Inverted ICL. (Courtesy of Brian Shafer, MD. Chester County Eye Care, Perelman School of Medicine, University of Pennsylvania,Pennsylvania, USA)

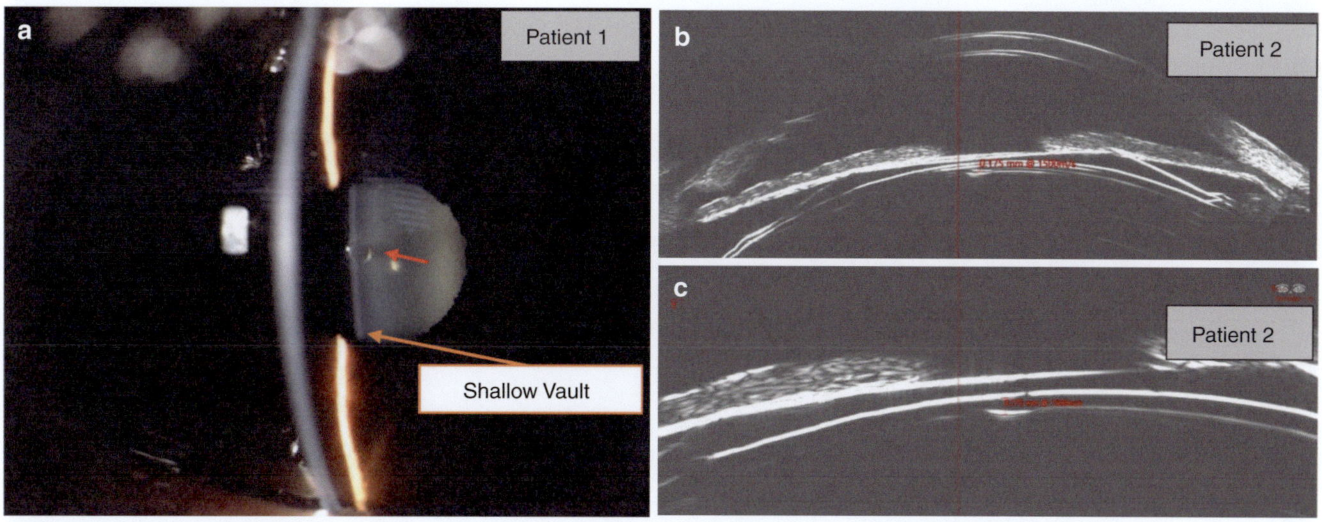

Fig. 15.4 Shallow vault. (*Courtesy of Suphi Taneri, MD, Augenzentrum am St. Franziskus Hospital Münster, Münster, Germany*. Courtesy of Dan Ohman, MD, Department of Ophthalmology, Orebro University Hospital, Orebro, Sweden)

Case: Cataract noted 6 years following ICL implantation for high myopia, visual acuity remained stable 20/25 compared to the early postoperative state and the patient is asymptomatic (Fig. 15.5).

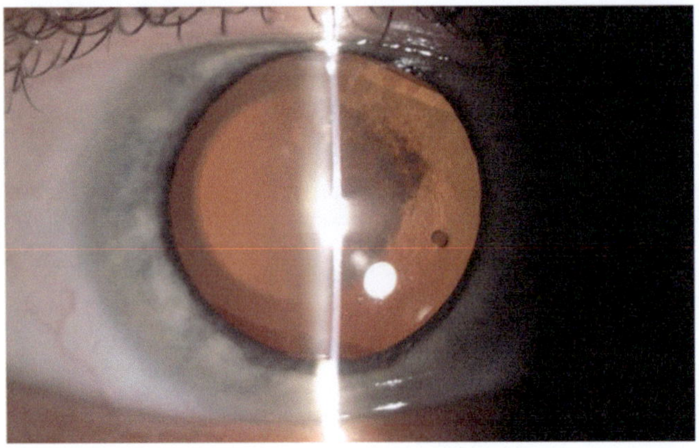

Fig. 15.5 Lens opacity. (*Courtesy of Suphi Taneri, MD, Augenzentrum am St. Franziskus Hospital Münster, Münster, Germany*)

Management: Observation vs. ICL explantation.

Core message: If the patient has a cataract and is asymptomatic, surgeon can elect to observe or explant the ICL, especially if it has a shallow vault.

Case: 5 Year following ICL, patient presented to clinic with progressive decline in his vision (Fig. 15.6). VA 20/60.

Exam: Anterior diffuse subcapsular opacity (Fig. 15.6a, b).

Management: ICL explanation with cataract extraction and posterior chamber IOL implantation.

Case: A 32-year-old patient presented for progressive blurry vision 8 years following a non-complicated ICL implantation (Fig. 15.7).

Exam: Slit lamp exam showed central anterior subcapsular opacity and a large superior surgical iridotomy (Fig. 15.7a); anterior chamber OCT showed a shallow vault with anterior capsular touch and anterior subcapsular cataract ***(red Arrow)*** (Fig. 15.7b).

Management: ICL explanation, phacoemulsification with IOL implantation were performed.

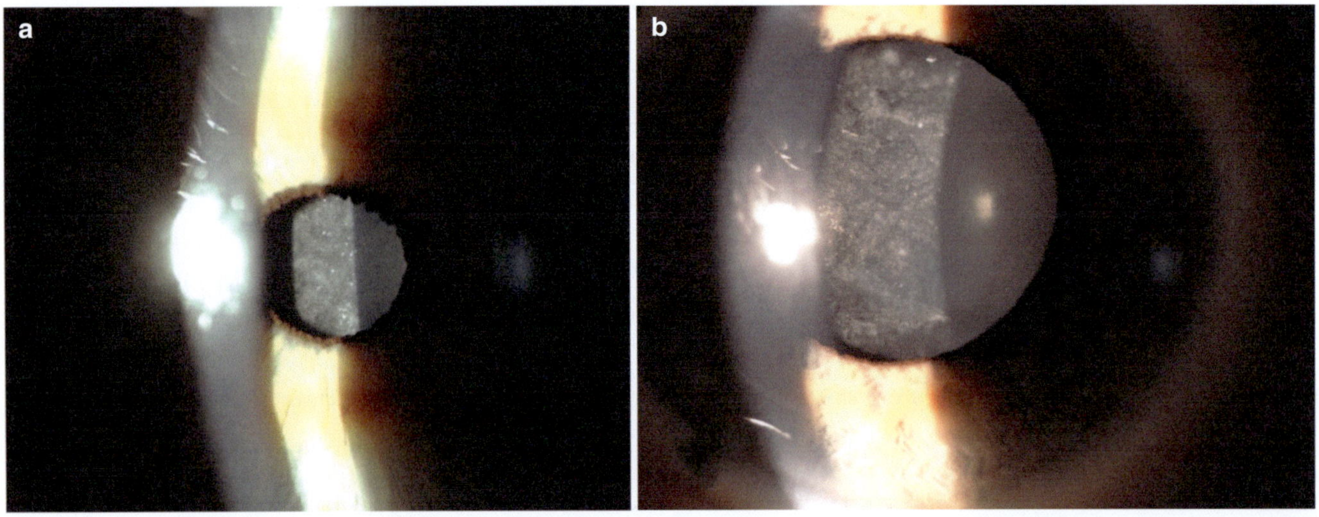

Fig. 15.6 Anterior subcapsular cataract

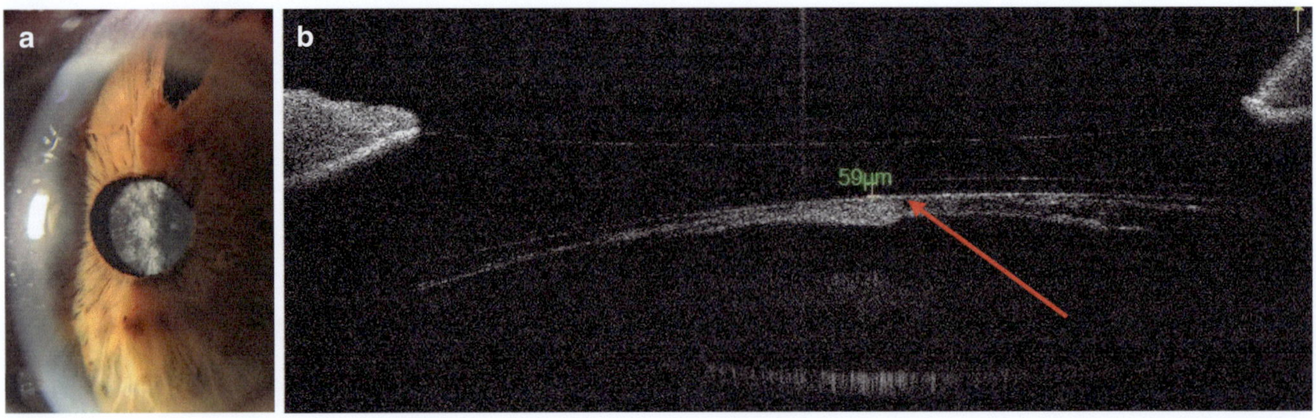

Fig. 15.7 ICL-lens touch. (*Courtesy of Jimmy Hu, MD. New York Eye and Ear Infirmary at Mt. Sinai, New York, USA*)

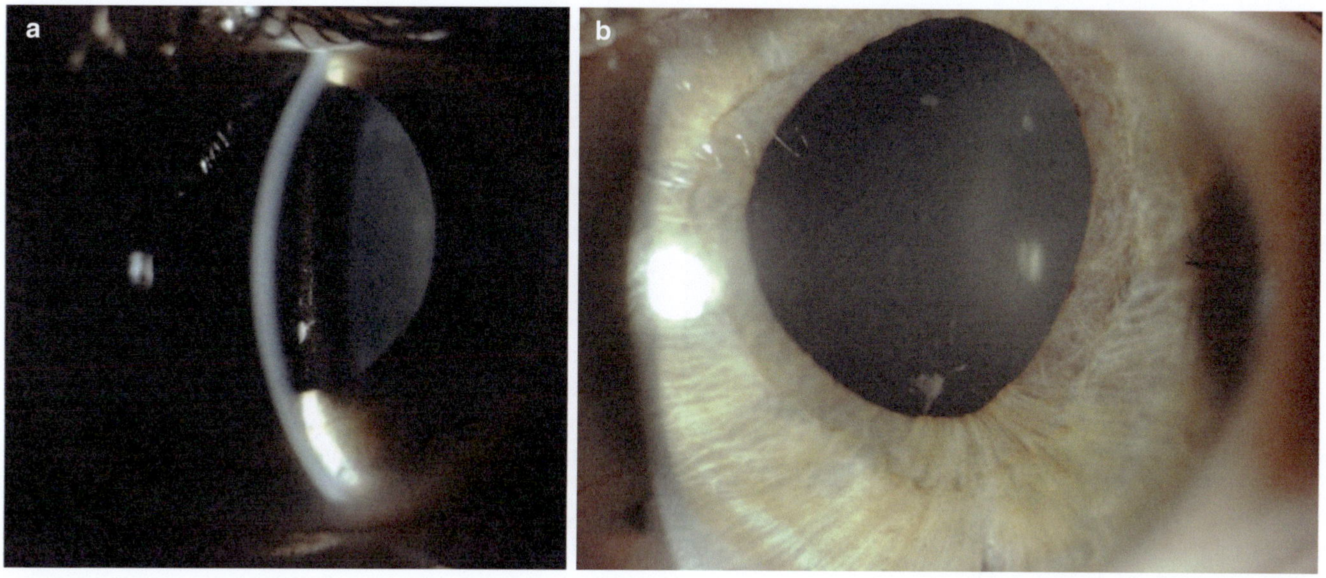

Fig. 15.8 ICL induced angle closure

Core message: When detected, a very shallow vault with ICL-lens touch should be explanted and replaced with a larger diameter lens.

Case: Few hours following ICL implantation (ICL V4, without a central hole), patient presented to the ED with pain, photosensitivity, and blurry vision. IOP was 55 mmHg. Patient had two previous peripheral iridotomies (Fig. 15.8).

Exam: Fixed dilated pupil and completely occluded angle with irido-corneal touch. High ICL vault is noted with pigment deposits on the ICL (Fig. 15.8a).

Management: Aqueous suppressants, pilocarpine, and enlarging the iridotomies failed to resolve the pupillary block. ICL was later explanted. When IOP normalizes a smaller size ICL was placed in a third surgery. Post operatively, the pupillary sphincter was noted to be ruptured and remained in a mid-dilated state (Fig. 15.8b).

Core message: Pupillary block and malignant glaucoma are hard to differentiate following ICL implantation. ICL should be explanted when there is no response to medical treatment.

Case: Few months following an uneventful toric ICL implantation **(lens axis rotated 10 degrees counterclockwise)**. A patient presented with a blurry vision when he was awake in the morning. Patient was reported to be restless overnight. UCVA was 20/100 but BCVA remained 20/20 but with an astigmatism correction >3D (Fig. 15.9).

Exam: Dilated exam showed that the toric ICL axis was 120 degrees ***(red arrow)*** **(total rotation of 70 degrees clockwise, compared to original position).**

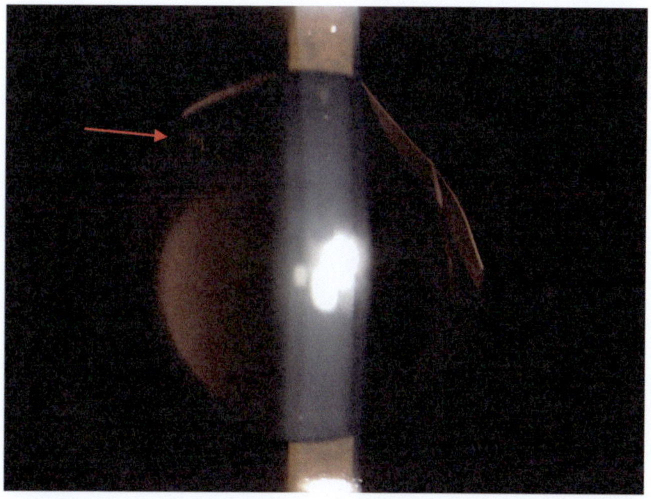

Fig. 15.9 ICL malrotation

Management: Surgical intervention was necessary to realign the axis to its recommended positioning.

Core message: ICL rotation is a known complication that can occur at any time postoperatively. In case of recurrence, ICL may be exchanged with a larger size.

Case: A Patient with keratoconus had both ICRS and ICL implanted (Fig. 15.10).

Core message: In stable keratoconus, if the corneal astigmatism becomes regular following ICRS insertion, ICL can be implanted to correct the residual refractive error.

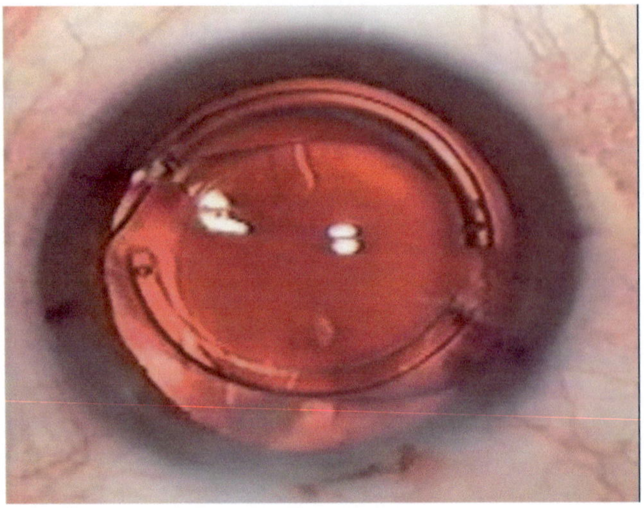

Fig. 15.10 Combined procedures. (*Courtesy of Arun Gulani, MD, Gulani Vision Institute, Florida, USA*)

Iris-Fixated Phakic IOL

See Fig. 15.11.

Case: Postoperative appearance of a noncomplicated iris-fixated phakic intraocular lens used to correct high myopia. Peripheral iridotomy is noted supero-temporally patient's uncorrected visual acuity was 20/20 (Fig. 15.12).

Case: Dilated pupil during a follow-up exam in a patient with iris-fixated IOL implantation (Fig. 15.13).

Core message: Iris-fixated phakic IOL does not contraindicate dilating the pupil.

Case: Poorly centered iris-fixated IOL in a patient with 20/25 uncorrected visual acuity (Fig. 15.14).

Management: Observation and regular specular microscopy is recommended.

Core message: Iris-fixated phakic IOL should be removed in case of lens-cornea touch, decreasing endothelial cell count or change in visual acuity.

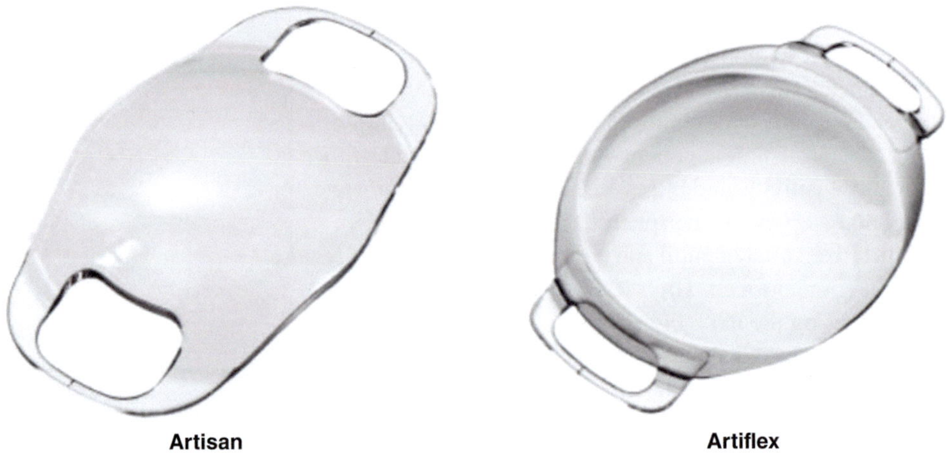

Fig. 15.11 Available types of iris-fixated IOL. (**a**) Artisan. (**b**) Artiflex

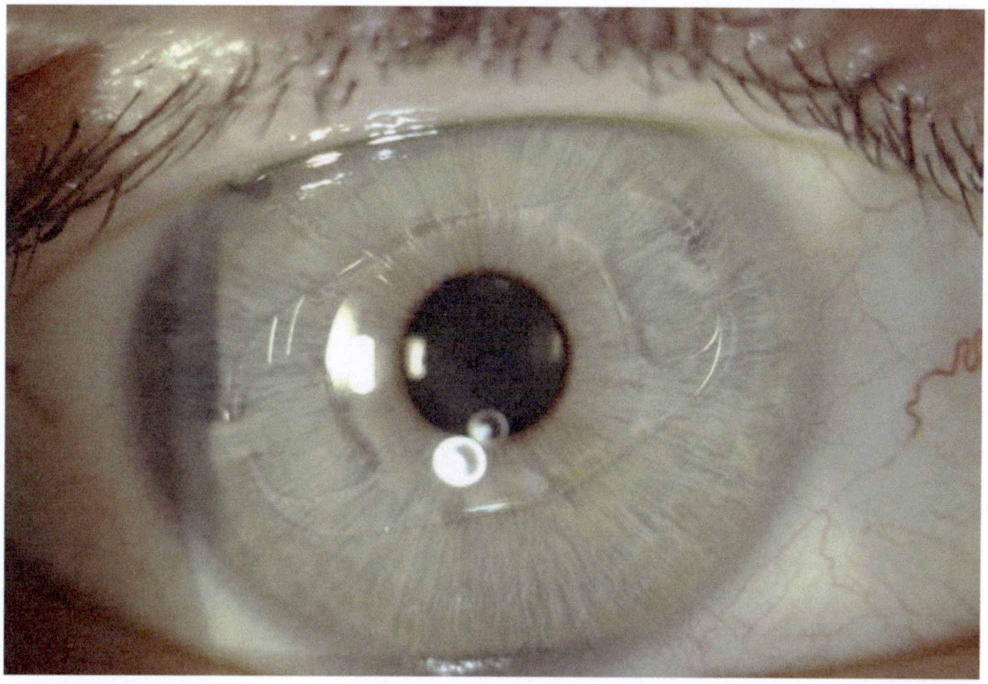

Fig. 15.12 Iris claw phakic IOL

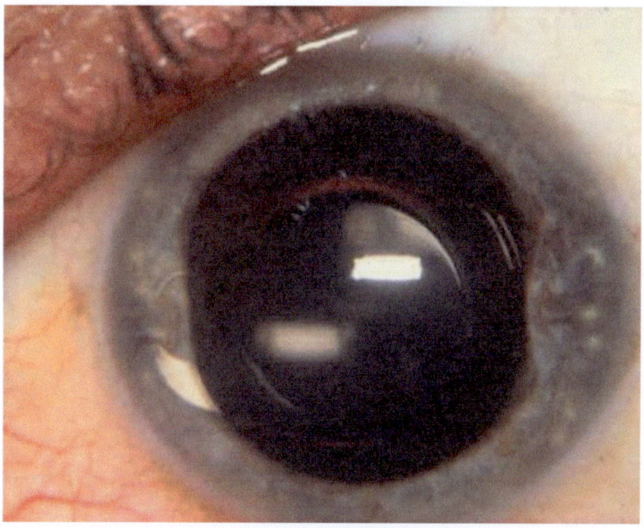

Fig. 15.13 Pupillary dilation in iris-fixated IOL. (*Courtesy of Arun Gulani, MD, Gulani Vision Institute, Florida, USA*)

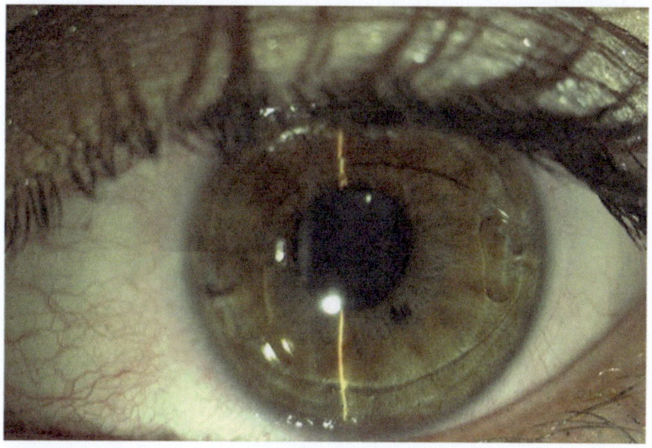

Fig. 15.14 Poor centration

Case: Patient with a history of good vision following iris-fixated IOL presented with sudden blurry vision (Fig. 15.15).

Exam: An inferiorly dislocated iris-fixated IOL can be noted; the superior claw is noted to be well attached.

Management: Since the iris is not atrophic, a repositioning was performed successfully. Otherwise, removal and exchange with an ICL at a later time is also possible.

Case: Patient presented with progressive blurry vision years following iris-fixated IOL (Fig. 15.16).

Exam: Inferior corneal edema extending into the visual axis, there is no lens-cornea touch.

Management: IOL explanation is necessary.

Core message: Specular microscopy and pachymetry should be performed regularly in patients with iris-fixated and AC IOL.

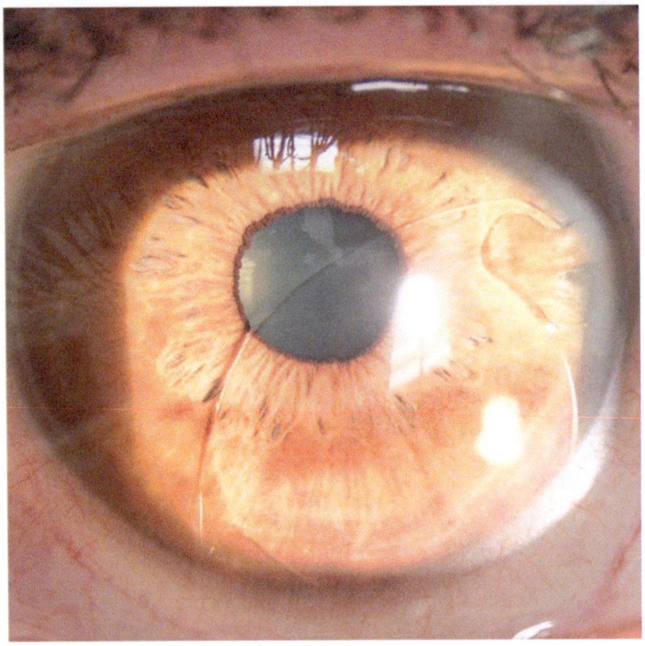

Fig. 15.15 Dislocated iris-fixated IOL. (*Courtesy of Majid Moshirfar. MD. Hoopes Vision, Draper UT; John A. Moran Eye Center, Department of Ophthalmology and Visual Sciences, University of Utah School of Medicine, Murray, Utah, USA*)

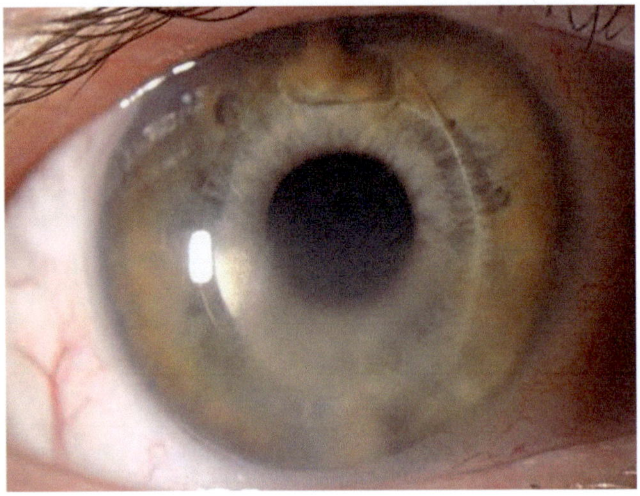

Fig. 15.16 Endothelial decompensation. (*Courtesy of Majid Moshirfar. MD. Hoopes Vision, Draper UT; John A. Moran Eye Center, Department of Ophthalmology and Visual Sciences, University of Utah School of Medicine, Murray, Utah, USA*)

Angle Supported Phakic IOL

Case: Patient with anterior chamber angle-supported IOL presented for a routine exam (Fig. 15.17).

Management: Observation and regular specular microscopy.

Take-Home Message

- Malrotation of toric ICL should be suspected when the astigmatism increases postoperatively and the BCVA is 20/20.
- Larger size ICL should be used when there is a shallow vault with Lens-ICL touch and when there is a recurrence of a malrotation.
- ICL should be explanted in angle closure that is unresponsive to medical treatment.
- ICL toric axis should be <30 degrees clockwise or counterclockwise to decrease the risks of malrotation.
- Iris-fixated IOL are rarely used nowadays in phakic patient due to the high success rate of ICL.
- AC phakic lenses have fallen out of favor due to higher endothelial cell loss compared to ICL.
- When there is evidence of endothelial cell injury following Iris-fixated IOL or AC IOL, IOL should be explanted. Endothelial keratoplasty can be delayed as in many cases the corneal edema resolves and the endothelial cell count stabilizes.

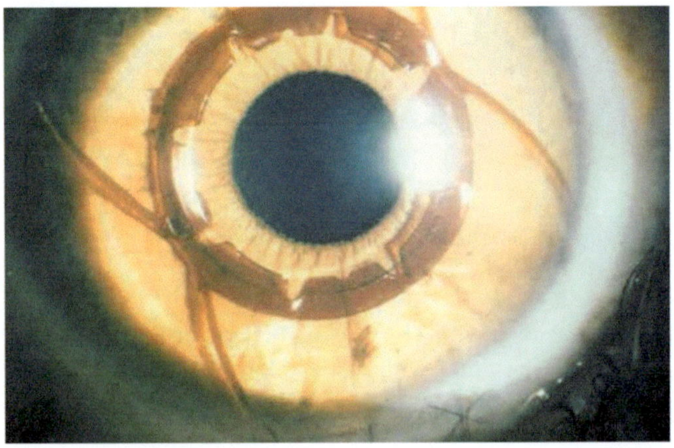

Fig. 15.17 Anterior chamber angle-supported phakic IOL. (*Courtesy of Arun Gulani, MD. Gulani Vision Institute, Florida, USA*)

16 Incisional Surgery

Lulwa El Zein, Samir A. Melki, and Jason Brenner

See Table 16.1.

Case: Patient presented >20 years following an RK surgery with a fluctuating vision. BCVA was 20/20 with a hyperopic astigmatism manifest refraction (Figs. 16.1 and 16.2).

Exam: 16 RK incisions are noted on the cornea.

Management: Observation with glasses or contact lens correction. CXL may be considered by some surgeons to reduce diurnal fluctuations.

Table 16.1 Current use and complications of different corneal incisional surgeries

Procedure	Description of procedure	Corneal effect	Current use	Complications
Radial keratotomy	8–16 radial incision outside the visual axis	Flattening of the incision and 90 degrees away meridian	Abandoned	Neovascularization, vision fluctuation, loss of BCVA, irregular astigmatism, late hyperopia, corneal flattening, wound gape, endothelial disruption beneath the incisions, glare, and halos
Tangential keratotomy	Tangential incisions made at 7 mm optical zone and these are usually coupled with radial keratotomy incisions	Flattening of the incision and steepening of the 90 degrees away meridian	Abandoned	Usually associated with radial keratotomy and shares the same complications
Arcuate keratotomy	Arcuate incisions at 7–9 mm optical zone with 95% depth of the cornea		Combined with cataract surgery, LASIK, PRK, or following penetrating keratoplasty	Irregular astigmatism, under or over correction, infection and perforation
Limbal relaxing incisions	Incisions are made just anterior to the limbus at 600-micron depth or 50 microns less than the thinnest pachymetry		Combined with cataract surgery, LASIK or PRK	
Hexagonal keratotomy	6 linear incisions forming and hexagon centered on the visual axis	Inconsistent results, irregular astigmatism	Abandoned	Glare, photophobia, polyopia, vision fluctuation, overcorrection, irregular astigmatism, corneal edema, corneal perforation, keratitis, wound healing abnormalities, and anterior displacement of the central cornea

L. El Zein (✉)
Department of Ophthalmology, Mayo Clinic, Rochester, MN, USA

S. A. Melki · J. Brenner
Boston Vision, Department of Ophthalmology, Harvard Medical School, Boston, MA, USA
e-mail: Melki@bostonvision.com; brenner@bostonvision.com

S. A. Melki et al. (eds.), *Refractive Surgery Atlas*, https://doi.org/10.1007/978-3-031-60661-8_16

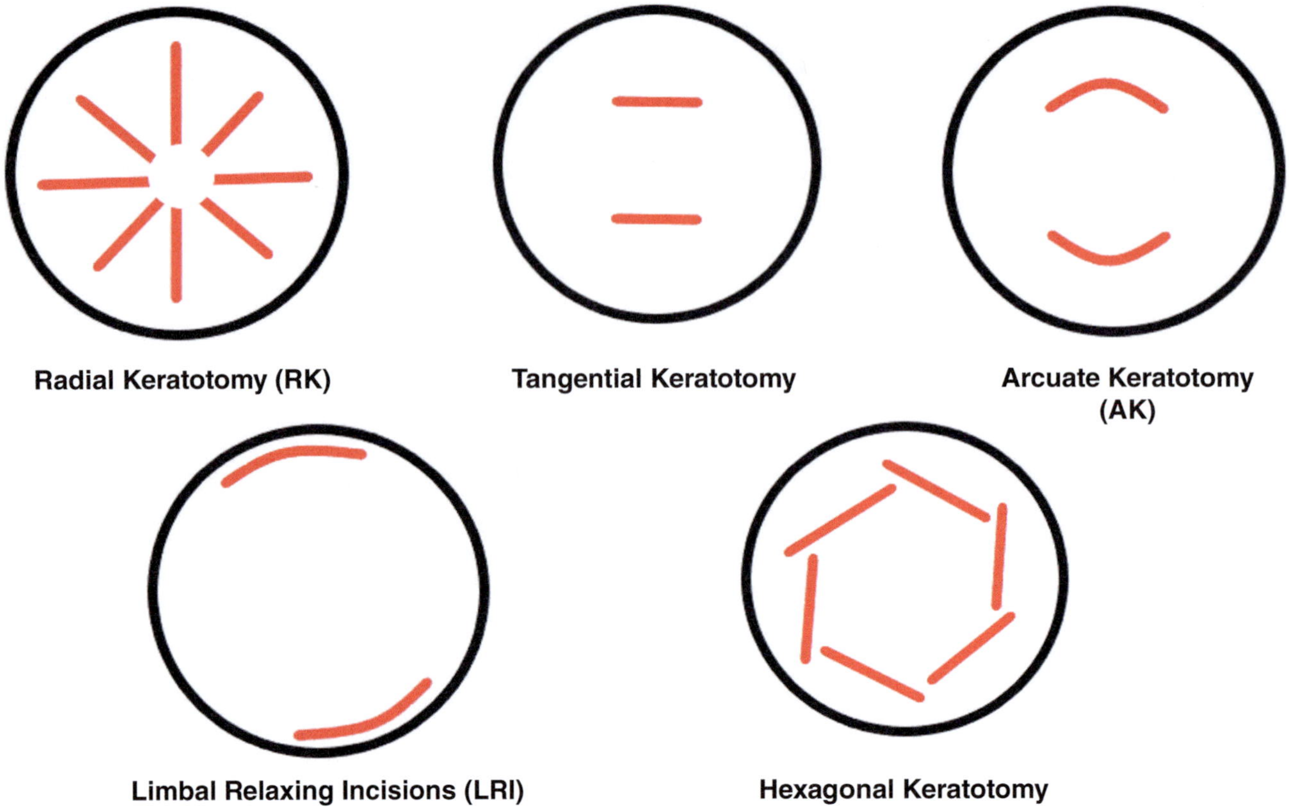

Fig. 16.1 Different incisional techniques. (**a**) **Radial Keratotomy (RK)** (**b**) **Tangential Keratotomy**. (**c**) **Arcuate Keratotomy (AK)**. (**d**) **Limbal Relaxing Incisions (LRI)**. (**e**) **Hexagonal Keratotomy**

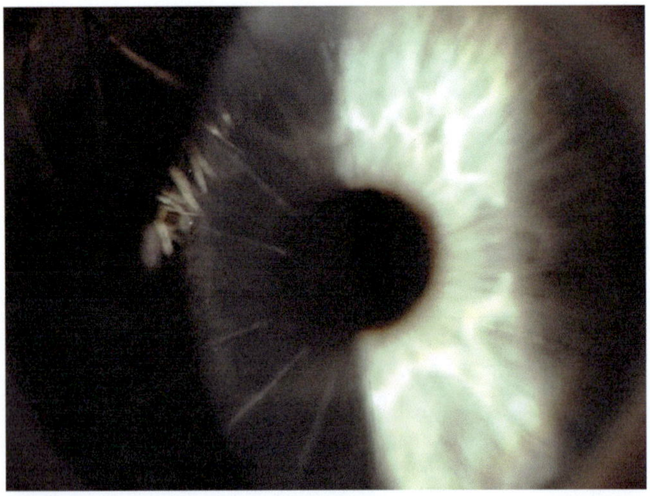

Fig. 16.2 Radial keratotomy

Core message: Hyperopic refraction and fluctuating refraction are common complications after RK.

Case: Patient presented with a cataract 25 years following RK (Fig. 16.3).

Exam: Fluorescein staining showing a filling defect at the 8 keratotomy incisions.

Management: Proceed with phacoemulsification and IOL implantation. The American society of cataract and refractive surgery (ASCRS) IOL calculator can be used for more accurate IOL power calculations. The light adjustable lens is a good option for these patients.

Core message: Corneal stroma never heals completely following RK incisions, it will always represent a weak spot where the cornea may rupture following a blunt trauma or surgical incisions. Surgeons should place the keratotomy incisions closer to the limbus and in between the incisions, if possible, to avoid wound dehiscence.

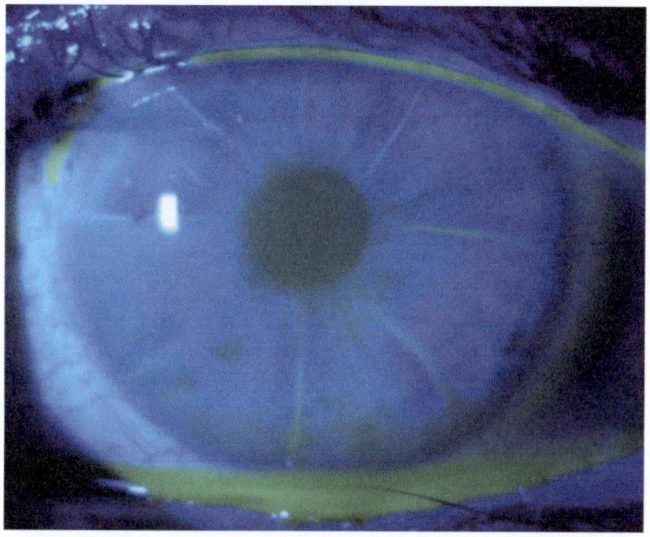

Fig. 16.3 Cataract following radial keratotomy. (*Courtesy of Suphi Taneri, MD. Augenzentrum am St. Franziskus Hospital Münster, Münster, Germany*)

Case: Patient presented with blurry vision years following RK surgery (Fig. 16.4).

Exam: Diffuse corneal scarring is noted along the radial ***(red arrow)*** and tangential ***(yellow arrow)*** keratotomy incisions extending into the visual axis (Fig. 16.4a).

Management: Deep anterior lamellar keratotomy was performed (Fig. 16.4b).

Case: Patient presented with progressive blurry vision following RK surgery, BCVA was 20/60 (Fig. 16.5).

Exam: Central corneal scarring with iron deposits in a cornea with 8 RK incisions (Fig. 16.5a).

Management: PTK was performed. Remnant of the scar persisted centrally but it was less prominent and the patient recovered a BCVA of 20/25 (Fig. 16.5b).

Case: Irregular RK incisions noticed on the cornea of patient during a routine exam ***(red arrow)*** (Fig. 16.6).

Management: Observation.

Case: Patient with previous RK incisions is examined 1 day following cataract surgery (Fig. 16.7).

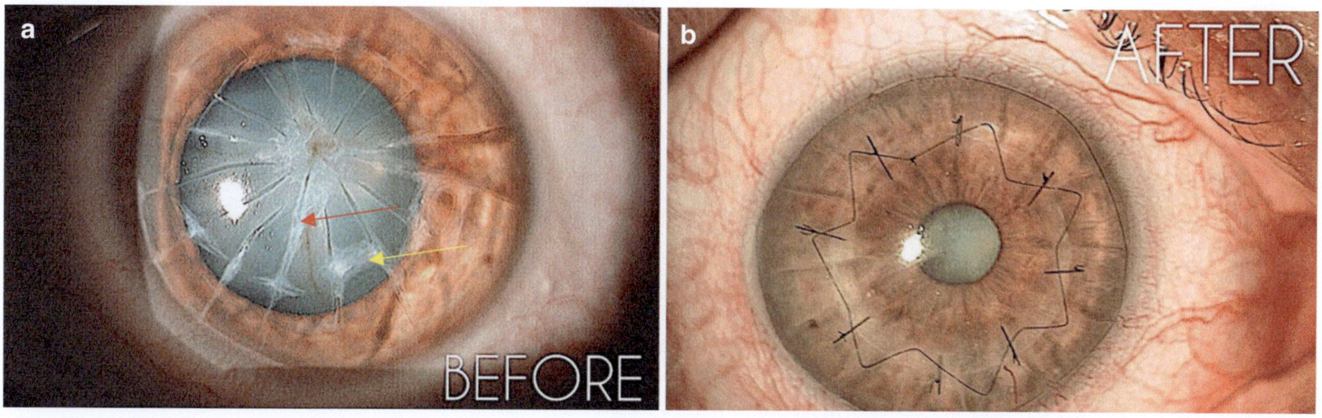

Fig. 16.4 Scarring following radial keratotomy. (*Courtesy of Arun Gulani, MD. Gulani Vision Institute, Florida, USA*)

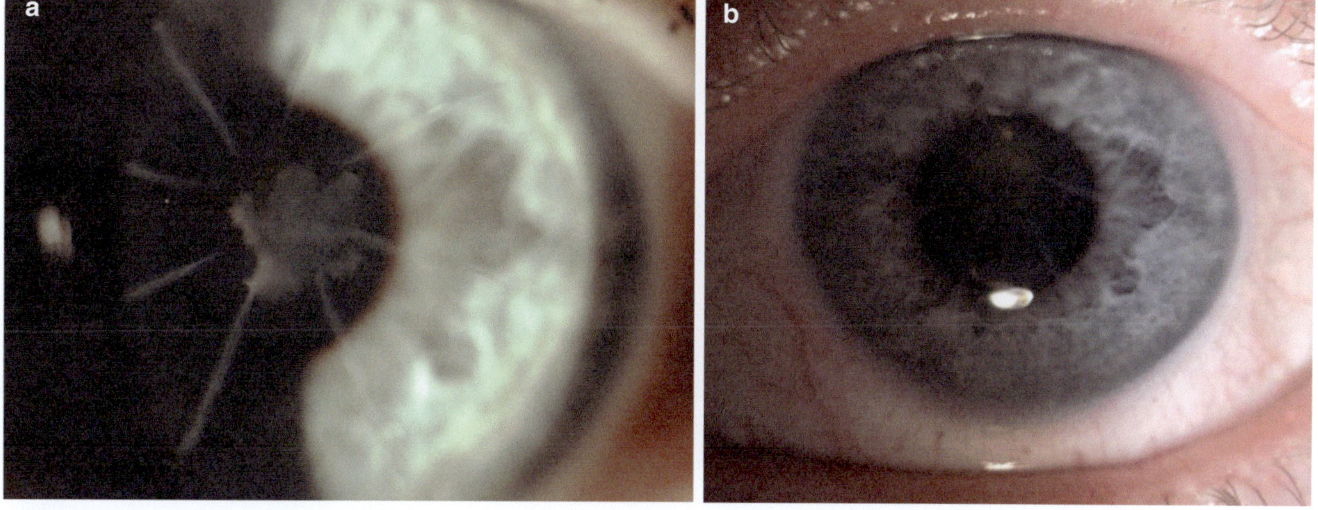

Fig. 16.5 PTK following radial keratotomy

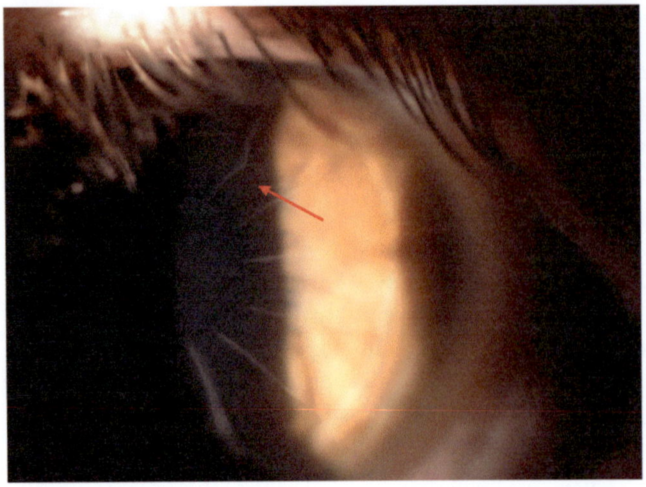

Fig. 16.6 Irregular incisions

Exam: Fluorescein staining shows a seidel positive sign revealing leakage from a dehiscence of a previous RK incision (Fig. 16.7a, b). One 10–0 nylon suture was already placed at the time of surgery **(red arrow)**.

Management: Two additional sutures were placed, and the leakage stopped (Fig. 16.7c).

Case: A patient who was recently operated with a vitrectomy and scleral buckle for retinal detachment presented with central perforated corneal ulcer. He had RK incisions 30 years ago (Fig. 16.8).

Exam: Slit lamp photo (Fig. 16.8a) and operative microscope photo (Fig. 16.8b) showing the RK incisions, a corneal perforation located along two of the radial incisions ***(red arrows)*** and shallow anterior chamber.

Management: Urgent penetrating keratoplasty was performed.

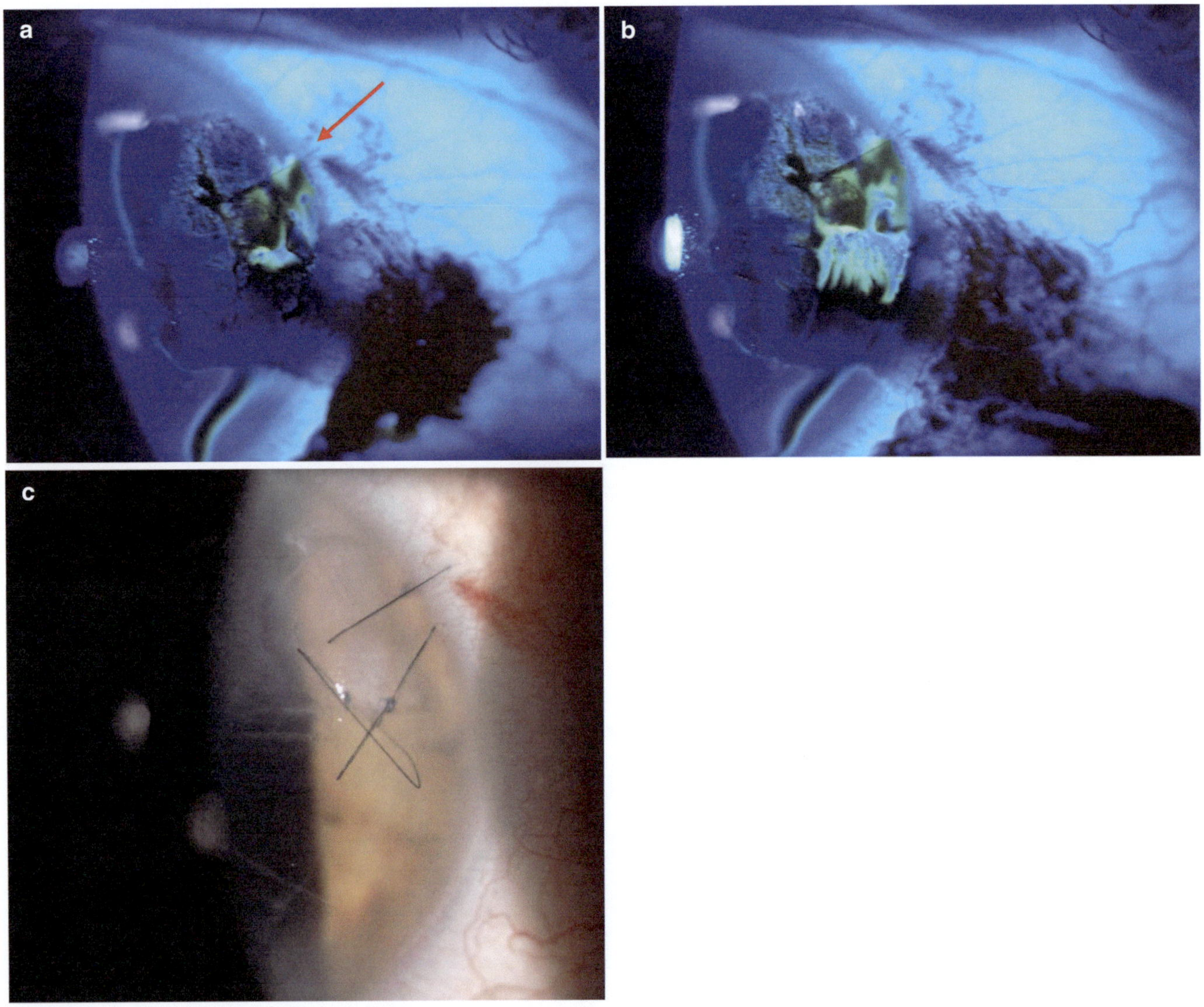

Fig. 16.7 Wound dehiscence

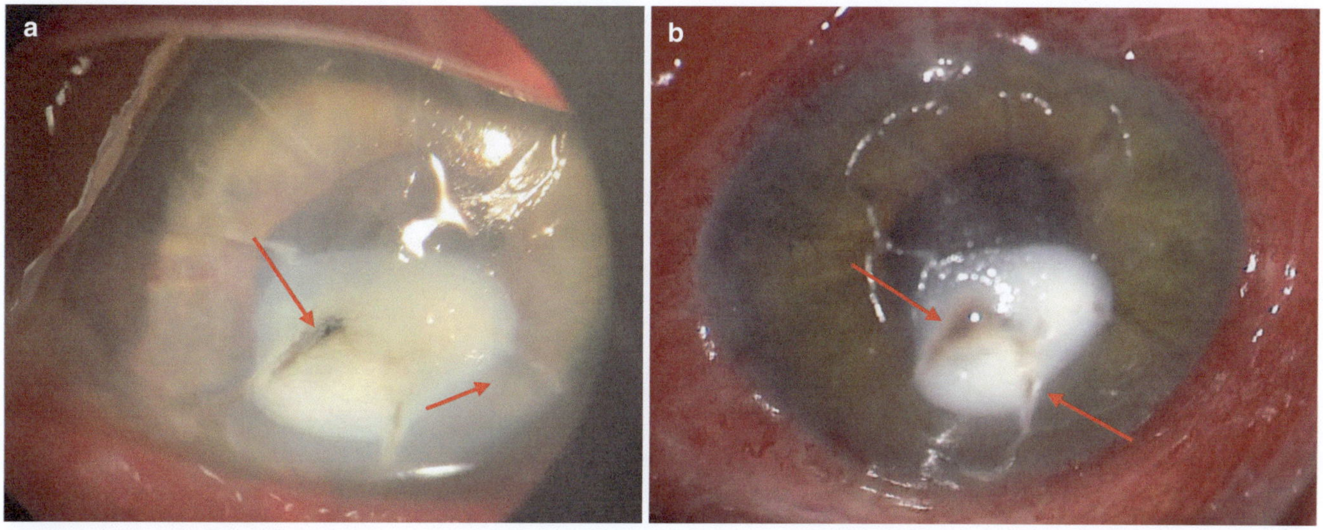

Fig. 16.8 Infectious keratitis in RK

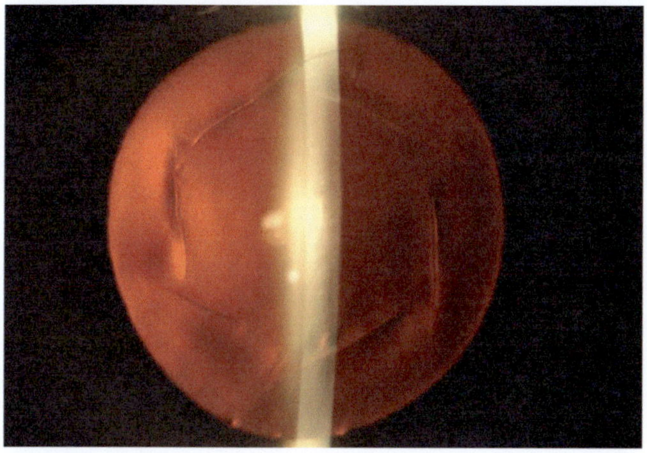

Fig. 16.9 Hexagonal keratotomy. (*Courtesy of Arun Gulani, MD. Gulani Vision Institute, Florida, USA*)

Core message: Patients with ulcers following RK should be followed closely as the cornea may perforate easily. If a penetrating keratoplasty is planned, surgeons should aim to include the keratotomy incisions inside the trephination zone to avoid having radial wound gaping at the keratotomy sites.

Case: Hexagonal incisions noted with retro-illumination in a patient presenting for routine exam (Fig. 16.9).

Core message: Hexagonal keratotomy is a historic refractive surgery. It is not recommended as it is not predictable and increases the risk of corneal rupture.

Case: Patient presented years following a hexagonal keratotomy with constant blurry vision (Fig. 16.10).

Exam: Hexagonal incisions are present <6 mm from the center of the cornea. Tangential keratotomy incisions are also noted ***(yellow arrows)***. Topography showed a high and irregular astigmatism of 23.5 D (Fig. 16.10a).

Management: ICRS were implanted and the corneal astigmatism decreased to 1.5D (Fig. 16.10b).

Core message: ICRS implantation can delay keratoplasty in patients with irregular corneas and a clear visual axis.

Case: Patient presented with intolerance to scleral lenses 10 years following a penetrating keratoplasty (PK). His BCVA was 20/125 (Fig. 16.11).

Exam: Topography showed a steep cornea with an irregular high astigmatism with a mean corneal astigmatism of 15.9D located at 15 degrees (Fig. 16.11a).

Management: Manual AK incisions were performed with relaxing incisions at 70% depth of the thinnest corneal pachymetry. The double 45-degree of arc incisions were centered at 15-degree axis and 1 mm interior to the graft border ***(red arrows)*** (Fig. 16.11c, d). One month postoperatively, corneal astigmatism decreased to 10.1D and BCVA with glasses was 20/25 using 6 D astigmatism correction (Fig. 16.11b).

Core message: AK is unpredictable following PK but it is effective in decreasing the corneal astigmatism.

Case: Patient had a femtosecond cataract surgery complicated with loss of suction during LRI creation. Postoperatively, the BCVA was 20/400 with a very high corneal astigmatism (Fig. 16.12).

Exam: The relaxing incision can be seen involving the visual axis (Fig. 16.12a, b) and it was deep, passing through the descemet membrane (Fig. 16.12c).

Management: Contact lens failed to improve the patient's vision. He was referred eventually for penetrating keratoplasty.

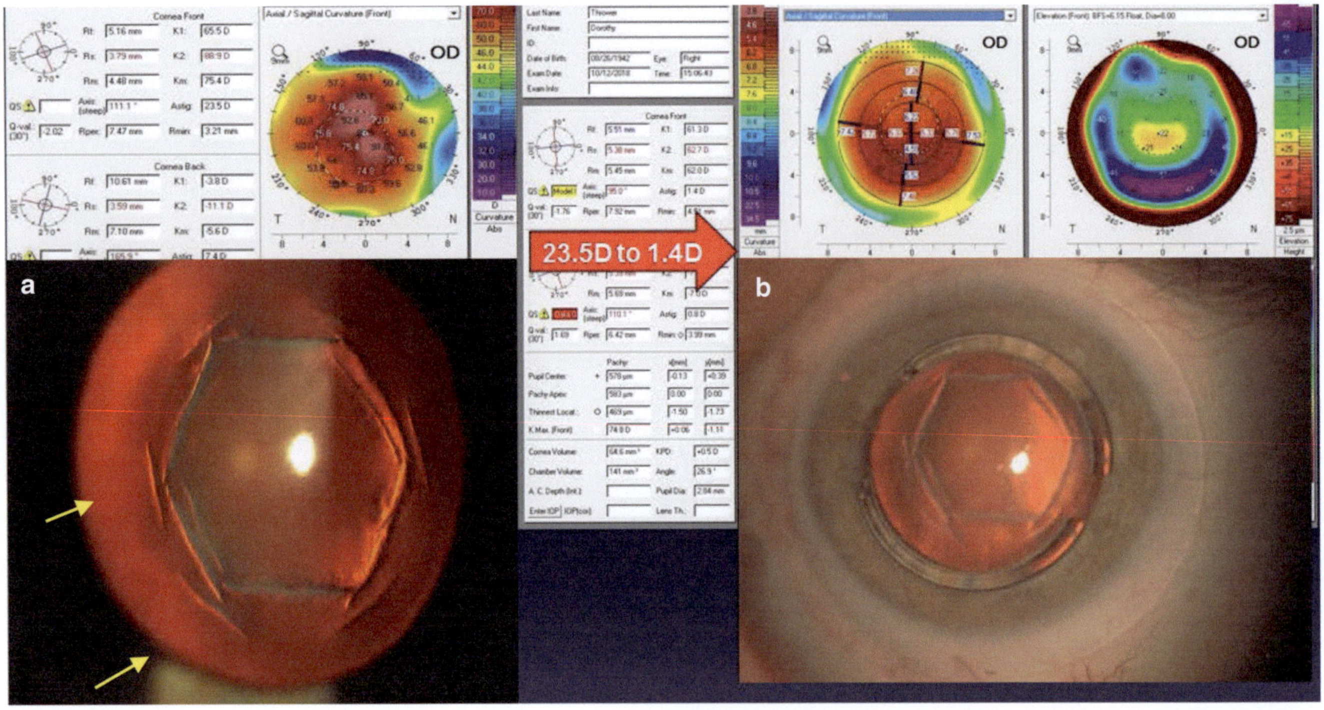

Fig. 16.10 ICRS following hexagonal keratotomy. (*Courtesy of Arun Gulani, MD. Gulani Vision Institute, Florida, USA*)

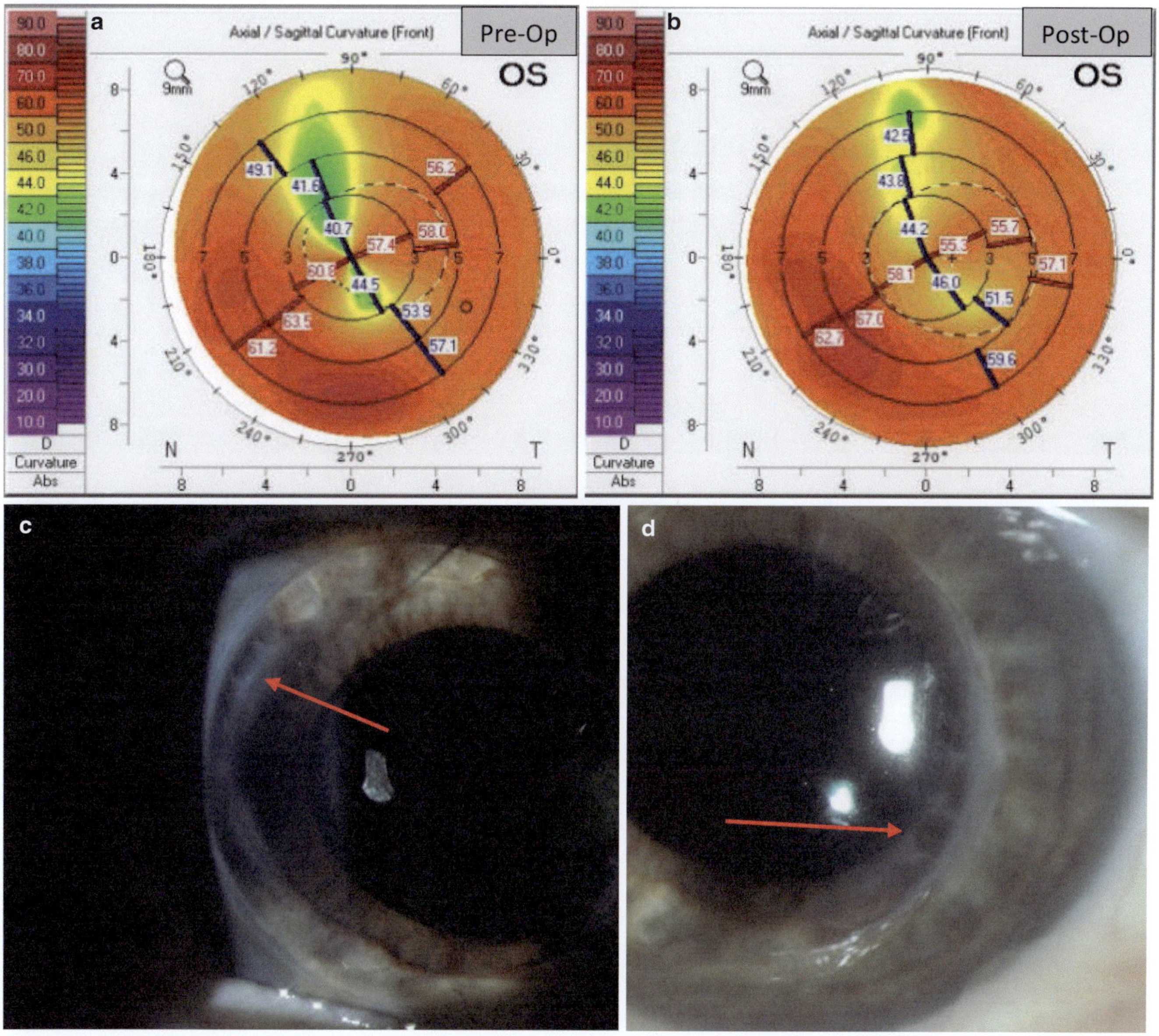

Fig. 16.11 Arcuate keratotomy post penetrating keratoplasty

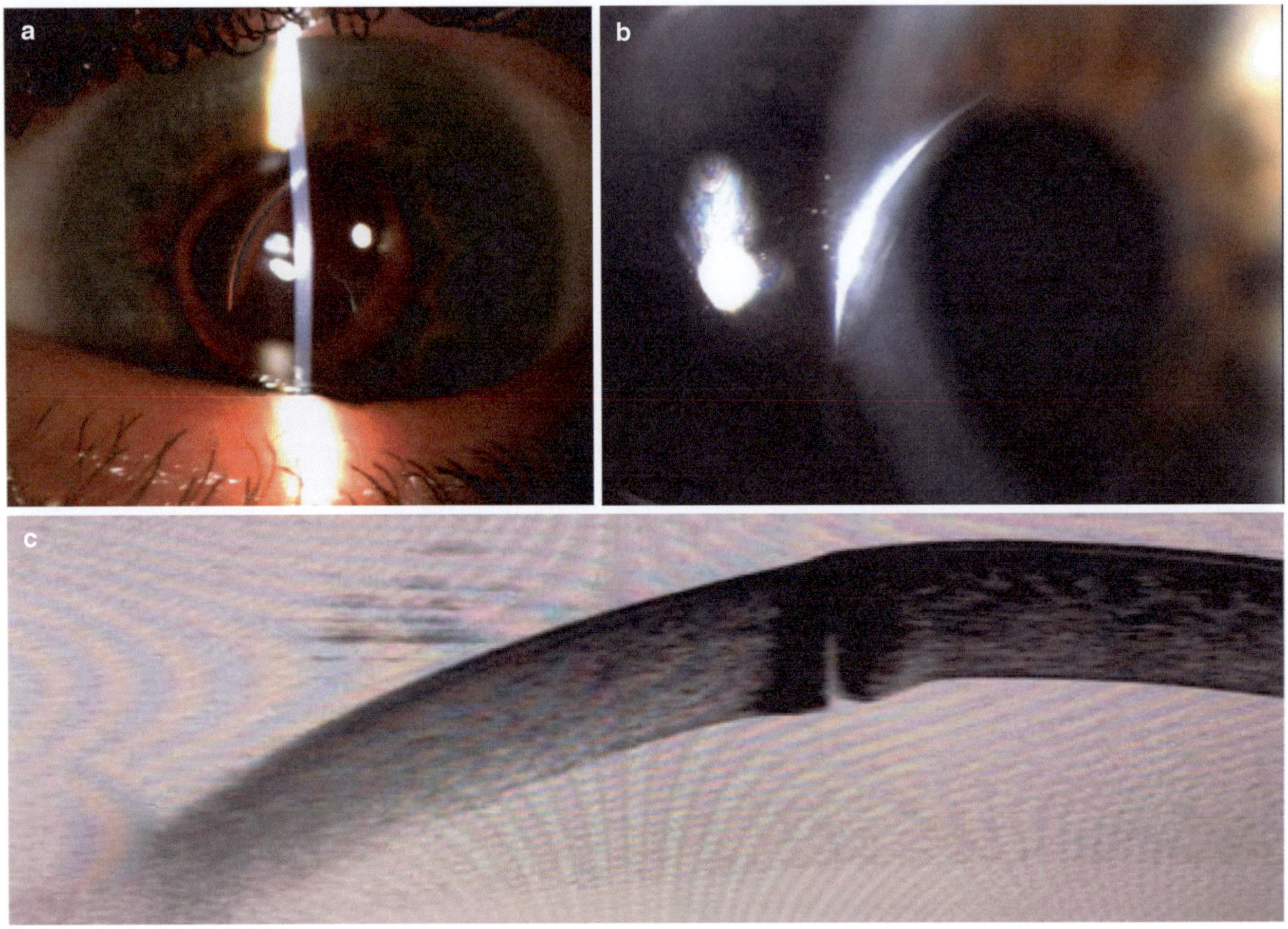

Fig. 16.12 ICRS following hexagonal keratotomy

Take-Home Message

- Radial keratotomy, tangential keratotomy and hexagonal keratotomy are historical surgeries. Incisions never heal completely, and many patients who have undergone these procedures have progressive flattening, irregular astigmatism, and corneal scars.
- During cataract surgery, more posterior limbal incisions or a scleral tunnel should be performed to avoid cutting into the RK scars and causing wound dehiscence.
- Incision keratotomy complications and residual refractive error can be managed on a case-by-case basis. PTK, PRK, DALK and PK have been proposed to improve these patients' vision.
- There is no AK algorithm for corneas with irregular astigmatism following penetrating keratoplasty. Surgeons should perform the incisions 1 mm inside the graft, 60–90% deep, and up to 60 degrees of arc.
- LRI post penetrating keratoplasty is unpredictable, there is a risk of perforation and reversal of astigmatism axis. However, it is an effective way to delay the need for a repeated keratoplasty.
- AK, LRI and ICRS are minimally invasive procedures that can be performed in patients with irregular corneas and intolerant to contact lenses in order to delay PK surgery.

17 Topographic and Tomographic Abnormalities

Shady T. Awwad, Yara Bteich, and Jad F. Assaf

Segmental Tomography: A Holistic Approach to Corneal Imaging after Refractive Surgery

Myopic Mechanical LASIK Vs Femto-LASIK Vs PRK

Case: OCT segmental tomography (Fig. 17.1a) with the anamorphic display using MS-39 Dual Placido anterior segment optical coherence tomography (AS-OCT) (CSO, Costruzione Strumenti Oftalmici, Florence, Italy) (Fig. 17.1b) following mechanical LASIK for the correction of myopia.

The flap created by the metal blade of the mechanical microkeratome is characterized by a meniscal interface **(arrows)** that is hypo-reflective in the center **(asterisk)** and hyperreflective in the periphery with tapered vertical incisions on both flap edges **(arrows).**

The bilaminar Bowman's layer (BL) is present postoperatively except at the periphery due to refraction and reflection of the AS-OCT signals, which hinder its resolution **(BL)** in Fig. 17.1b.

Case: AS-OCT following LASIK for the correction of myopia (Fig. 17.2a, b).

Hexa-map corneal tomography display from an eye following myopic Femto-LASIK reveals the edges of the optical zone (OZ) through the anterior tangential curvature map with normal posterior curvature. We also note that following LASIK for myopia correction, the central cornea is flatter relative to the periphery leading to an oblate surface with

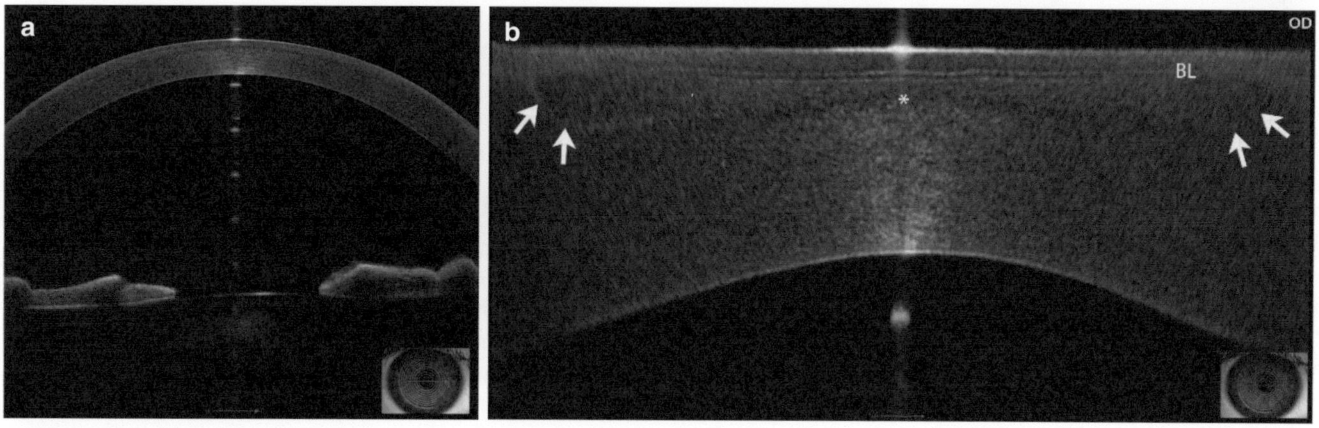

Fig. 17.1 Myopic mechanical LASIK

S. T. Awwad (✉) · Y. Bteich
Department of Ophthalmology, American University of Beirut Medical Center, Beirut, Lebanon

J. F. Assaf
Faculty of Medicine, American University of Beirut Medical Center, Beirut, Lebanon

S. A. Melki et al. (eds.), *Refractive Surgery Atlas*, https://doi.org/10.1007/978-3-031-60661-8_17

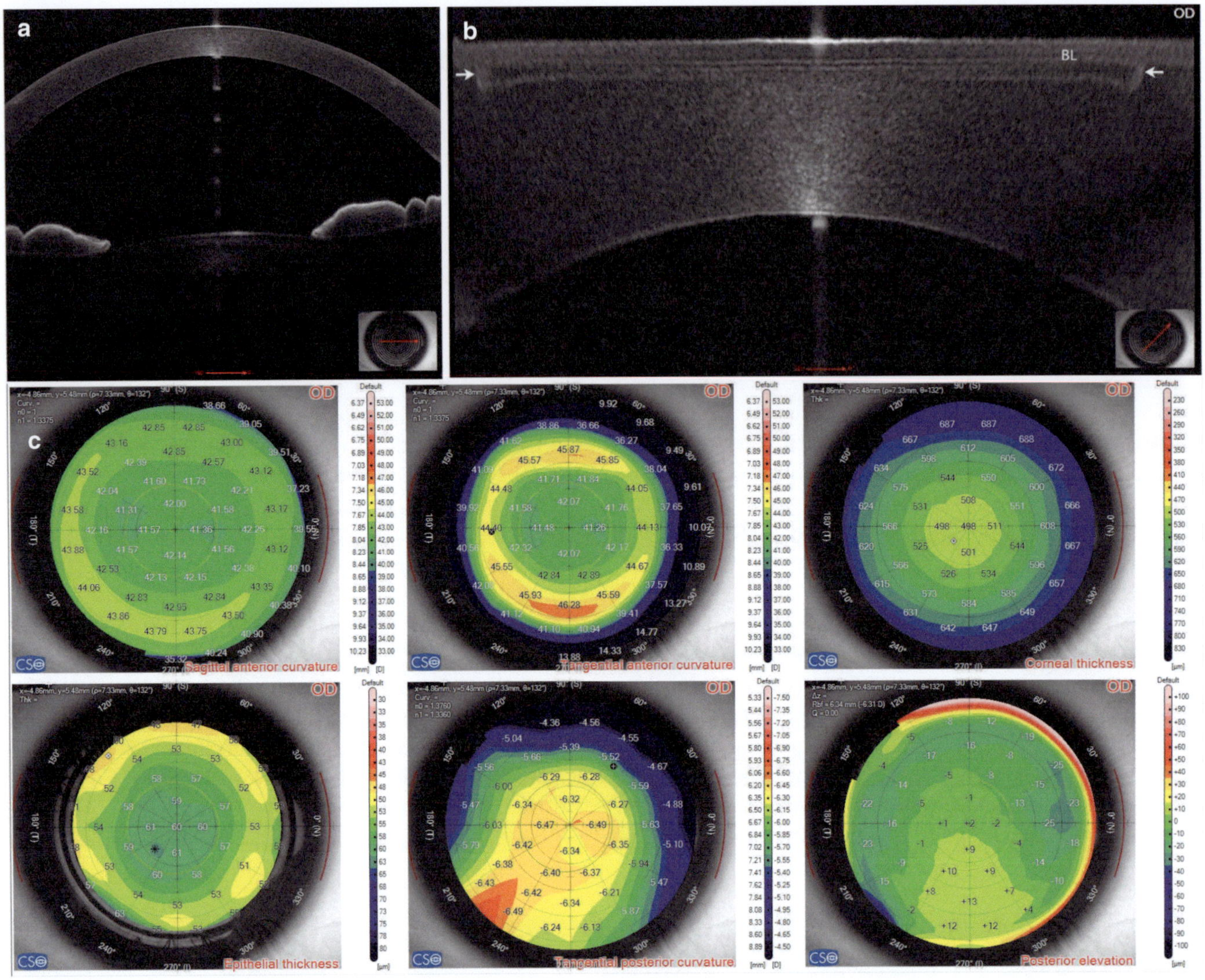

Fig. 17.2 Myopic Femto-LASIK

thicker central epithelium (Fig. 17.2c). This is also evident in the anamorphic display of the OCT section (Fig. 17.2b) showing a thicker epithelium in the center, a finding that can give an idea about the patient's refractive surgery history. The bilaminar *BL* is also present postoperatively ***(BL)*** in Fig. 17.2b.

Core message: The anamorphic or applanated display is particularly useful in differentiating between the two techniques as it flattens the cornea against its anterior curvature, providing a clearer view of its structure and any anomaly that may be present.

Case: AS-OCT section of an eye with a history of PRK for correction of myopia (Fig. 17.3a, b). The bilaminar structure underlying the epithelium (Bowman's layer) is absent and is replaced by a one-layer structure (basement membrane) and there is no evidence of flap creation in the stroma as shown on the applanated view (Fig. 17.3b).

Hyperopic Mechanical LASIK Vs PRK

Case: Hexa-map tomography of an eye with a history of hyperopic mechanical LASIK (Fig. 17.4a). There is marked epithelial remodeling characterized by an epithelial thickness that is thinner in the center relative to the periphery partially contributing to regression of the hyperopic treatment. This is coupled with a steeper central cornea compared to its periphery as the excimer laser pulses are applied to the mid-periphery, resulting in a hyper-prolate shape.

As in the case of myopic mechanical LASIK, the segmental OCT section (Fig. 17.4b) shows a meniscal flap **(arrows)** that is better visualized on anamorphic display. Additionally, we can see a bilaminar layer indicating the presence of the BL ***(BL)***.

Case: the BL of an eye with a history of PRK for the treatment of hyperopia is present only in the very center as

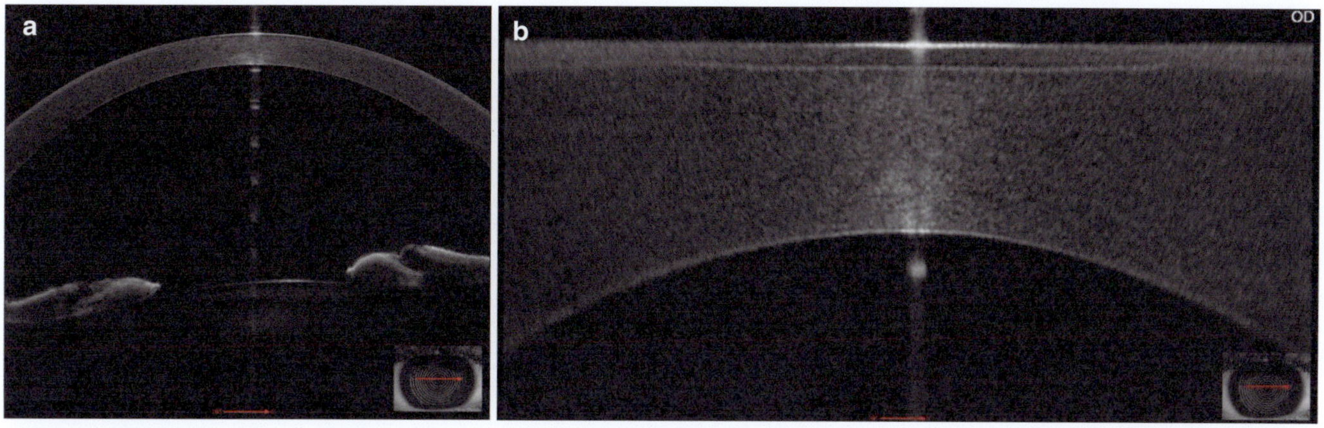

Fig. 17.3 Myopic PRK

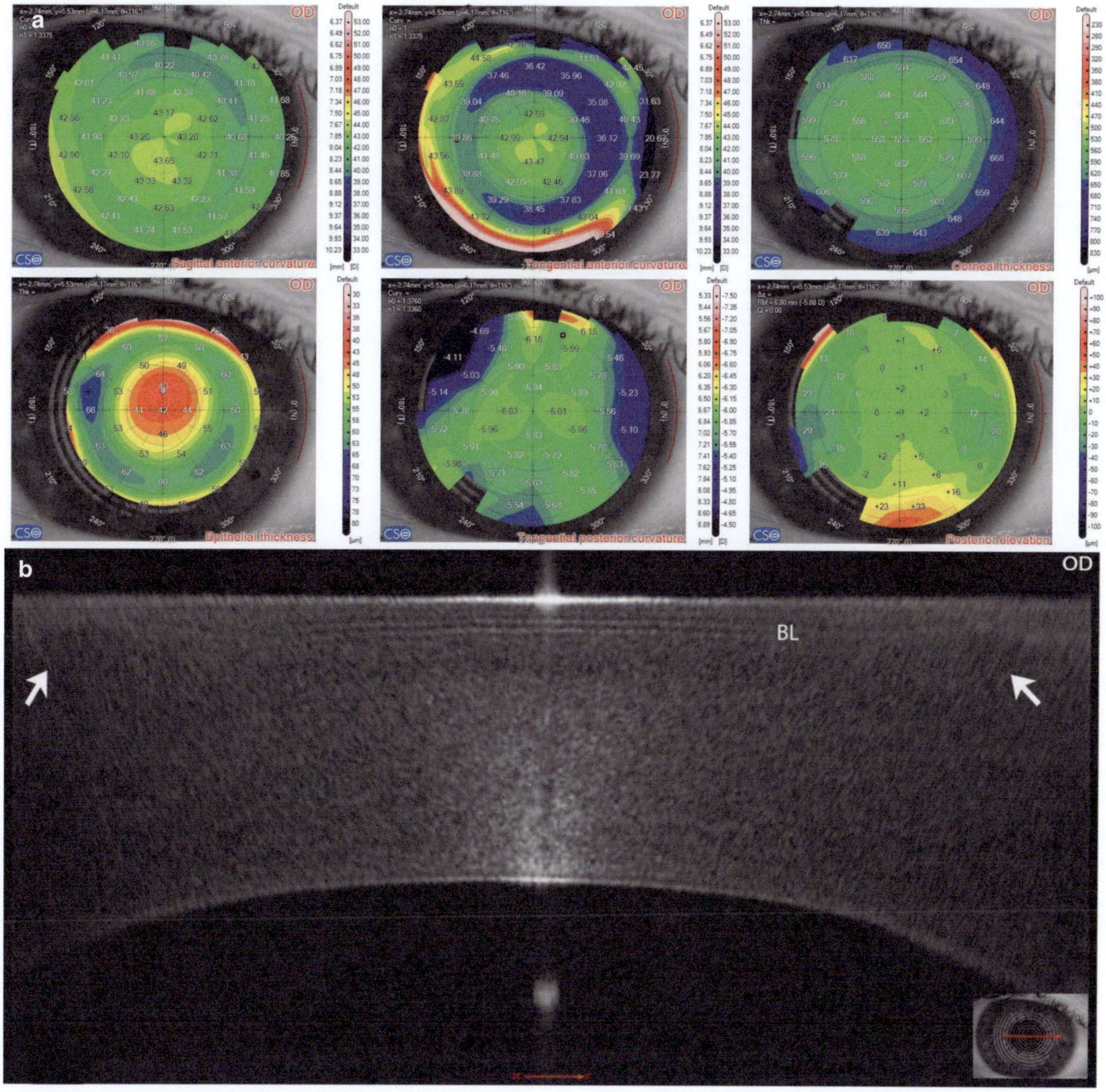

Fig. 17.4 Hyperopic mechanical LASIK

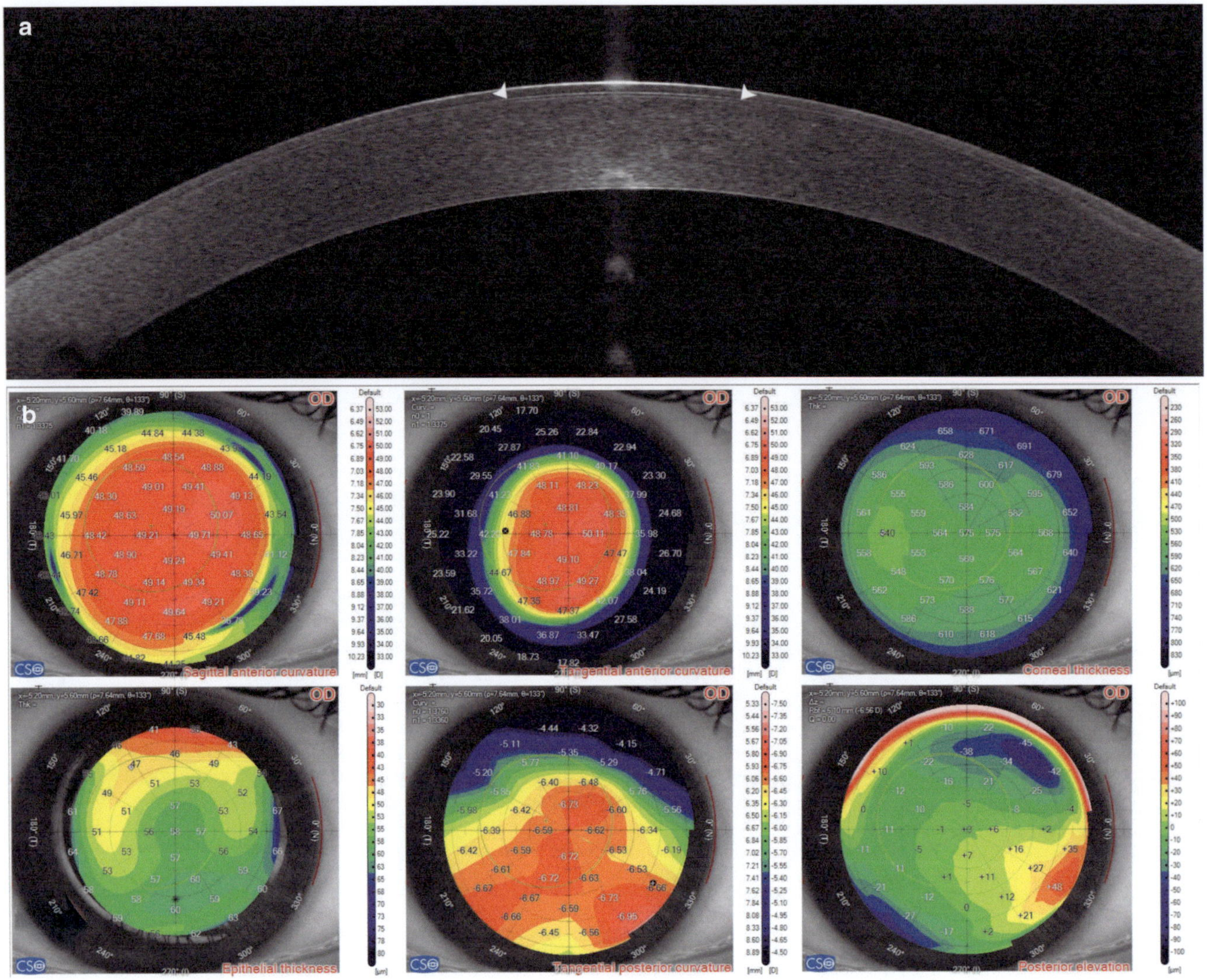

Fig. 17.5 Hyperopic PRK

the treatment spares the center. We can see the fusion of the BL in the mid-periphery marking the beginning of the central OZ **(arrowheads)** (Fig. 17.5a). Therefore, eyes with mild hyperopic PRK correction might sometimes be confused with virgin eyes on AS-OCT as the Bowman layer's bilaminar structure often disappears in the periphery due to light scatter and refraction.

Hexa-map tomography of the latter eye shows a large homogeneous and well-centered OZ with minimal epithelial remodeling as shown by the epithelial maps which can explain the absence of regression in this case (Fig. 17.5b).

Hyperopic LASIK + PRK

Case: This patient initially presented with a history of hyperopic mechanical LASIK with inferior steepening and decentered ablation. PRK with minimal tissue ablation was then performed over the LASIK flap, resulting in a well-centered treatment with regular astigmatism as compared to the baseline. This is clear on anterior and posterior tangential curvature maps (Fig. 17.6a).

The applanated view of a cornea showing a flap characterized by a meniscal interface **(white arrows)** and BL **(black arrow)** only in the center with a thinner central epithelium rela-

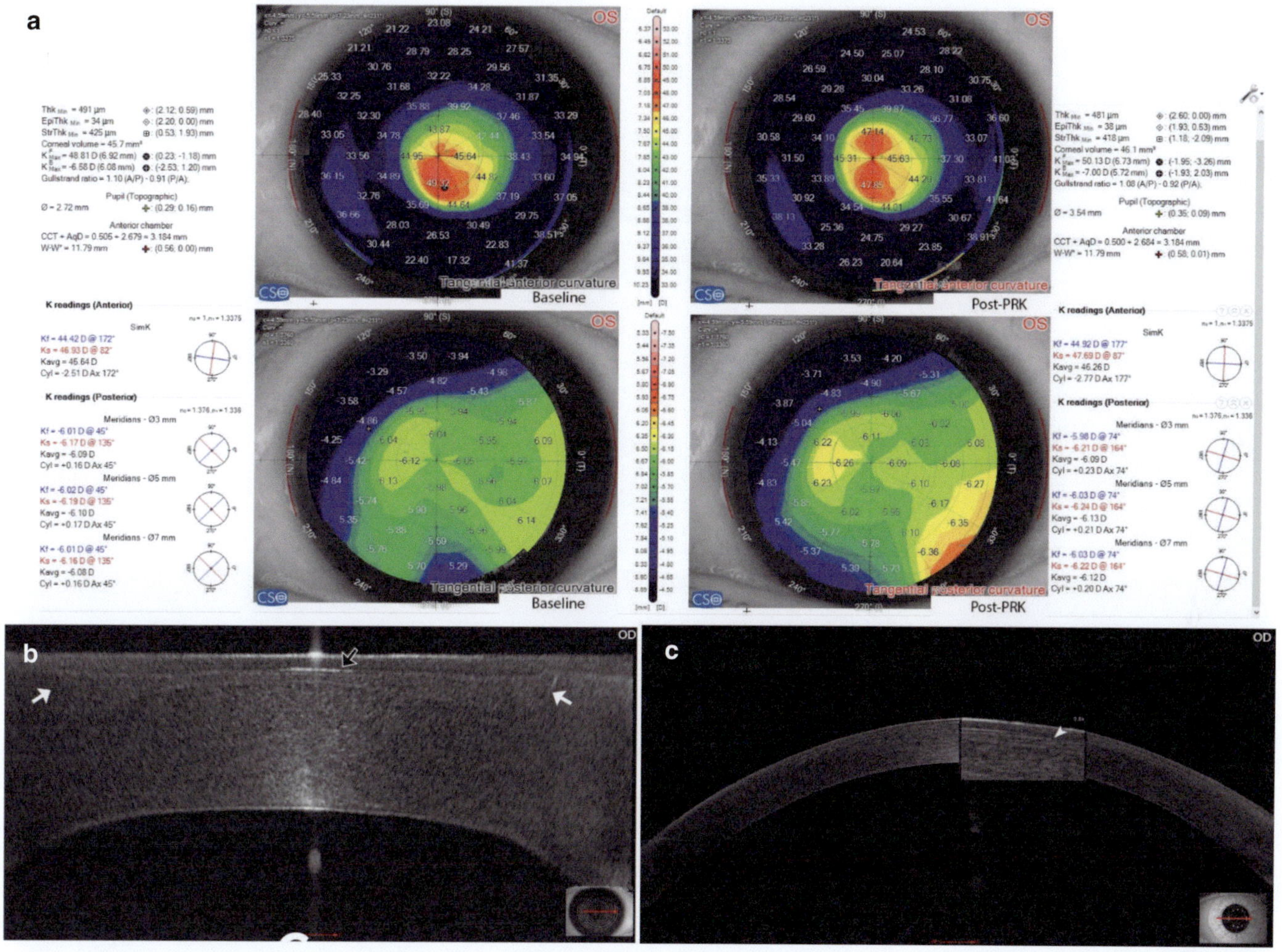

Fig. 17.6 Hyperopic LASIK + PRK

tive to the periphery, indicating a history of hyperopic PRK as well as mechanical LASIK (Fig. 17.6b). These characteristics are hard to distinguish on regular, non-applanated topography, which mainly shows fusion of the BL at the periphery, marking the beginning of the optical zone **(arrowhead)** (Fig. 17.6c).

Femtosecond Lenticule Extraction

Case: Anamorphic display of an eye after lenticule extraction (Fig. 17.7a). Compared to the flap-related procedures described earlier, there is no vertical interface at the periphery except at the site of incision for lenticule extraction. We also note some undulations at the level of the BL **(arrows).** Postoperatively, the cap has less room to stretch in contrast to the LASIK flap, which explains these undulations.

The topography map from AS-OCT for this case shows mild decentration of the OZ temporally that is offset by the large and homogenous nature of the OZ, allowing the patient to achieve good visual acuity and quality (Fig. 17.7b).

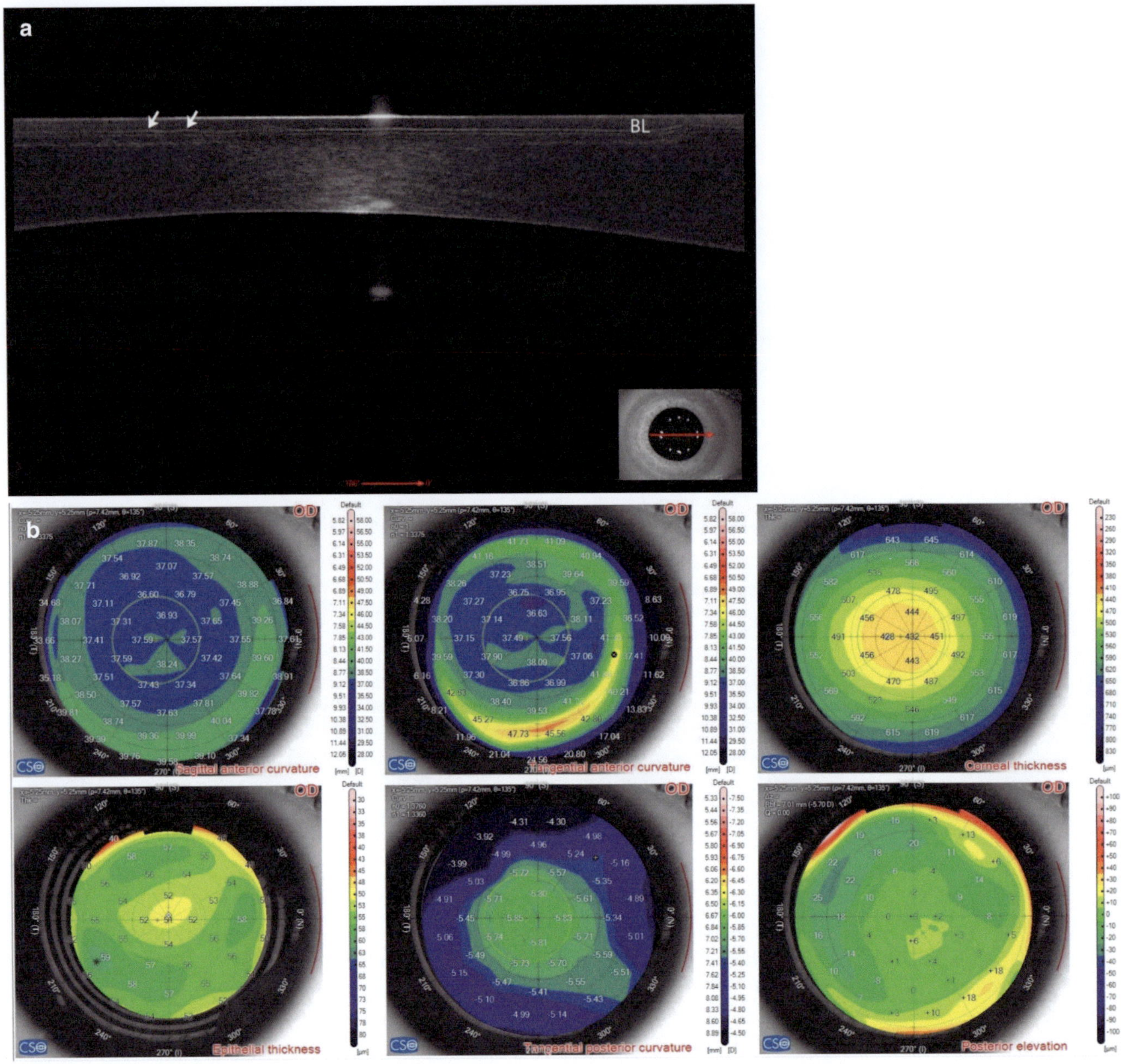

Fig. 17.7 Femtosecond lenticule extraction

Interface Fluid Syndrome

Case: A 75-year-old man with a history of LASIK refractive surgery and anterior-chamber intraocular lens (AC-IOL) inserted in the left eye following posterior dislocation of the previous one presented to our clinic with decreased vision. His previous AC-OCT showed an AC-IOL **(arrow)** and LASIK flap (**arrowheads**) (Fig. 17.8a).

Additional ophthalmic history includes compromised endothelial function based on low cell count and density on specular microscopy and cystoid macular edema (CME) managed by the retina specialist with topical steroids and NSAIDs QID.

Exam: Upon examination, the cystoid macular edema had resolved, and intraocular pressure (IOP) measured by Goldmann applanation was 16 mmHg. AS-OCT was done and showed fluid collection in the corneal flap interface **(arrowheads)**, confirming the diagnosis of interface fluid syndrome (Fig. 17.8b).

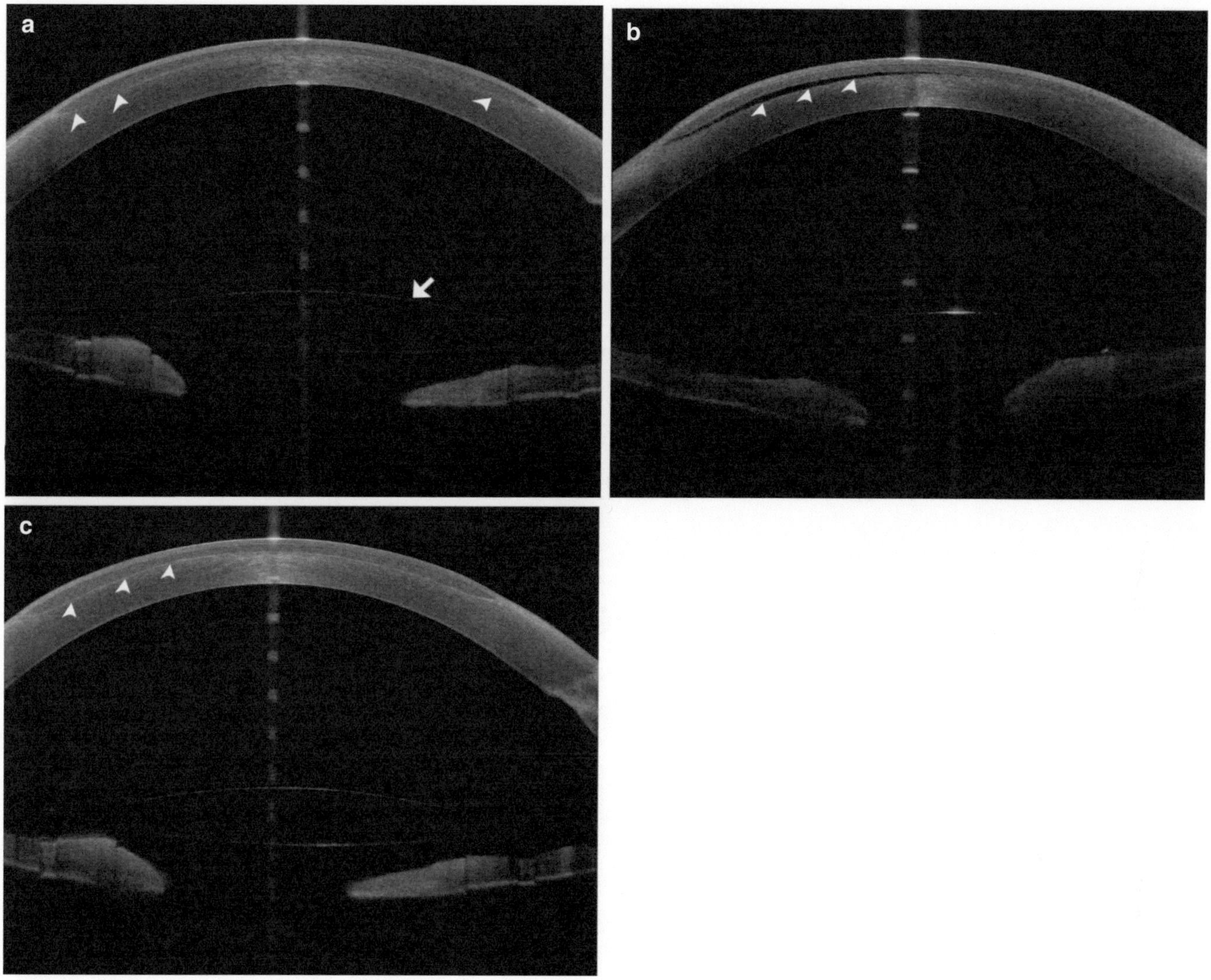

Fig. 17.8 Pressure-induced interlamellar stromal keratitis

This accumulated fluid is responsible for the falsely low IOP on Goldman applanation, while IOP measured outside the flap margin using a handheld tonometer was 32 mmHg.

Management: The patient received pressure-lowering medication and steroid medication was discontinued as CME had already resolved. This led to a fast recovery of the condition as shown by the resolution of the fluid in the interface **(arrowheads)** (Fig. 17.8c).

Core message: The dysfunction in the endothelial cell layer impairs the capacity of the sodium-potassium pumps to efflux fluid from the stroma to the anterior chamber. Additionally, the presence of a steroid-induced increase in IOP redirects the fluid to the low-resistance corneal flap interface.

Case: Patient being treated for uveitic glaucoma s/p valve surgery, presented with worsening vision. Patient had a LASIK procedure years ago (Fig. 17.9).

Exam: Slit lamp exam showed descemet folds and endothelial failure. IOP was within normal limits in the central and peripheral cornea. Corneal OCT showed diffuse interface fluid.

Management: DMEK was performed. Corneal swelling decreased and interface fluid disappeared.

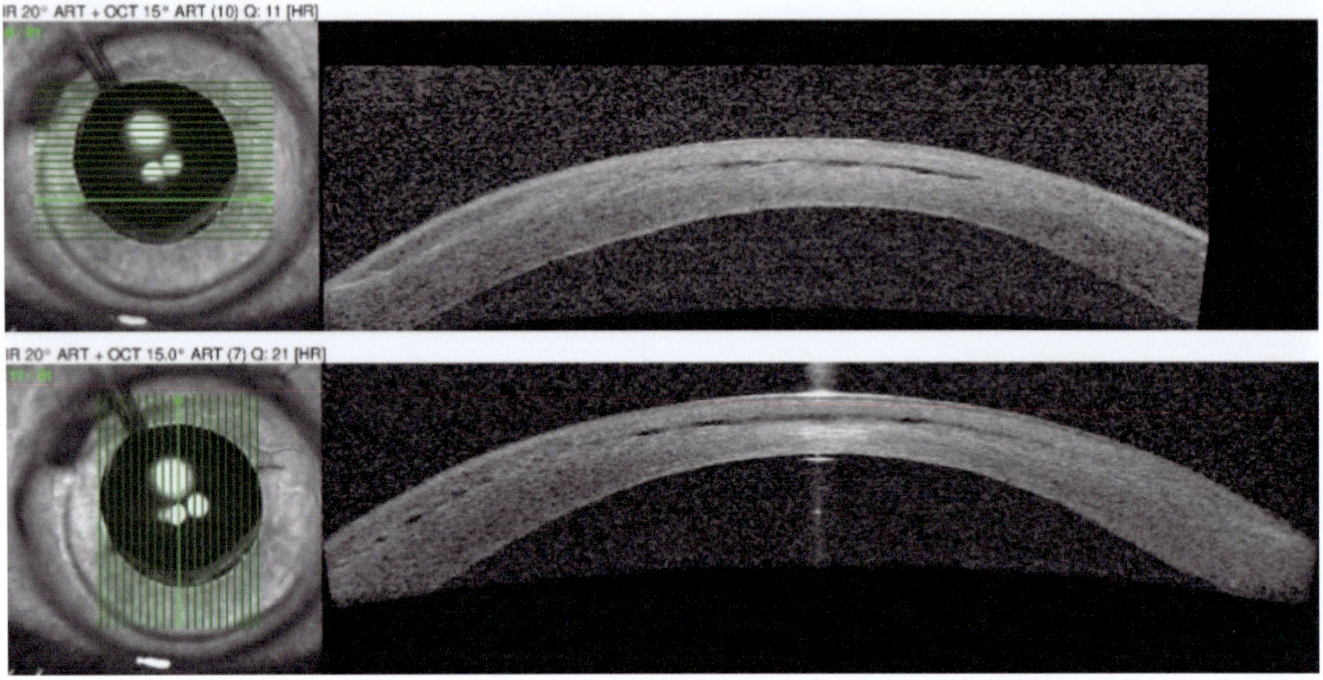

Fig. 17.9 Interface fluid syndrome following endothelial failure. (*Courtesy of Joshua H. Hou, MD. University of Minnesota, Minnesota, USA*)

Intra Stromal Ring Segments

Case: Following ICRS implantation in a female patient with keratoconus, BCVA improved from 20/50 preoperatively to 20/25 1 week following the procedure (Fig. 17.10).

Exam: INTACS ICRS were placed at 6 mm from the pupillary center (Fig. 17.10a) and at a 2/3 depth of the cornea (Fig. 17.10b).

Topography: There was a decrease in the central and peripheral corneal steepness following ICRS implantation (Fig. 17.10d) compared to the preoperative values (Fig. 17.10c).

Case: Case where melt over one of the PMMA segments was managed by removal and replacement with a corneal allogenic intrastromal ring segment (CAIRS) (white arrow CAIRS, black arrow PMMA segment) (Fig. 17.11).

Exam: Slit lamp photo shows one CAIRS and one INTACS (Fig. 17.11a). After the exchange, the anterior curvature map shows stability as compared to keratometry values before ASN (Fig. 17.11b).

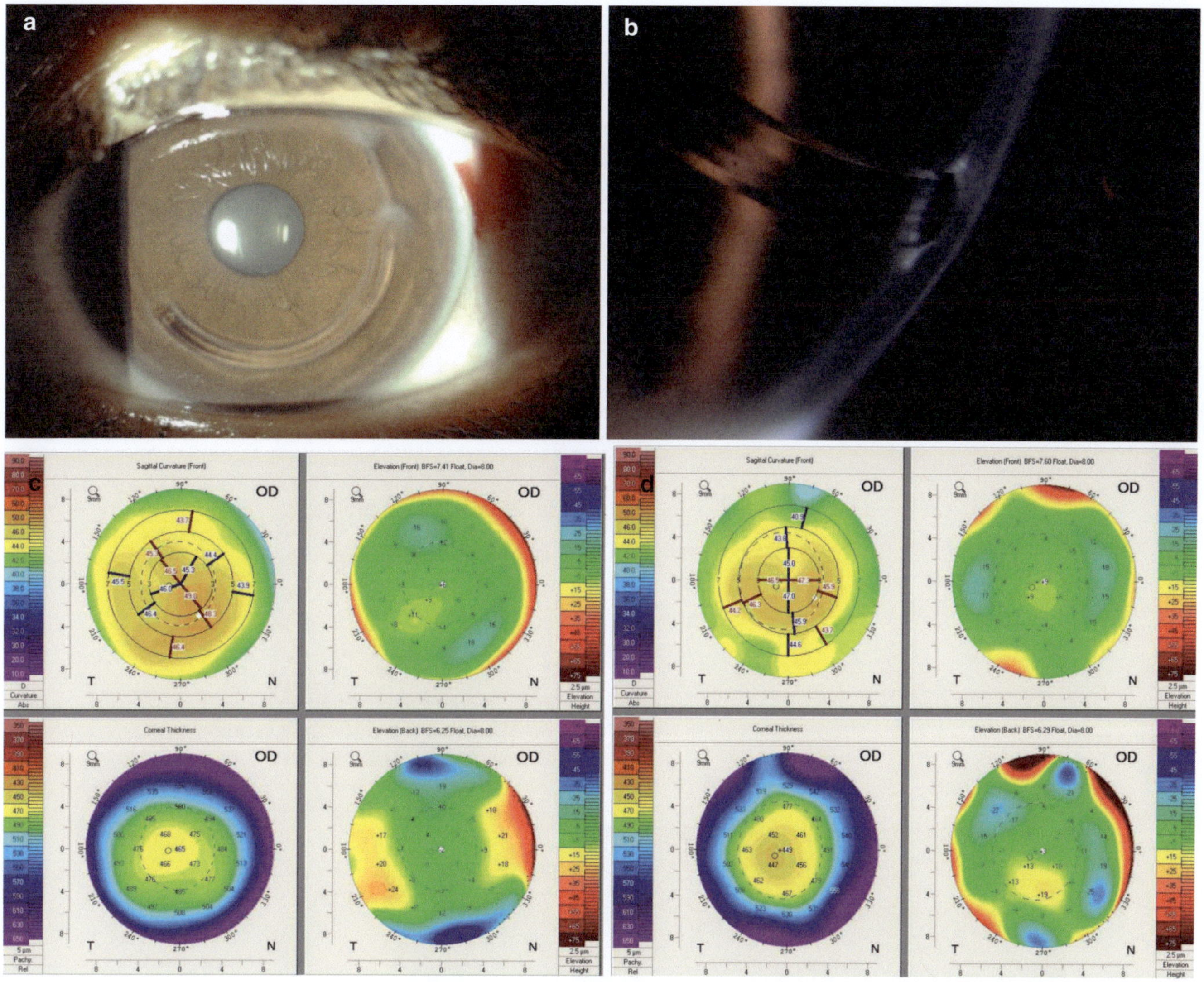

Fig. 17.10 Corneal ICRS. (*Courtesy of Samir Melki MD*)

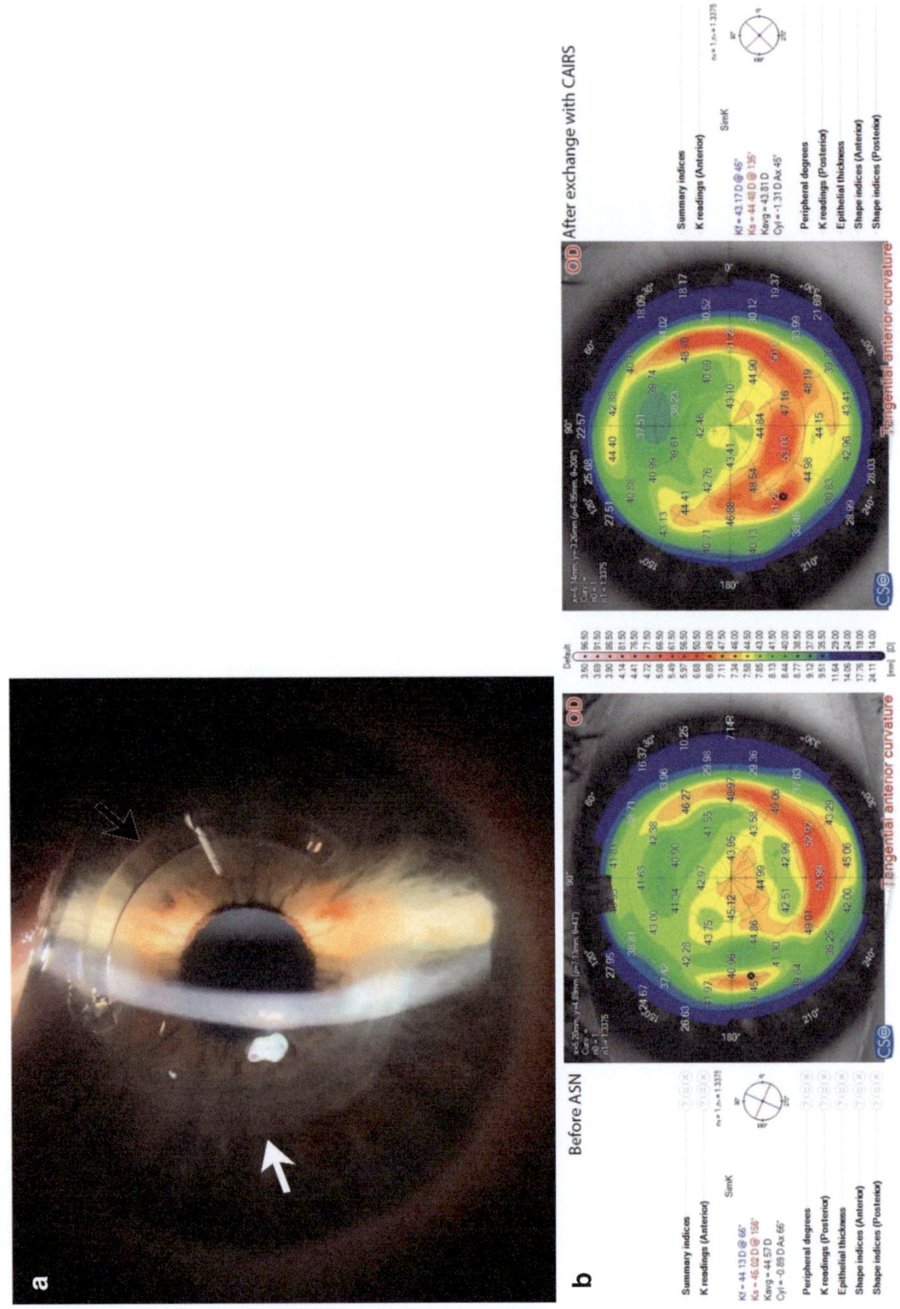

Fig. 17.11 Topography changes in CAIRS

Post-Myopic LASIK Ectasia

Case: Tomography maps showing signs of early corneal ectasia with a flat optical zone in a patient with a history of LASIK for the correction of myopia. The right eye maps reveal early anterior steepening in the mid-inferior optical zone that is much more pronounced in the posterior curvature. The discrepancy between anterior and posterior maps can be at least partially explained by the epithelial thickness map which shows a thin layer over the protrusion suggesting an early change that deviates from the typical post-myopic LASIK pattern of a thicker epithelium in the center. The relatively thinner central epithelium reduces the apparent magnitude of the protrusion on the anterior surface. The stromal elevation (anterior elevation minus the epithelial layer) shows a protrusion at the same location that is less prominent than the posterior best-fit sphere elevation (Fig. 17.12a).

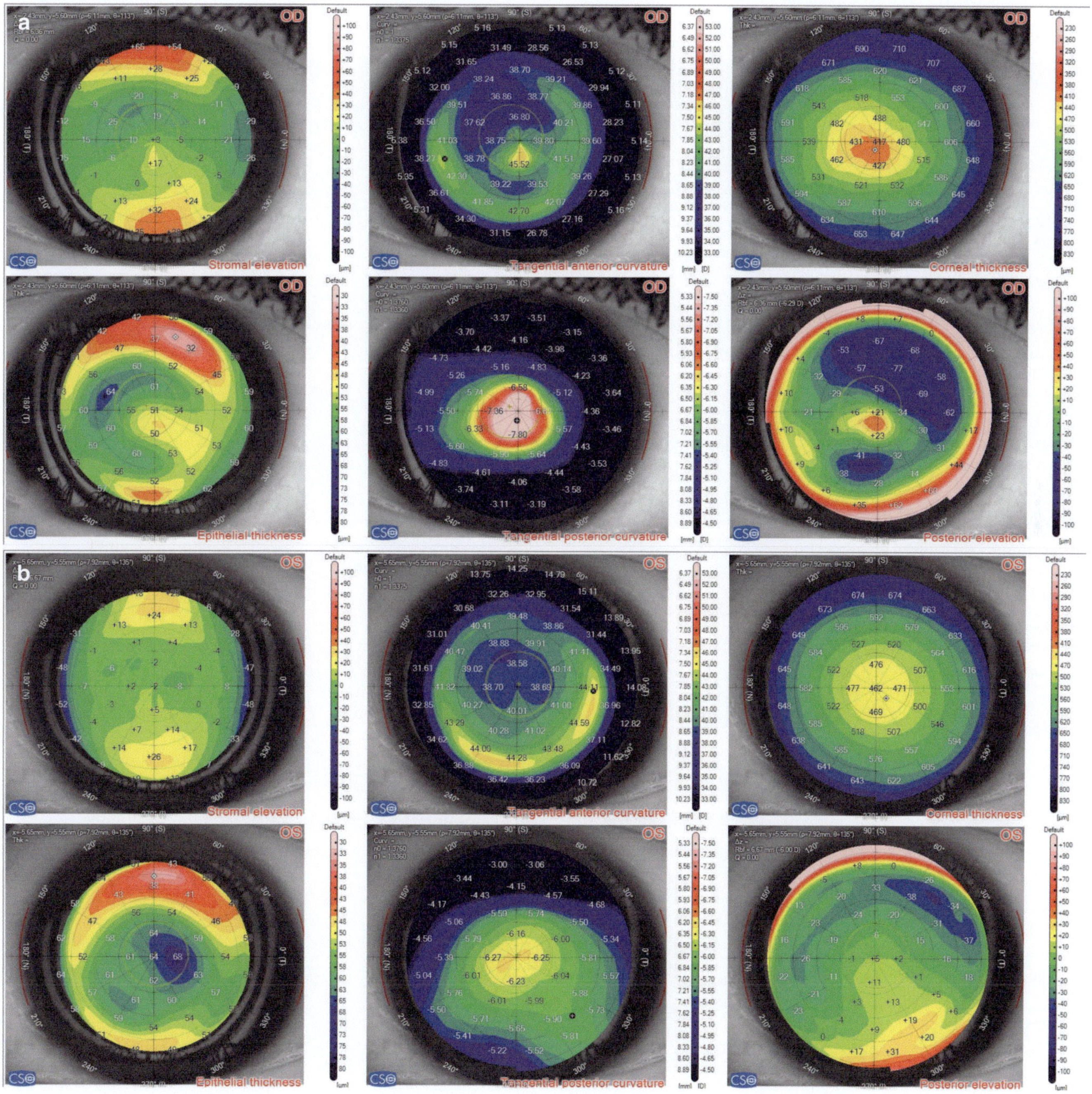

Fig. 17.12 Topography maps in post-myopic LASIK ectasia

These changes were not observed in the other eye with normal keratometry anteriorly and posteriorly as well as regular epithelial thickness as would be expected for post-myopic LASIK (Fig. 17.12b).

Core message: The case presented emphasizes the role of OCT and epithelial mapping in detecting early signs of corneal ectasia following laser vision correction. Topography maps alone may not always reveal the full extent of changes in corneal curvature, and discrepancies between anterior and posterior maps can be better understood through epithelial thickness maps.

Severe Irregular Subepithelial Haze after PRK

Case: The patient's history is significant for PRK 6 years prior to presentation with a best-corrected vision of 20/80 in the right eye.

OCT segmental tomography showing severe and irregular subepithelial haze with variable thickness and density: thicker superiorly (75 µm) and thinner inferiorly (25 µm) at the 45-degree axis (Fig. 17.13a).

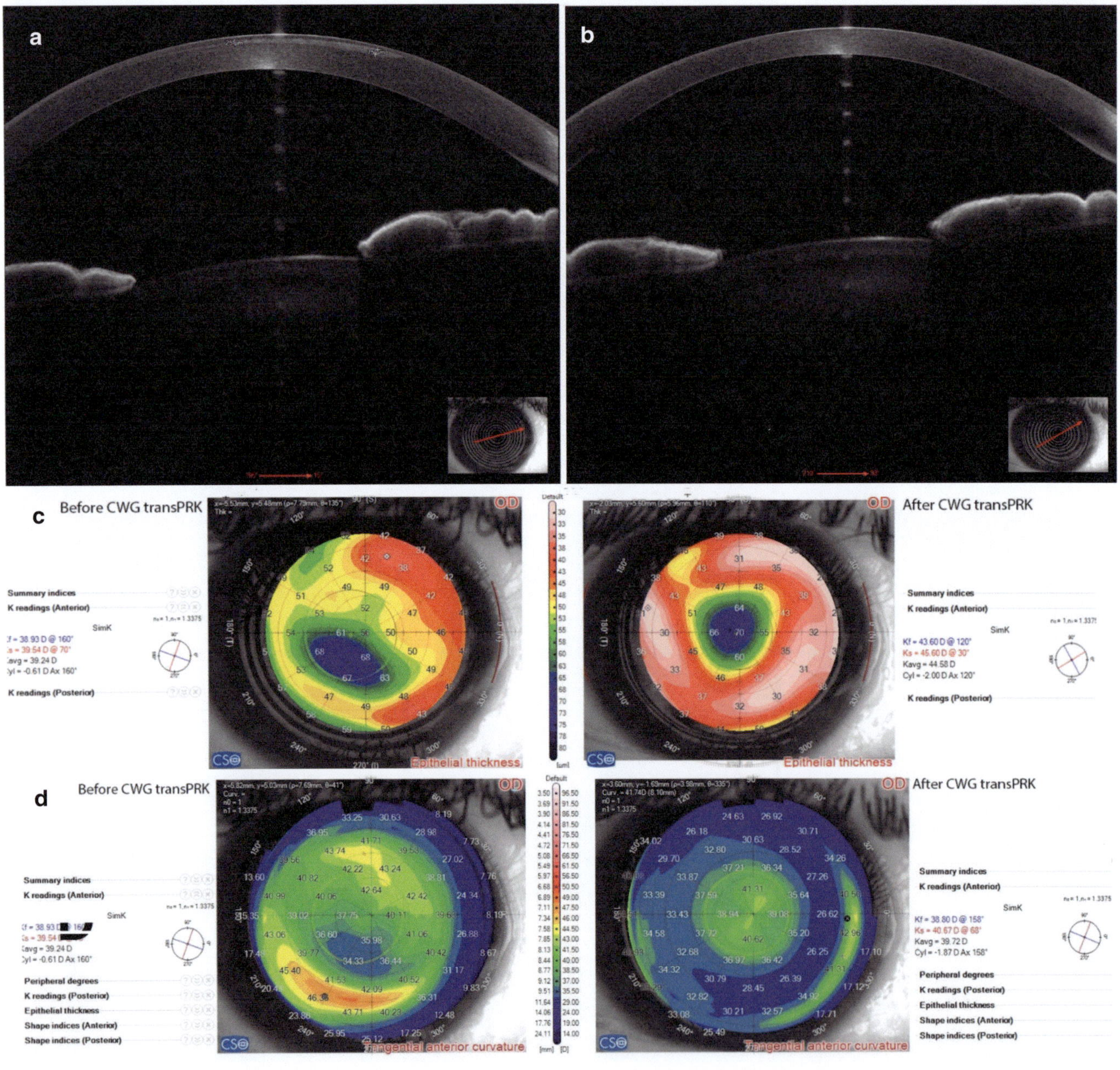

Fig. 17.13 Epithelial and tengential maps in corneal haze

Exam: The epithelium has remodeled in a way to partially compensate for surface irregularities with a thicker profile over the flat inferotemporal area and a thinner profile over the steep superonasal part (Fig. 17.13c). Therefore, the decreased vision was not only a result of haze development but also due to haze-induced irregularity.

Management: Consequently, corneal wavefront-guided (CWG) transepithelial PRK followed by phototherapeutic keratectomy (PTK) with fluid masking to eliminate the haze and smoothen the surface was performed. The AS-OCT section (Fig. 17.13b), epithelial map (Fig. 17.13c), and tangential anterior curvature map **(D)** improved 1 month following the procedure respectively. There is epithelial remodeling, which will likely continue beyond 1 month postoperatively, resolution of haze, and regularization of the corneal surface. As a result, significant improvement in BCVA was observed.

Radial Keratectomy with Big Angle Kappa and De-Centered Spherical Aberration

Case: Anterior tangential curvature map of the left eye of a 48-year-old woman with a history of radial keratotomy (RK) presenting with blurry vision (Fig. 17.14a). The figure shows a small decentered optical zone with severe flattening. It is obvious from the pupil border as displayed on the map that its centroid is superotemporal and away from the center of measurements, which is the corneal vertex. Hence, the patient has a large angle kappa chord. Therefore, the RK treatment was probably centered on the pupil instead of on the visual axis, resulting in a decentered optical zone.

Total corneal aberrometry using dual Placido and OCT tomography showed pupil-centered vs keratoscopy-centered (vertex-centered) aberrations (Fig. 17.14b). We can see that

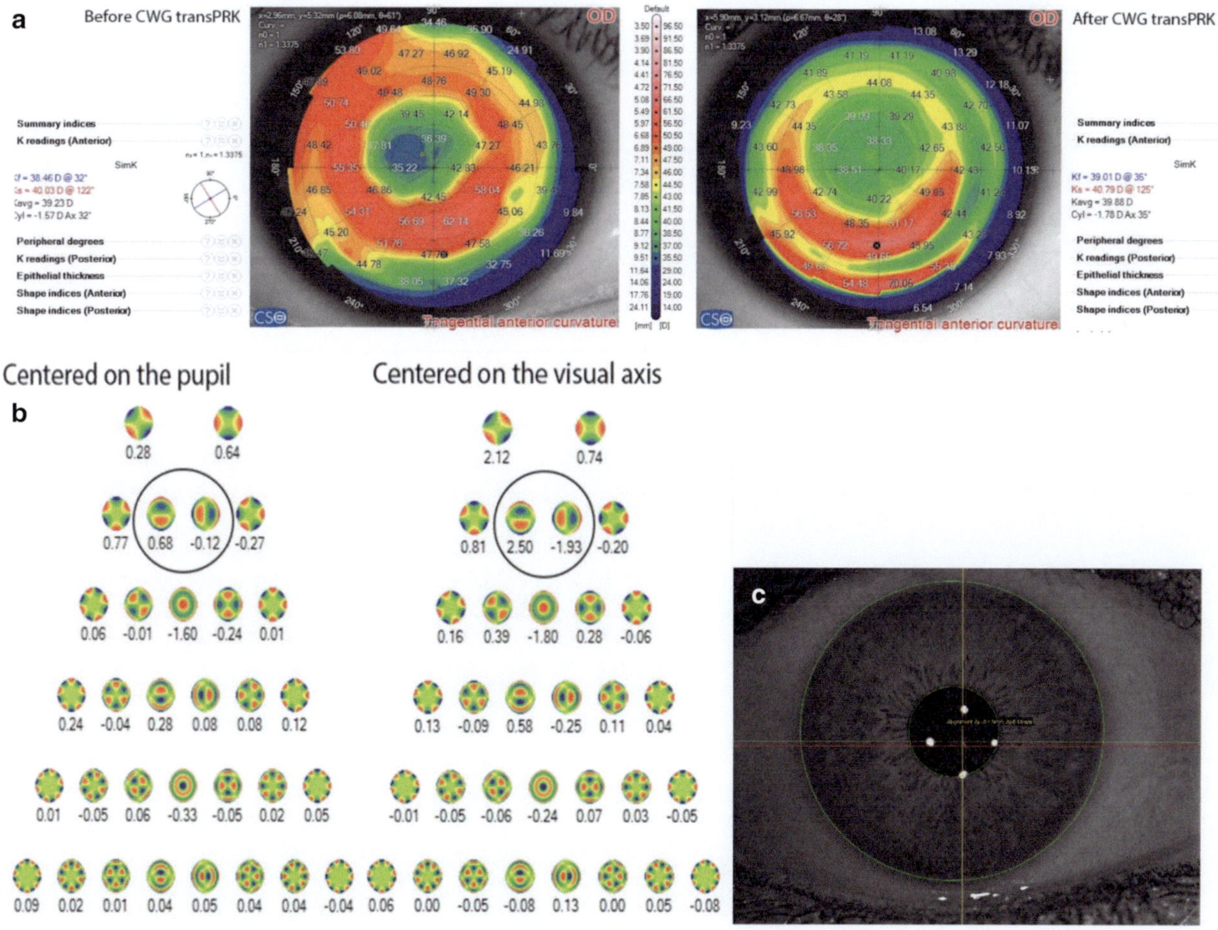

Fig. 17.14 Large angle kappa and spherical aberration

when centered on the pupil, the main aberration is spherical aberration, while coma is mild. However, when centered on the corneal vertex, coma increases dramatically. This underlies the importance of evaluating aberrations based on the corneal vertex when performing any kind of vision correction. This is even more impactful in eyes with big angle kappa that represents the distance between the pupil centroid and the corneal vertex, as in this case (Fig. 17.14c). Infrared image from the Galilei dual Placido and scheimpflug tomographer showed the large angle kappa (Fig. 17.14c).

Management: Corneal wavefront-guided transepithelial PRK was performed, resulting in enlargement of the optical zone (Fig. 17.14a) and improvement in the aberration profile, both coma and spherical aberration, and significant improvement of the hyperopic error.

Epithelial Ingrowth Post-LASIK

Case: A patient with worsening vision was followed for an epithelial ingrowth post-LASIK (Fig. 17.15).

Exam: The increase in the ingrowth is mirrored by the increase in astigmatism and irregularities on topography, which shows steepening at the superonasal side (Fig. 17.15a).

AS-OCT imaging revealed a hyperintense signal under the flap edge **(arrowhead)** (Fig. 17.15b1). Additionally, a fistula tract connecting the epithelial ingrowth area to the intact flap edge was noted on the slit lamp (Fig. 17.15c).

Management: Removal of the ingrowth by flap lifting and scraping improved CDVA as a result of corneal regularization (Fig. 17.15b2).

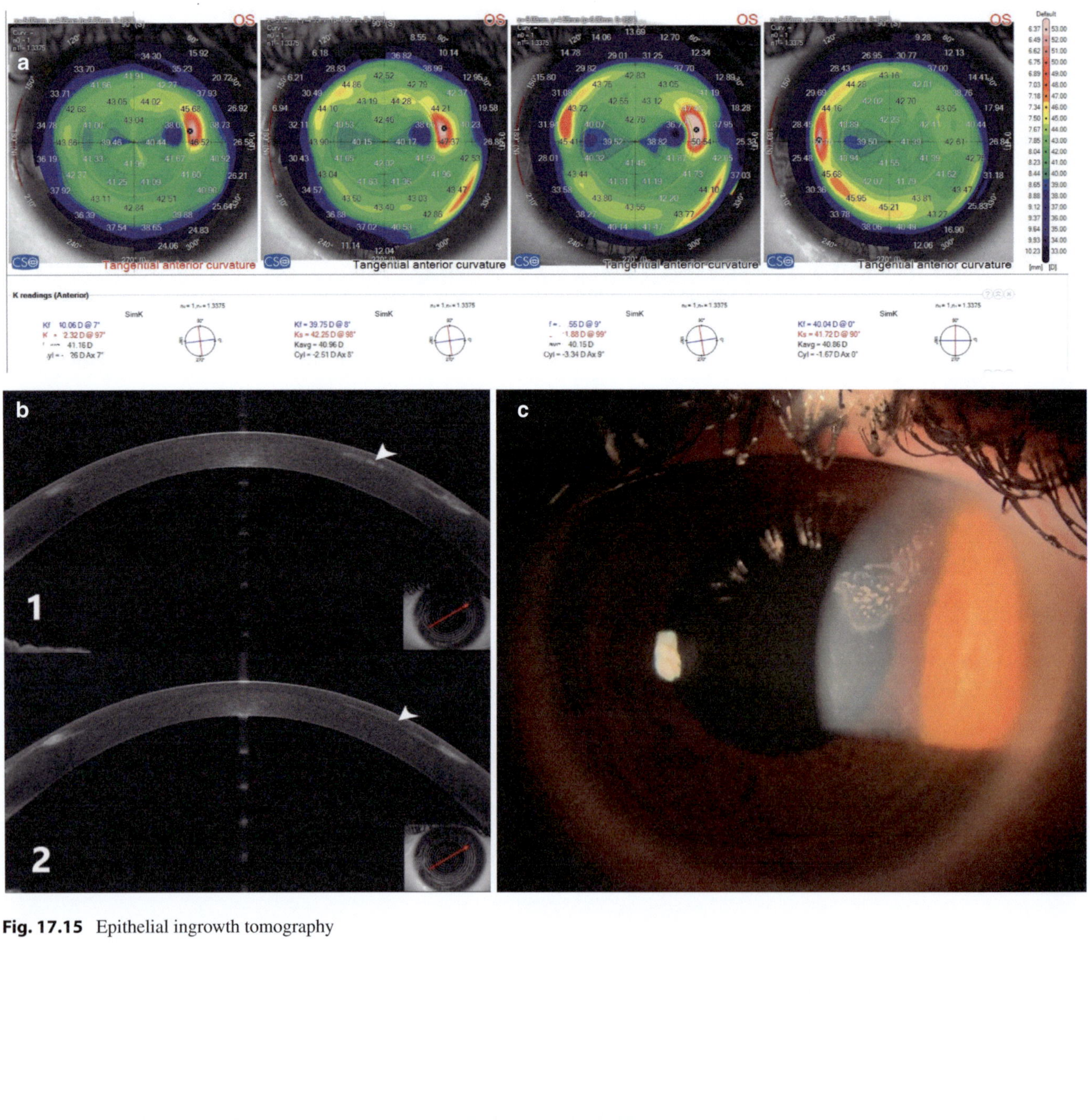

Fig. 17.15 Epithelial ingrowth tomography

Epithelial Mapping in Pre-Operative Refractive Surgery Evaluation

Case: Quad-map from the Galilei dual placido and scheimpflug tomographer showing anterior curvature in a laser vision correction candidate showing significant inferior steepening of >4D with an average index of steepening (I-S) of 2.69D. The posterior curvature is normal, showing a regular bowtie pattern of astigmatism without any hotspots (Fig. 17.16a).

Epithelial maps from MS39 dual Placido and OCT tomographer confirmed the presence of an isolated steepening in the anterior surface of the cornea, but epithelial maps showed a marked increase in epithelial thickness in the inferior region (Fig. 17.16b).

Management: Epithelial map helped ruling out keratoconus, and patient was able to proceed with refractive surgery.

Core message: Epithelial warpage can create falsely abnormal topographies that might affect sphero-cylinder refraction.

Case: High-definition OCT as part of refractive surgery evaluation of a patient with high myopia and astigmatism reveals anterior inferior steepening in the right eye together with a thin pachymetry profile, all suspicious of keratoconus (Fig. 17.17a). The tangential posterior curvature is normal with a regular bowtie pattern of astigmatism, but the epithelium is diffusely thin centrally (42 µm) with an irregular pattern (Fig. 17.17a). This denotes contact lens warpage and a dry ocular surface with a thin tear film and a dehydrated thin epithelial layer, leading to an irregular and overall thin epithelial thickness.

Management: Contact lenses were discontinued for 2 weeks, and aggressive treatment of the patient's dry ocular surface was initiated. Repeat imaging showed regularization of the anterior curvature and epithelial map and an improvement in vision to 20/20 BCVA (Fig. 17.17b). This case was then managed by an intraocular collamer lens.

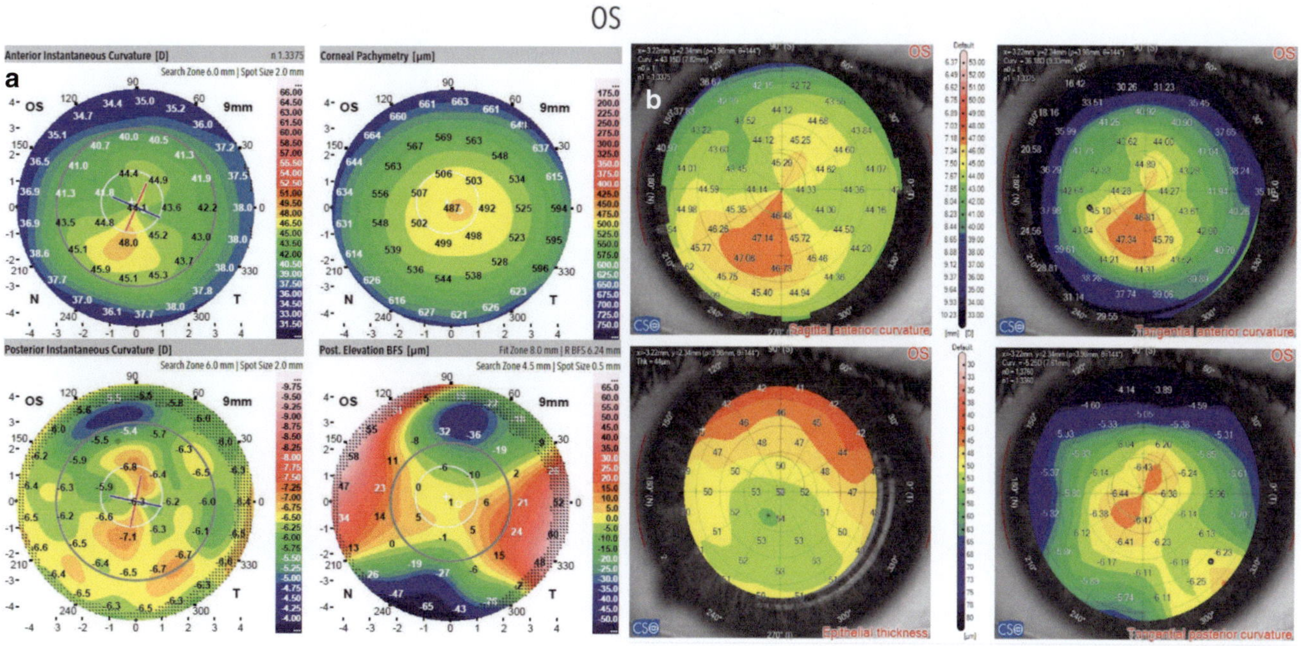

Fig. 17.16 Epithelial thickening inducing anterior curvature abnormality

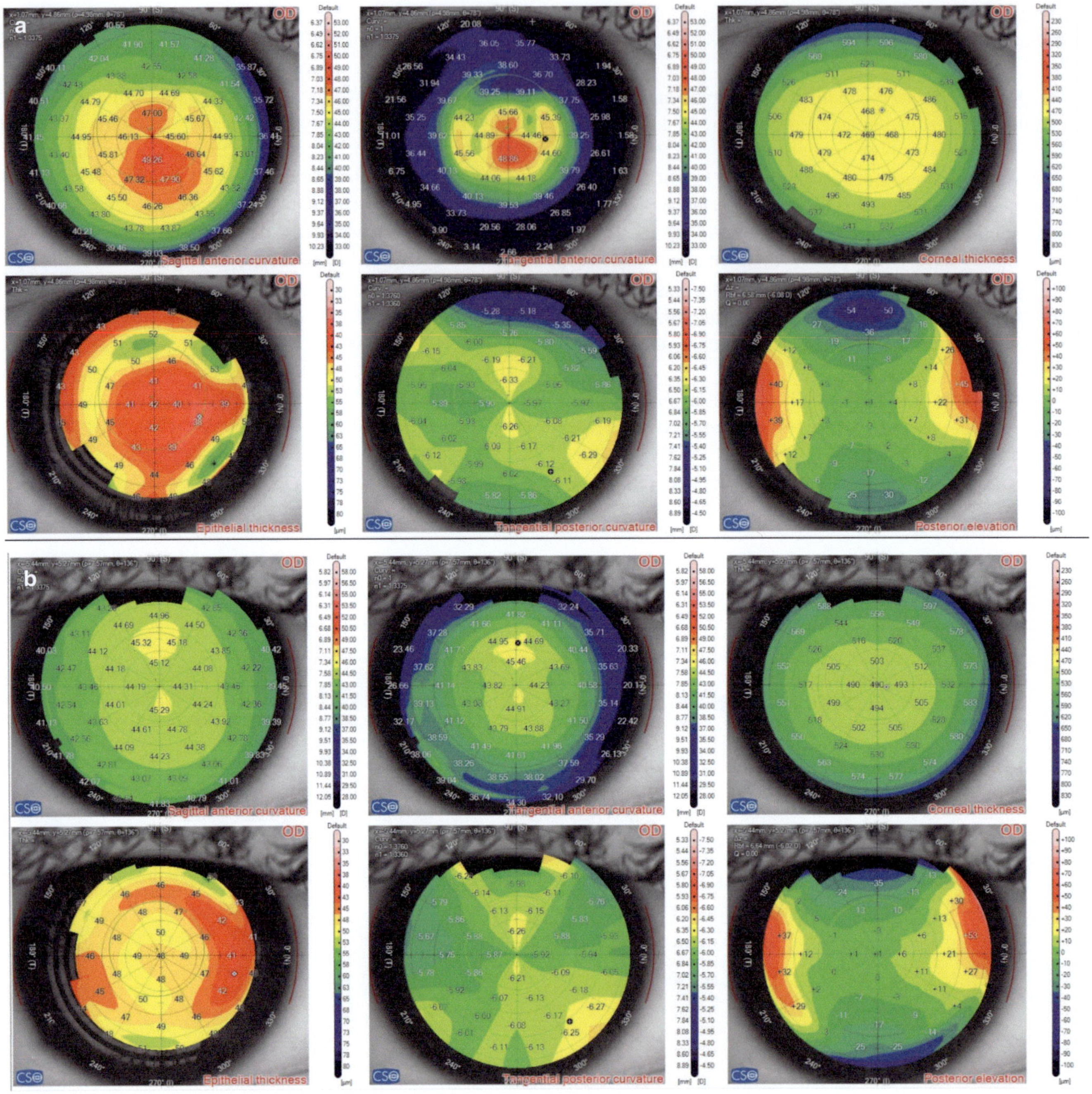

Fig. 17.17 Epithelial thinning and warpage reflecting dry ocular surface simulating keratoconus

Take-Home Message

- From Placido topography to Scheimpflug tomography to dual Placido and OCT-based tomography, anterior segment imaging has evolved to include the anterior corneal surface, posterior corneal surface, and everything in between, from epithelial maps, stromal elevations, and corneal structures as displayed by OCT sections. This provides the clinician and surgeon with more detailed information for treatment planning and outcome evaluation. It is thus crucial to adopt a comprehensive and holistic approach during the analysis of corneal tomography to cover all aspects of this expanding field.
- Epithelial mapping is a helpful tool in the preoperative evaluation of patients undergoing refractive surgery, and especially for early keratoconus screening. Corneal warpage can display a thickened epithelium, while early keratoconus typically presents with epithelial thinning over the ectatic area.
- Interface fluid syndrome can be induced by any pathology that disrupts endothelial function, and it has been reported in both LASIK and SMILE procedures. Etiologies associated with this syndrome include high intraocular pressure, uveitis, infectious keratitis, and endothelial decompensation.
- In case of acute stromal necrosis over an intra-stromal ring segment, early intervention by removal of the segment is crucial before expansion of the necrosis.

Ectasia After Small-Incision Lenticule Extraction: Management and Lessons Learned (Black-Box Thinking)

18

Renato Ambrósio Jr, Louise Pellegrino Gomes Esporcatte, Marcella Q. Salomão, Aydano P. Machado, and Guy M. Kezirian

Case Initial Presentation

A 26-year-old woman with fairly high myopia and intolerant to contact lenses presented with an interest in refractive surgery. Uncorrected distance visual acuity (UCVA) was counting fingers in both eyes. Best corrected distance visual acuity (BCVA) was 20/20 (−9.50/−0.50 × 160°) in the right eye (OD) and 20/20 (−9.50/−0.50 × 173°) in the left eye (OS). The silt lamp exam and fundoscopy were unremarkable.

Corneal front surface topography was within normal limits, with a symmetric bow tie in both eyes (Fig. 18.1). Simulated keratometry (Sim K keratometry) results were 42.7 × 19,5° × 43.4 in the OD and 42.8 × 164.1° × 43.8 in the OS. The central corneal thickness (CCT) was 520 and 522 μm in OD and OS, respectively.

The Belin/Ambrósio enhanced ectasia display from Pentacam (Oculus Optikgerate GmbH, Wetzlar Germany) demonstrated normal elevation maps for both eyes (Fig. 18.2). The deviation index (BAD-D) was 1.27 in OD and 1.07 OS. Ambrósio Relational Thickness (ART-max) was 359 and 352 μm in OD and OS, respectively.

Segmental tomography with corneal OCT by RTVue (Optovue Inc., Fremont, CA, USA) revealed the thinnest point of 504 μm in OD and 502 μm in OS. The epithelial thickness map had a pattern of mild thinning towards the temporal inferior quadrant in both eyes (Fig. 18.3).

The Laser-Assisted Lenticular Extraction with a small incision (LALEX) was considered the best suitable procedure, considering the correction level, the patient's age, and the corneal tomographic data. The calculated residual stromal bed (RSB) thickness based on the CCT was 250 μm in OD and 257 μm in OS. Small Incision Lenticular Extraction (SMILE) in both eyes with the 500 kHz Visumax femtosecond laser (Carl Zeiss Meditec, Jena, Germany) for making the lenticule in each eye (Fig. 18.4). The lenticule dissection and extraction was uneventfully performed using the technique described by Reinstein without complications.

Normal symmetrical bow-tie was observed with the Atlas Scale (Fig. 18.1a) and the Ambrosio 2 Scale (Fig. 18.1b).

The Belin/ambrosio enhanced ectasia display of both eyes. The BAD-D of OD (Fig. 18.2a) was 1.27 and ARTmax of 359, and (Fig. 18.2b) in OS had a BAD-D of 1.07 and ARTmax of 352.

The preoperative OCT of both eyes, showing normal pachymetry and epithelium maps of OD (Fig. 18.3a) and OS (Fig. 18.3b).

The ZEISS SMILE programming of OD (Fig. 18.4a) and OS (Fig. 18.4b).

R. Ambrósio Jr (✉)
Department of Ophthalmology, Federal University the State of Rio de Janeiro (UNIRIO), Rio de Janeiro, Brazil

L. P. G. Esporcatte · M. Q. Salomão · A. P. Machado
Department of Ophthalmology, Federal University of São Paulo, São Paulo, Brazil
e-mail: marcella@barravisioncenter.com.br

G. M. Kezirian
World College of Refractive Surgery and Visual Sciences, Scottsdale, AZ, USA
e-mail: guy1000@surgivision.net

S. A. Melki et al. (eds.), *Refractive Surgery Atlas*, https://doi.org/10.1007/978-3-031-60661-8_18

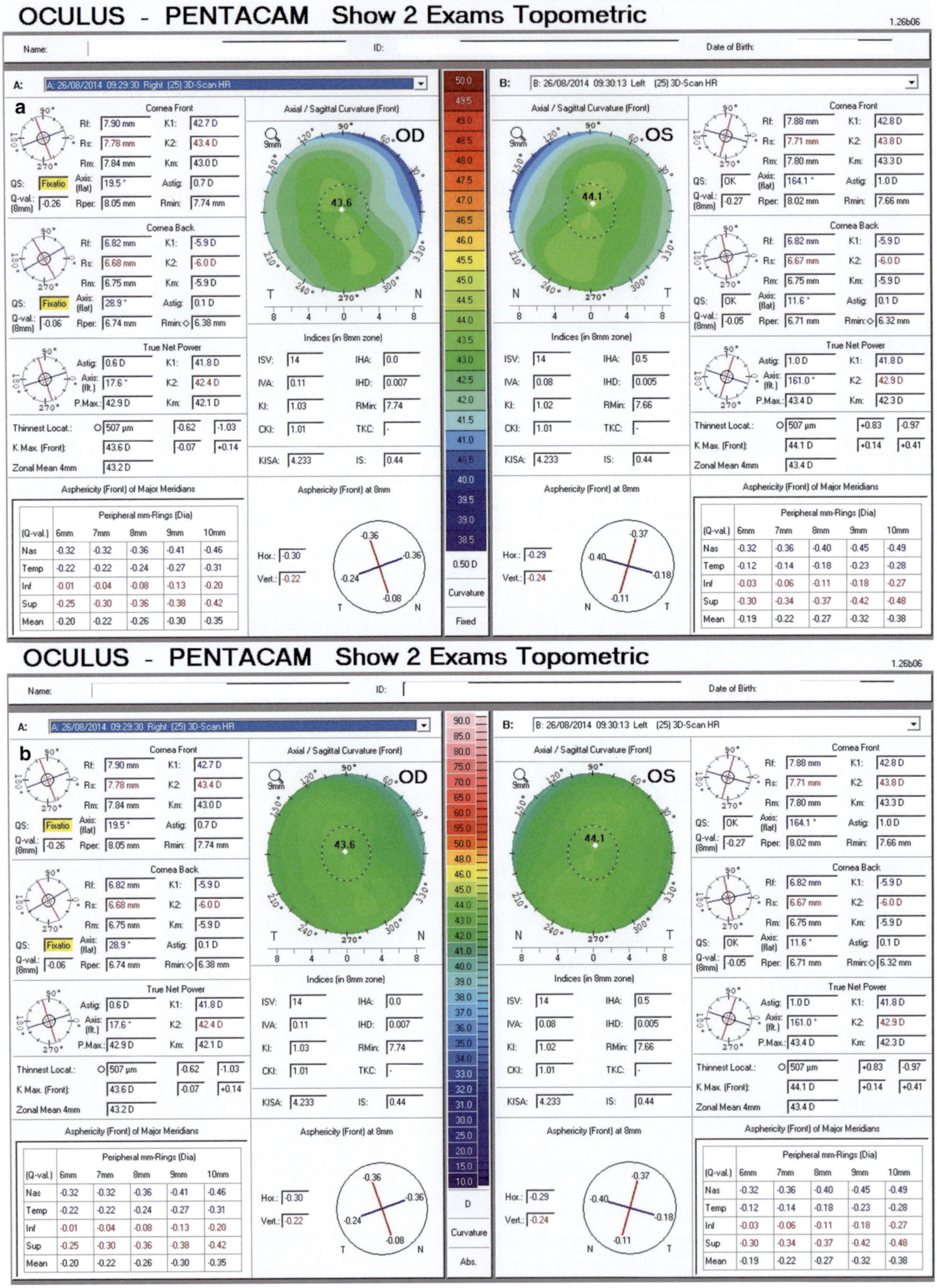

Fig. 18.1 Pentacam topometric maps preop

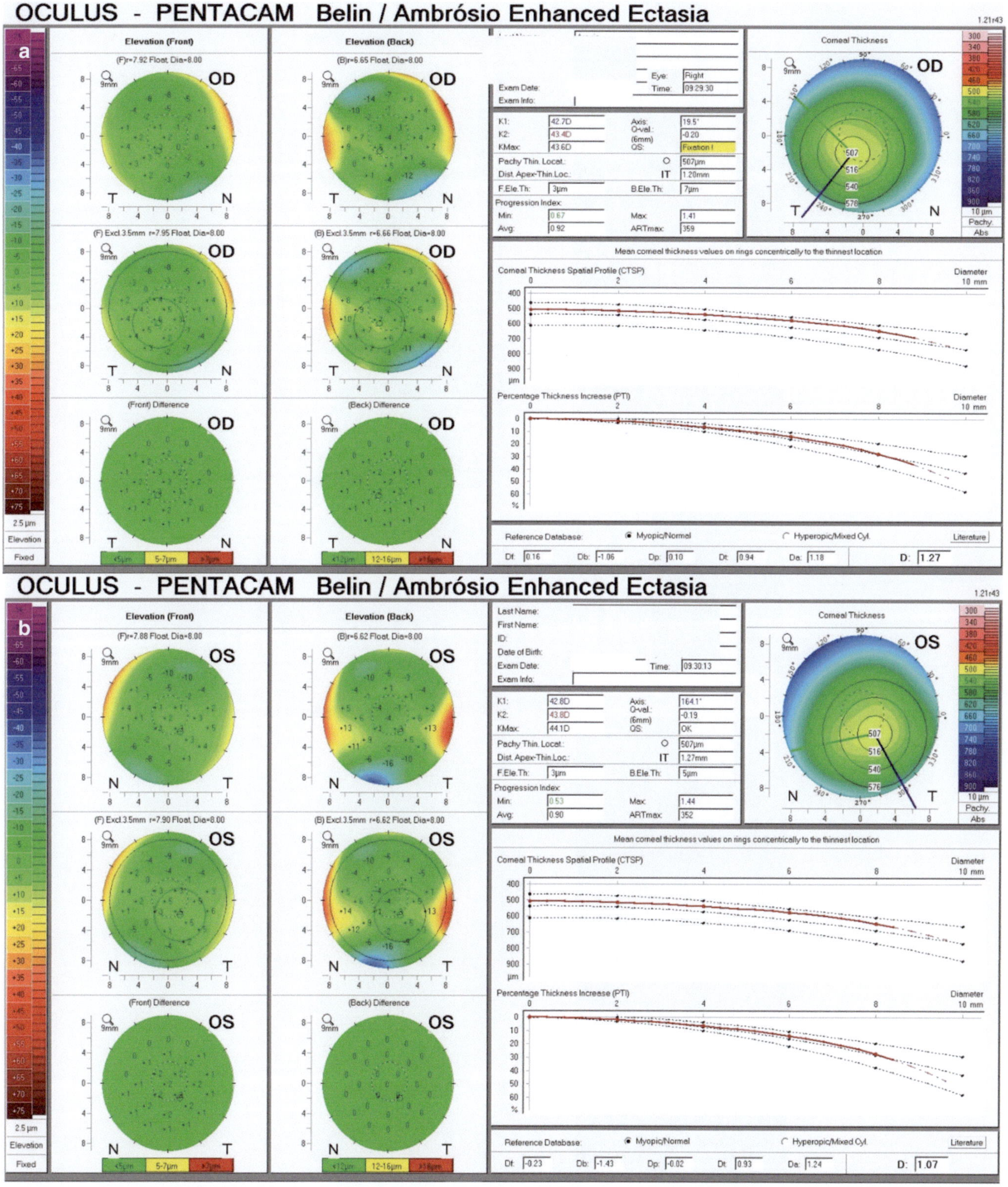

Fig. 18.2 Belin/ambrosio enhanced ectasia display

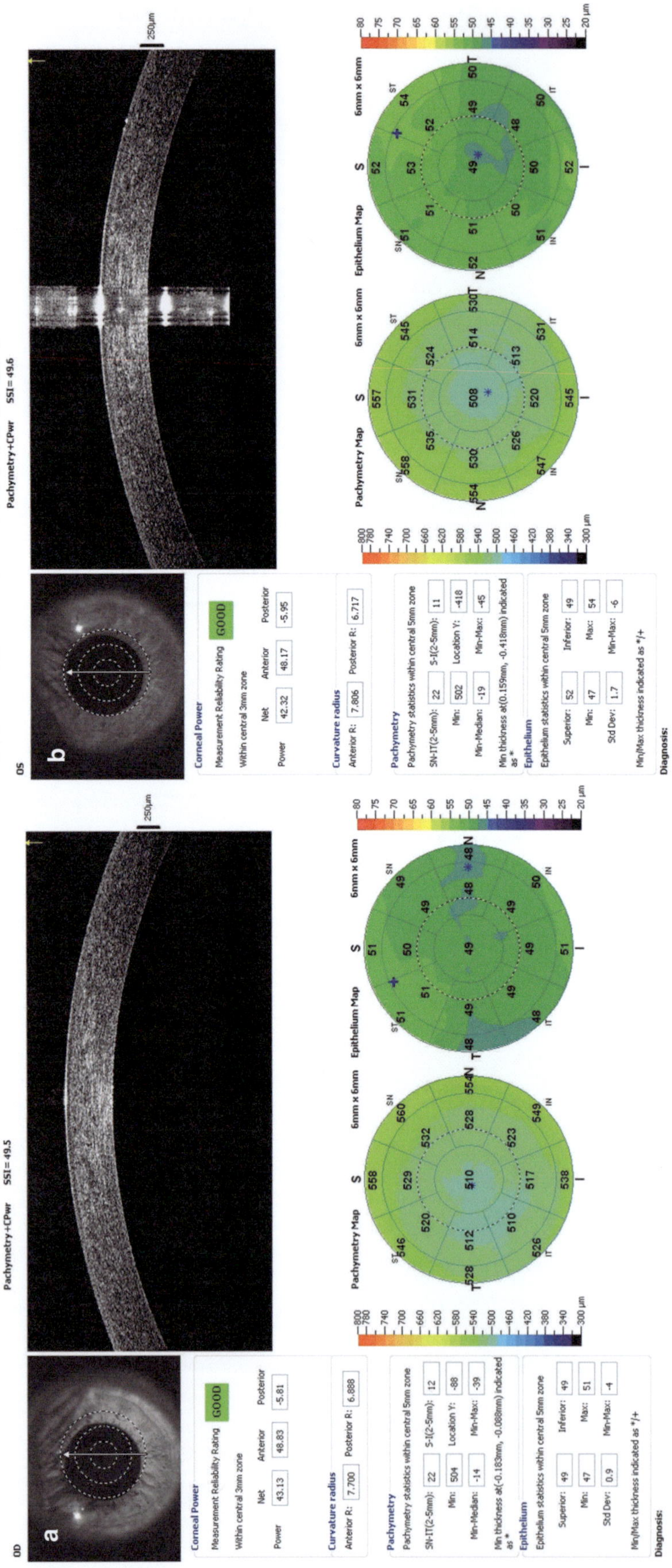

Fig. 18.3 Preoperative OCT

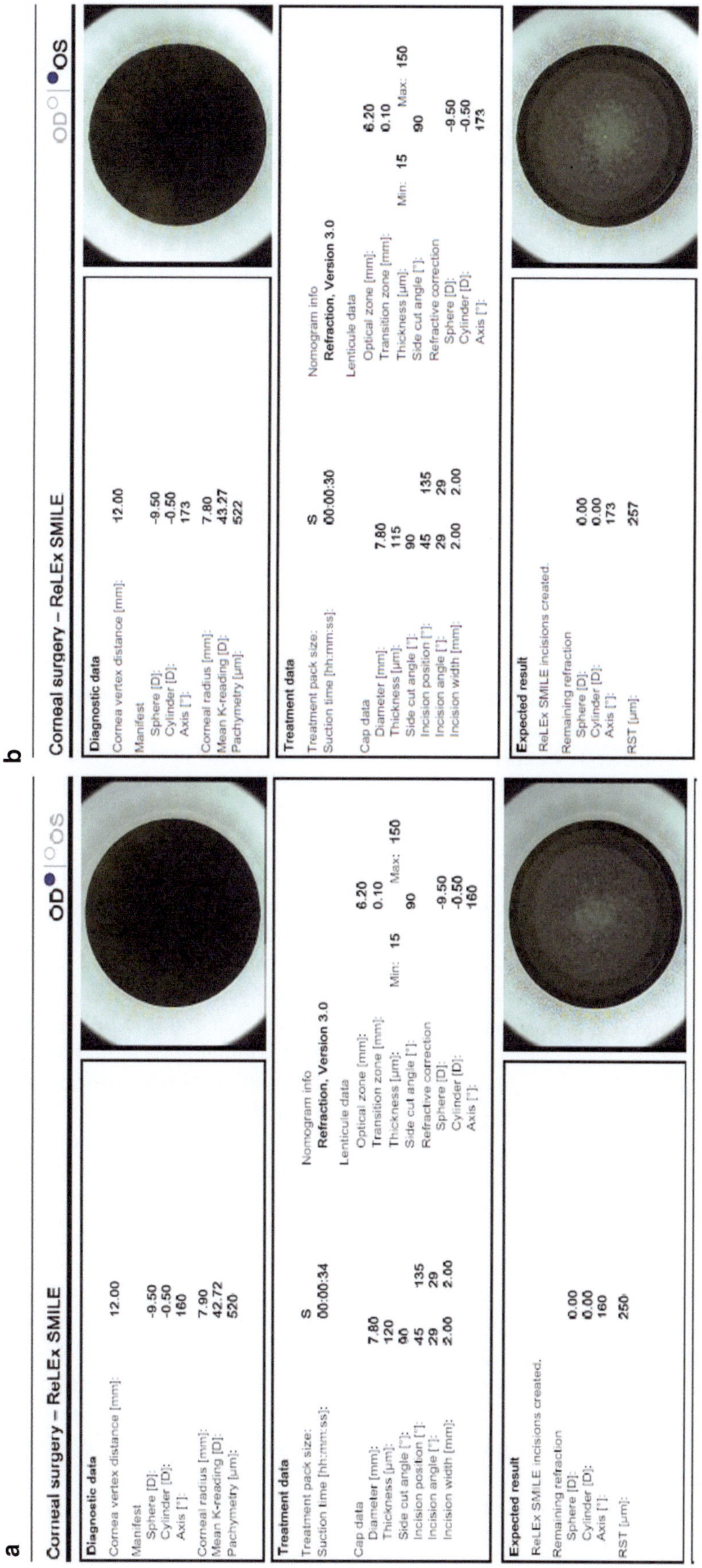

Fig. 18.4 SMILE surgical programming

Postoperative Management

The patient did well after the procedure, presenting with UCVA of 20/20 in both eyes 6 days after SMILE. She returned with no complaints for regular follow-ups at 1 month, 6 months, 1 year, and 2 years after the procedure when a dilated fundus exam was performed.

Four years after SMILE surgery, the patient returned due to progressive vision deterioration in the right eye. The UCVA was 20/100 in OD and 20/25 in the left eye. The BCVA was 20/25- (−2.00/−4.00 × 55°) in the OD and 20/20 (plano/−1.00 × 92°) in the OS. The topometric (Fig. 18.5) and posterior elevation (Fig. 18.6) evolutions demonstrate unquestionable ectasia progression in the right eye.

The OCT demonstrated a thinning pattern consistent with ectasia in OD (Fig. 18.7). The left eye had a thicker epithelial in the center, corroborating a stable, not ectatic pattern.

The diagnosis of iatrogenic ectasia after SMILE was confirmed OD. The management of such complications initiates with patient education and counseling. The patient admitted allergic episodes and eye rubbing before noticing decreased vision OD. Considering the status of the left eye, no surgery was indicated, but the clinical treatment starts with an emphatic orientation for avoiding eye rubbing. Ocular allergy control and ocular surface optimization included oral vitamin B2 (riboflavin) associated with omega-3 essential fatty acids, artificial tears with no preservatives, and topical antihistaminic drops.

A frank discussion was accomplished with the patient about her current condition and treatment options to halt the ectatic process and rehabilitate vision. Contact lens fitting and corneal transplantation were mentioned as possible solutions. Nevertheless, surgery is indicated considering the progressive nature of ectasia in OD. Also, a keratoplasty procedure should be the last option for patients with corneal ectasia.

The therapeutic surgical approach was performed in OD with a Femtosecond-Assisted Intracorneal Ring Segment implantation (FS-ICRS) (Keraring SI6 150°/250 µm) associated with crosslinking with no epithelial removal. After implanting the ICRS in the inferior-temporal region, a Dextran-free solution of Riboflavin 0.15% with HPMC was injected in the tunnel created by the Visumax femtosecond laser. The circular tunnel was created at 295 µm, and the incision at 126°. Epithelium-on Collagen Crosslinking (Epi-ON CXL) was performed with a fast protocol using UVA (365 nm) at 9 mW/cm^2 for 10 min with the Avedro KXL (Glaukos; Burlington, USA).

The patient had an uneventful recovery with mild discomfort shortly after the therapeutic procedure of FS-ICRS + Epi-ON CXL (Fig. 18.8). Eight months after the therapeutic surgery in OD, the UCVA was 20/50, and BCVA was 20/25 (−1.50/−1.50 × 104°). The tomographic evolution after the implant of the ICRS shows the corneal flattening in the differential map of anterior curvature and a mild increase in backward scattering on Scheimpflug densitometry (Fig. 18.9).

The patient returned for a routine clinical exam, including retinal evaluation, 3 years and 6 months after the therapeutic surgery. She was relatively happy with the result. Her UDVA was 20/40 in OD and 20/20 in the left eye. The BCVA was 20/20 (−1.50/−1.50 × 125°) in the OD and, in the left eye, 20/20+ (plano/−0.75 × 100°). The curvature map was stable with central flattening, no change in posterior elevation, and the Corneal Biomechanical Index (CBI) post-Laser Vision Correction (LVC) was 0.00 in the left eye (Fig. 18.10), demonstrating stability at the tomography and biomechanical assessments in the left eye.

The topometric (front corneal surface) evolution of the right eye has been observed since the preoperative visit **"D"** throughout the four-year follow-up period. In **"C"**, 6 months postoperatively, a slight decentralization of the flattening zone was noted. In **"B"**, 2 years postoperatively, a small central steepening was observed, which continued to progress until the four-year follow-up **"A"**. The differential map between **"A"** and **"B"** shows a central steepening of 4.6D between the four- and two-year mark after SMILE (Fig. 18.5).

Tomographic evolution of the posterior elevation of the right eye with a fixed best-fit sphere (BFS) for the first (preoperative) measurement **"D"**, demonstrating the progression of the ectatic disease over 4 years postoperatively. One year later, the posterior elevation progression was minimal **"C"**. The evidence of progression in the posterior elevation is marked after 4 years "**A"**, but could have been previously detected 2 years after surgery "**B"** (Fig. 18.6).

OCT 4 years after SMILE, with OD demonstrating the epithelial thinning pattern consistent with ectasia and thick central epithelial in OS, corroborating no ectasia progression (Fig. 18.7).

Slit-lamp biomicroscopy 1 week after FS-ICRS implantation associated with Epi-ON CXL OD (Fig. 18.8).

Pentacam topometric and corneal densitometry differential displays before **"B"** and 8 months after **"A"** ICRS + Epi-ON CXL OD (Fig. 18.9).

The postoperative of ARV (Ambrósio, Roberts & Vinciguerra) biomechanical and tomographic assessment display of OS shows the CBI post LVC of 0.00 (Fig. 18.10).

The retrospective evaluation of the preoperative ARV (Ambrósio, Roberts & Vinciguerra) biomechanical and tomographic assessment display demonstrates a borderline CBI (0.34) and a high tomography and biomechanical index (TBI) (0.73) (Fig. 18.11).

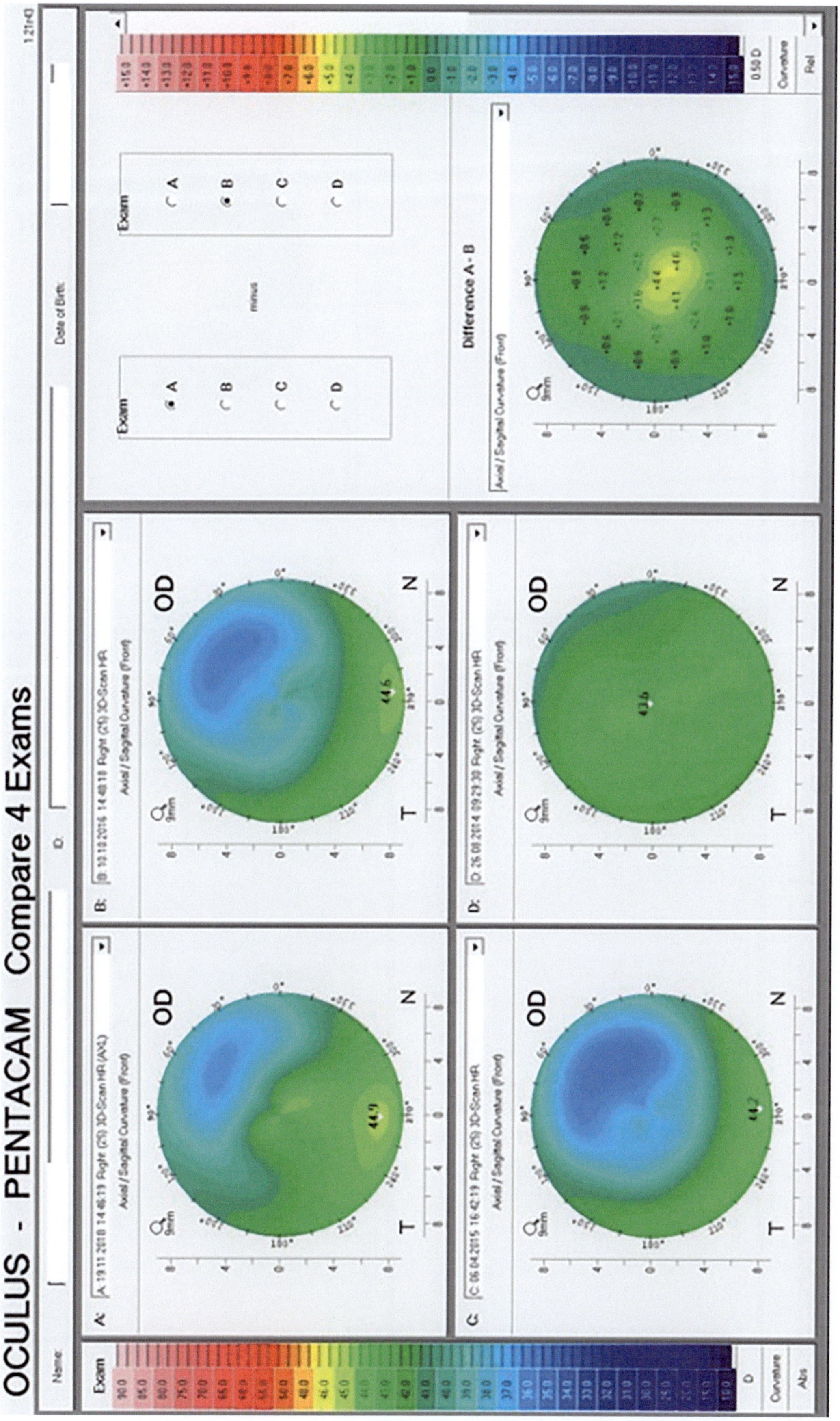

Fig. 18.5 Longitudinal topometric evaluation from pentacam of OD

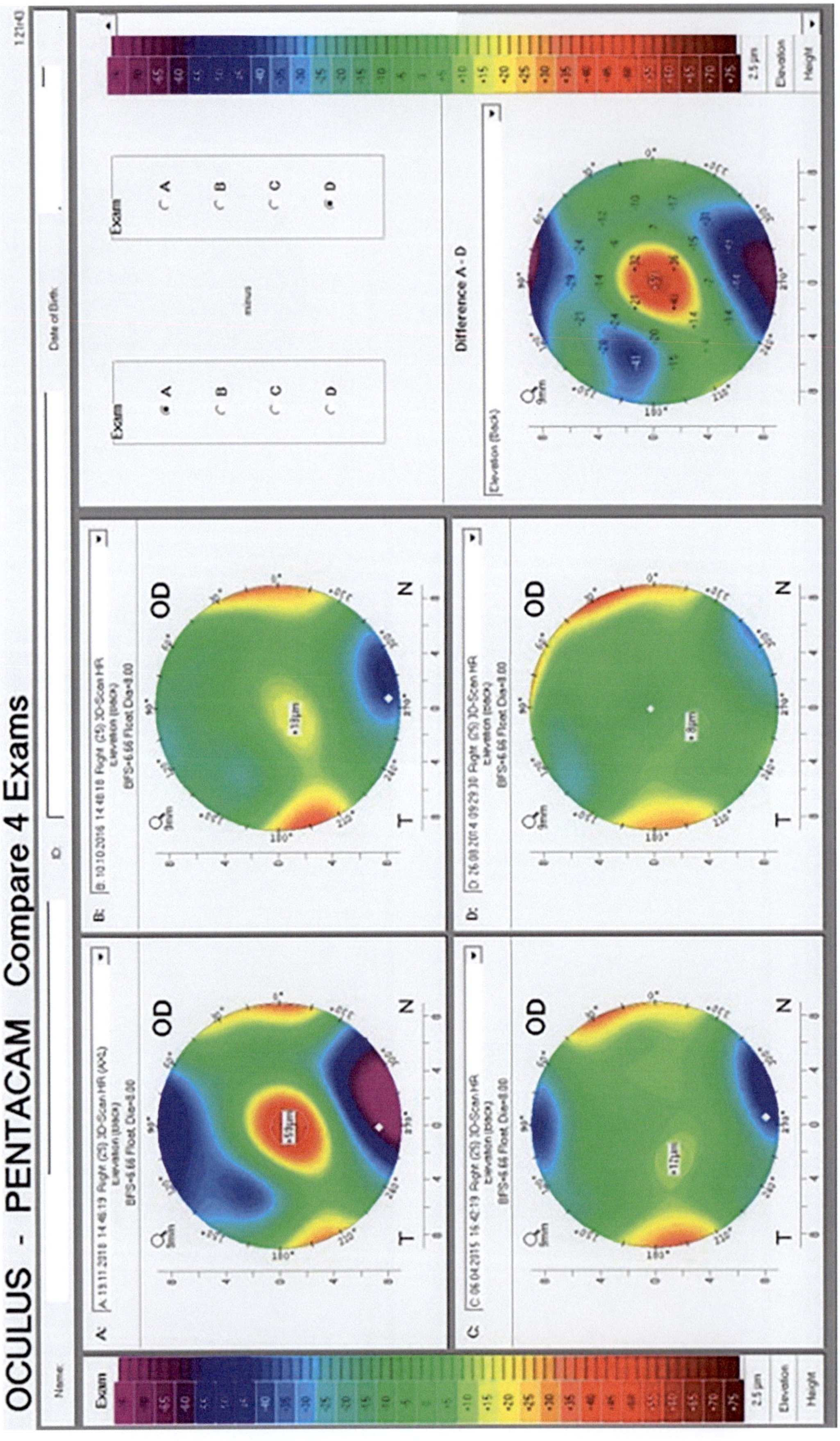

Fig. 18.6 Longitudinal tomographic evaluation of the posterior elevation OD

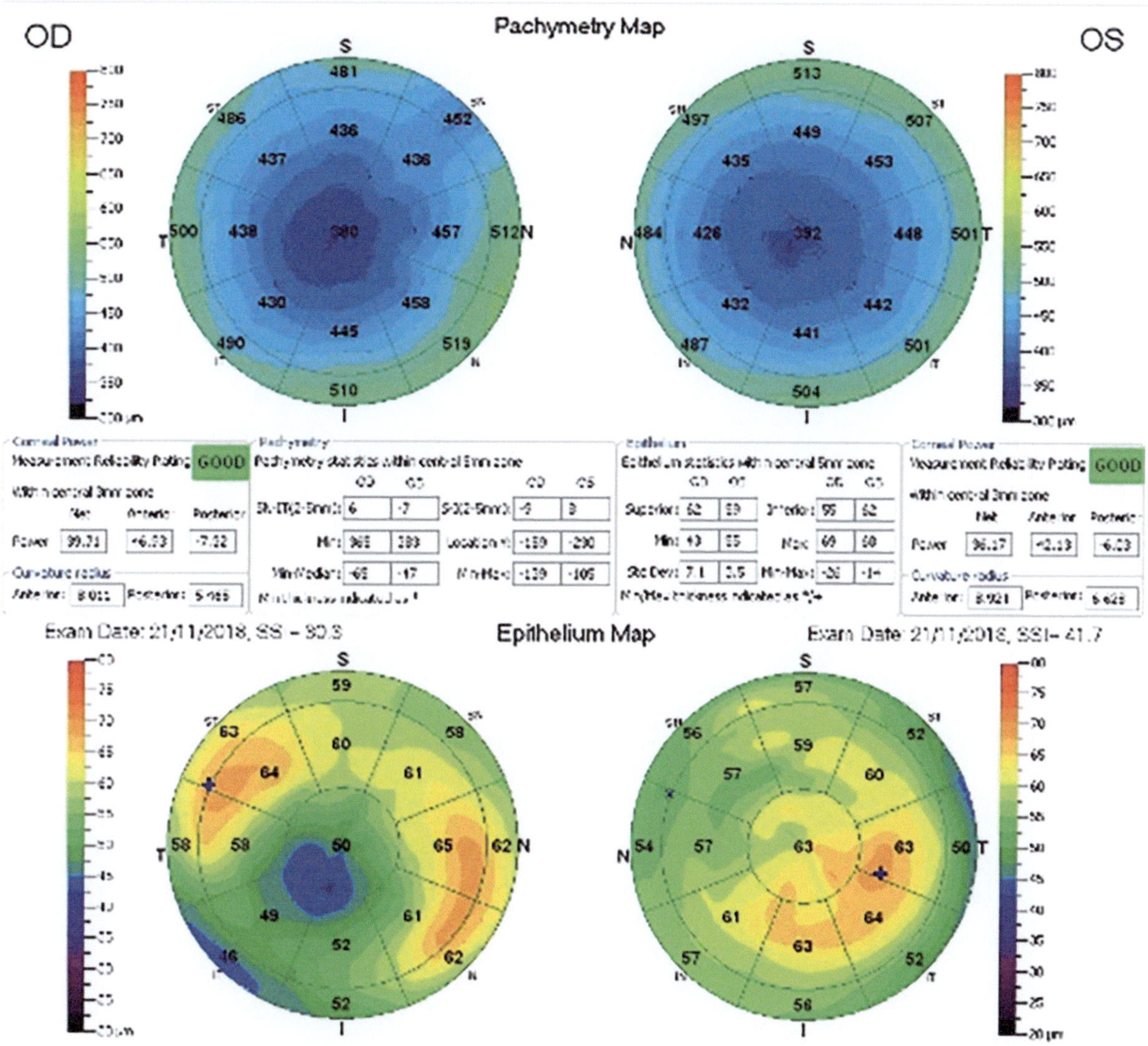

Fig. 18.7 OCT segmental tomography of OS

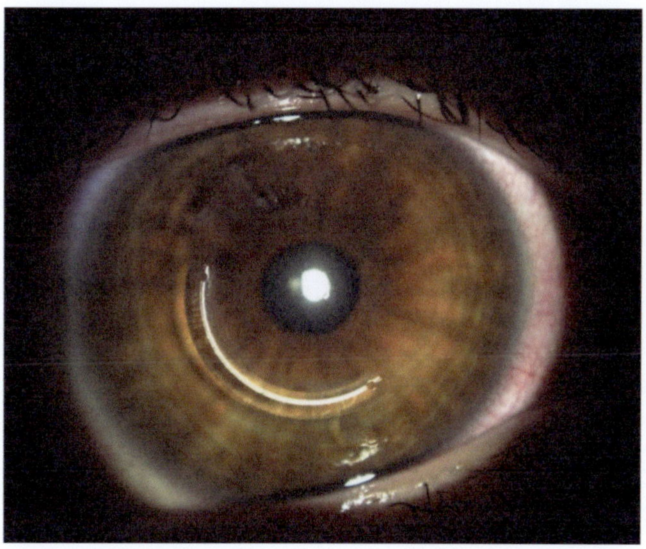

Fig. 18.8 Biomicroscopy

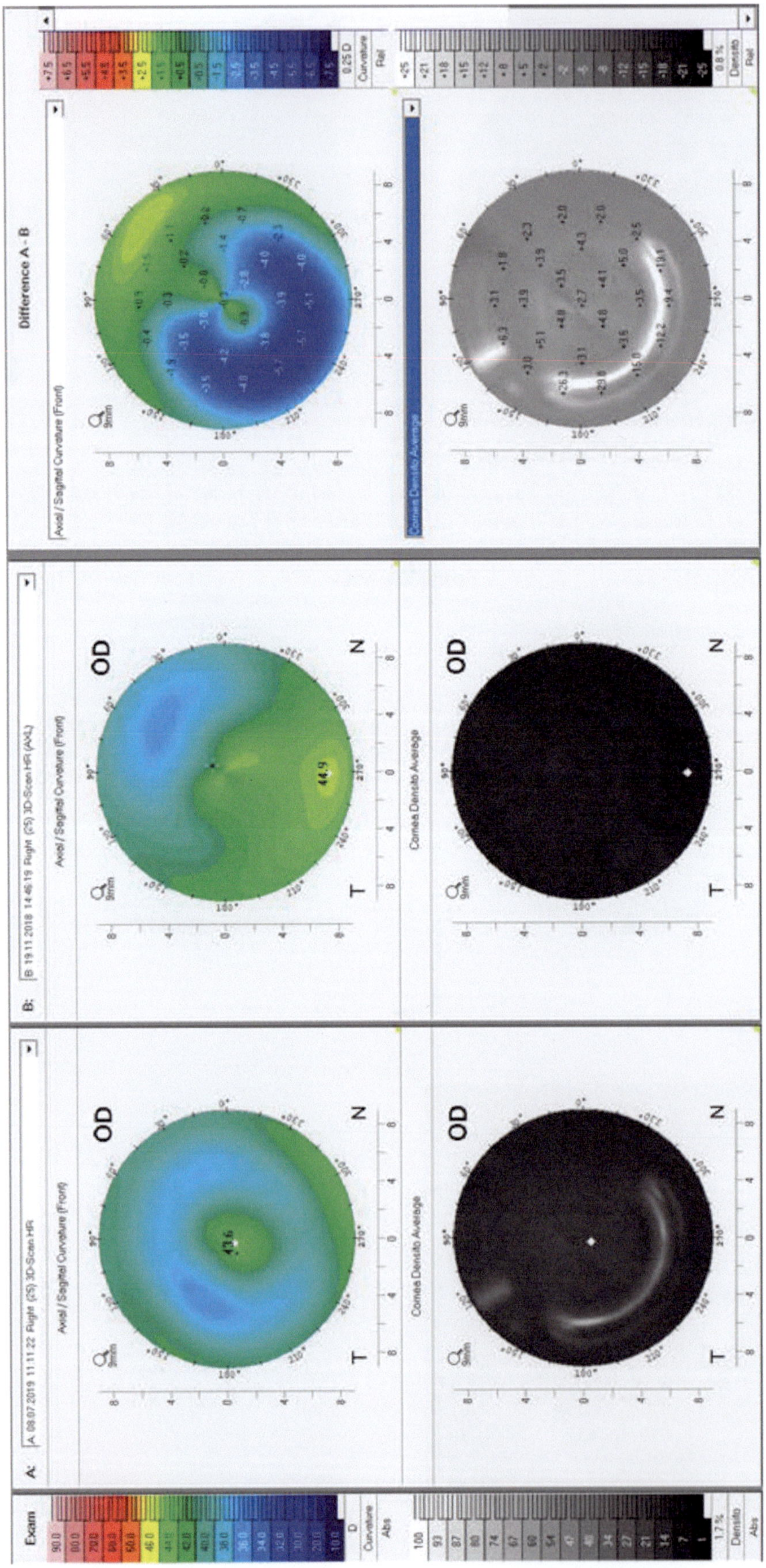

Fig. 18.9 Tomographic evolution after ICRS + Epi-ON CXL in OD

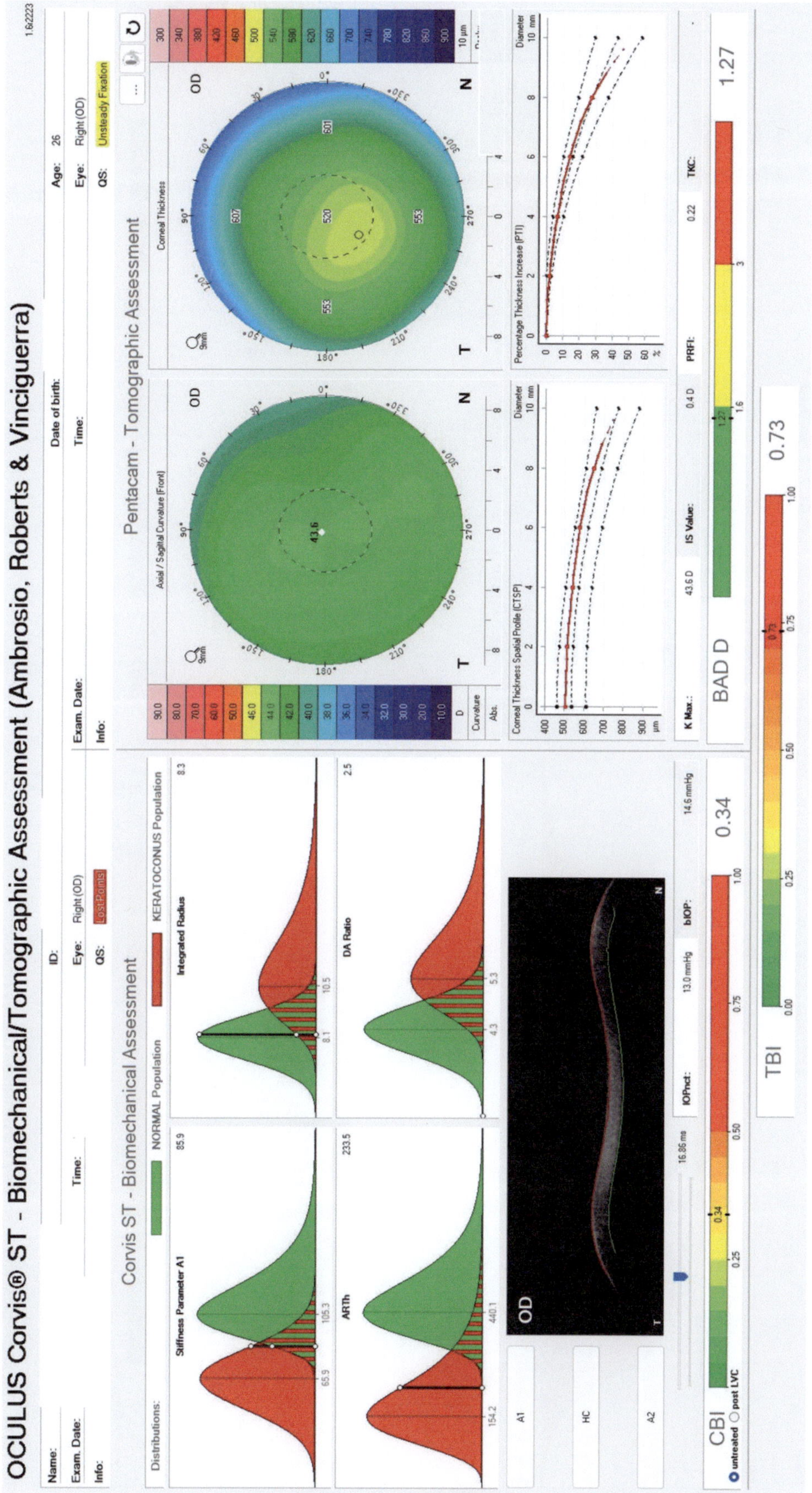

Fig. 18.10 Biomechanical and tomographic assessment display post-op OS

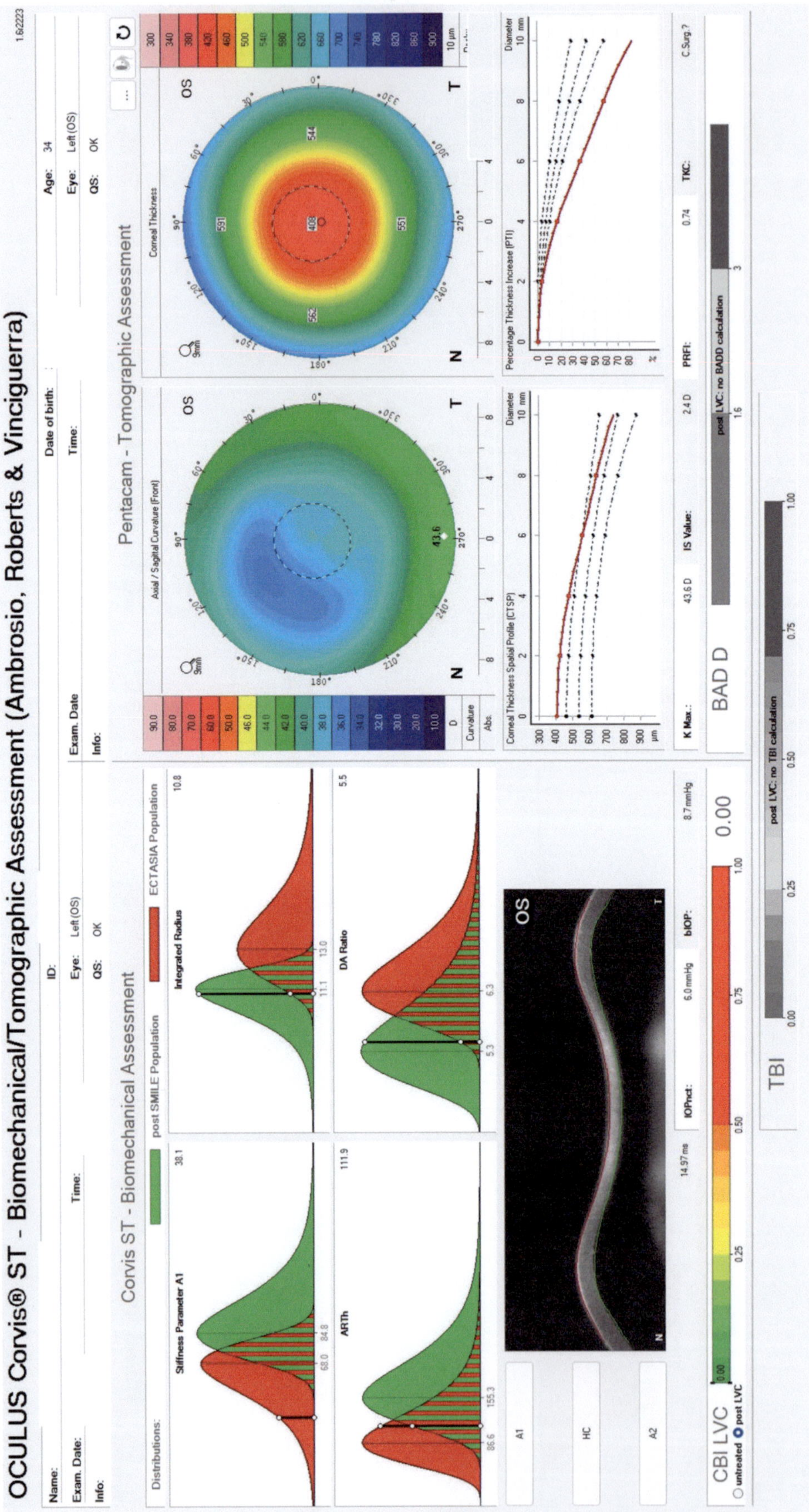

Fig. 18.11 Biomechanical and tomographic assessment display preop OD

$(A^2\ I)^2$ and Black Box Thinking: Growing Mindsets for Refractive Surgeons

The concept of "black-box thinking"draws from aviation, where the flight data recorder ("black-box") is recovered after accidents to investigate the root cause of the accident to improve processes and system design to avoid future recurrences.

Black box thinking can be applied to any field as a means to learn from failures and faults, facilitating progress and innovation. Morbidity and mortality conferences serve as an example of the black box thinking approach; however, they are infrequently utilized. Instead, errors and complications are often suppressed rather than communicated, due to concerns surrounding medicolegal liability or other factors [1].

Black box thinking, process generation, and system design are most applicable in fields where data are available, risks can be identified, and processes can be routinized. These features describe much of refractive surgery. The current case provides an excellent example of how after-the-fact analysis can lead to insights and understanding that may help avoid similar problems in the future using the black-box thinking model [1].

While we recognize the inherent complexity involved in diagnosing and treating conditions like corneal ectasia, fostering a culture of openness empowers refractive surgeons to consistently enhance safety and improve patient outcomes [2]. The unwavering pursuit of knowledge and the humility to acknowledge the limits of our understanding establish the foundation on which black box thinking thrives, propelling refractive surgery and all areas of medicine forward.

Two significant aspects offer valuable lessons in this case. The first aspect is related to the early detection of ectasia following LVC. Additionally, and more importantly, this case provides crucial information for preventing iatrogenic ectasia through a comprehensive retrospective evaluation of the patient's clinical data [3].

During the two-year follow-up period, clinical signs demonstrated mild ectatic progression. UCVA was 20/25 + 2 in the OD and 20/20 in the OS at this visit. The BCVA was 20/20–2 (−0.25/−0.50 × 160°) in the OD and 20/20 (plano/−0.25 × 75°) in the OS. The topometric evaluation had a mild central steepening (Fig. 18.5b). Also, a significant posterior elevation with 18 μm float was noted at the scan 2 years after surgery (Fig. 18.6b). The comparative change of posterior elevation was possible by fixing the reference surface to the best-fit-sphere (BFS) for the preoperative baseline exam, demonstrating a 10 μm increase (Fig. 18.6d). While these findings were overlooked, at this time point, a proactive education to advise against eye rubbing and treating ocular allergy would be indicated, along with oral riboflavin supplementation [4]. A close follow-up would have been mandatory to detect progression at an early stage, which would allow for considering CXL before a loss of BCVA.

A critical retrospective evaluation of the preoperative data would detect remarkable signs of ectasia risk before SMILE. The current understanding of ectasia risk assessment is based on the classic two-hit hypothesis for keratoconus, which involves the inherent patient predisposition (biomechanical susceptibility), and the impact of the environment [5, 6]. The biomechanical impact or effect from LVC is calculated based on the RSB and the percent of tissue altered (PTA). The thinnest point is preferable to the central (apex) pachymetric value. In this case, the RSB was calculated considering the CCT, while the thinnest point value from OCT or Scheimpflug would lead to an RSB lower than 250 μm in both eyes. In addition, the PTA would be over 50% in both eyes.

Considering the preoperative corneal data, there are relevant signs of ectasia susceptibility. The evaluation of tomographic data from Pentacam highlights an ARTmax lower than 390 μm in both eyes. The Pentacam Random Forest Index (PRFI) was 0.22 in OD and 0.19 in OS, higher than the optimized cut-off of 0.15. The term Random Forest refers to a method in machine learning that uses multiple decision trees to validate the outcome and is often used in regression and classification algorithms [7]. The OCT (segmental or layered) demonstrated a relatively thinner epithelium inferiorly, a described pattern consistent with mild ectatic change.

In addition, the preoperative data from Corvis ST (Oculus Optikgerate GmbH, Wetzlar Germany) was available for retrospective calculations of the CBI and the TBI [8, 9]. Both indices became available only in 2016, while the patient was operated in 2014. Figure 18.11 illustrates the display that integrates Scheimpflug tomography and biomechanical data [10]. The CBI was 0.34, and the TBI was 0.72 in OD, demonstrating a high susceptibility for ectasia before SMILE [11].

Such results would be contrary to the indication of a lamellar LVC for correcting −9.75D of spherical equivalent. The left eye had a preoperative TBI of 0.27—which would also be considered high for this patient's refractive treatment. Importantly, the stable outcome in OS illustrates that such good results are possible despite the increased risk for ectasia. Possibly, clinical treatment was effective in the left eye to avoid ectasia progression. Nevertheless, a phakic IOL would have been the most suitable procedure for this patient.

The available data for surgeons can be overwhelming. An excessive amount of data can lead to important findings being overlooked. Artificial intelligence (AI) can assist in detecting significant results by analyzing data from multimodal refractive imaging, enabling an enhanced assessment of the risk of ectasia progression prior to refractive surgery [12]. This allows for instantaneous evaluation of limitless data and real-time alerts to the surgeon regarding risks. The BrAIN (Brazilian Artificial Intelligence Networking in Medicine) software (https://sys.braincornea.com) offers a solution that integrates corneal structure data and the impact of the laser vision correction (LVC) procedure using a concept called relational tissue alteration (RTA). By harnessing the power of AI algorithms, we can amalgamate data from various imaging modalities, such as corneal topography, tomography, and biomechanical measurements, to gain a comprehensive understanding of corneal health and stability. Additionally, further analysis includes incorporating the impact of the corneal procedure to establish the risk of ectasia before laser vision correction.

The algorithm $(A2I)^2$ refers to the implementation of AI (the hows) in analyzing a wide range of data from various imaging modalities, as well as drawing upon ancient intelligence or philosophy to understand the underlying reasons (the "whys"). By consciously applying AI, we can optimize decisions related to refractive surgery. This personalized approach guarantees improved accuracy in assessing ectasia risk and empowers surgeons to further enhance visual outcomes. Ultimately, the combination of AI and ancient intelligence has the potential to revolutionize refractive surgery, leading to greater precision, reduced risks, and transformative patient care.

Take-Home Messages

- Refractive surgeons should embrace the philosophy of black-box thinking to prevent complications and optimize clinical outcomes.
- Corneal tomography should be considered before LVC, starting the analysis of the thinnest point instead of central thickness for calculating the RSB and PTA.
- The biomechanical impact on the integrity of the cornea of SMILE is likely lower than LASIK, but it does not eliminate the risk of ectasia.
- Identifying high-risk or susceptible cases for biomechanical failure to prevent iatrogenic keratectasia after LVC represents a major challenge for refractive surgeons.
- Enhanced multimodal imaging goes beyond, not over, the detection of mild (subclinical or fruste) keratoconus. The current task is to characterize ectasia susceptibility and to consider such properties with the impact of the LVC.
- Refractive surgeons should remain vigilant for signs of progressive ectasia postoperatively to properly manage such rare but severe complications.

References

1. Sayed M. Black box thinking, why Most people never learn from their mistakes, but some do. London: Portfolio Publishing; 2015.
2. Ambrosio R Jr. Post-LASIK ectasia: twenty years of a conundrum. Semin Ophthalmol. 2019;34:66–8.
3. Ambrosio R Jr. Multimodal imaging for refractive surgery: quo vadis? Indian J Ophthalmol. 2020;68:2647–9.
4. Ambrosio R Jr. Violet June: the global keratoconus awareness campaign. Ophthalmol Ther. 2020;9:685–8.
5. Esporcatte LPG, Salomao MQ, Lopes BT, et al. Biomechanical diagnostics of the cornea. Eye Vis (Lond). 2020;7:9.
6. Salomao MQ, Hofling-Lima AL, Gomes Esporcatte LP, et al. Ectatic diseases. Exp Eye Res. 2021;202:108347.
7. Ambrosio R Jr, Luz A, Lopes B, Ramos I, Belin MW. Enhanced ectasia screening: the need for advanced and objective data. J Refract Surg. 2014;30:151–2.
8. Ambrosio R Jr, Machado AP, Leao E, et al. Optimized artificial intelligence for enhanced ectasia detection using Scheimpflug-based corneal tomography and biomechanical data. Am J Ophthalmol. 2023;251:126–42.
9. Vinciguerra R, Ambrosio R Jr, Elsheikh A, et al. Detection of keratoconus with a new biomechanical index. J Refract Surg. 2016;32:803–10.
10. Vinciguerra R, Ambrosio R Jr, Elsheikh A, et al. Detection of post-laser vision correction ectasia with a new combined biomechanical index. J Cataract Refract Surg. 2021;47:1314–8.
11. Ambrosio R Jr, Ramos I, Lopes B, et al. Ectasia susceptibility before laser vision correction. J Cataract Refract Surg. 2015;41:1335–6.
12. Lopes BT, Ramos IC, Salomao MQ, et al. Enhanced tomographic assessment to detect corneal ectasia based on artificial intelligence. Am J Ophthalmol. 2018;195:223–32.

Index

S. A. Melki et al. (eds.), *Refractive Surgery Atlas*, https://doi.org/10.1007/978-3-031-60661-8

N

O

P

R

S